Study Guide to Accompany

# FUNDAMENTALS OF
# NURSING

## THE ART AND SCIENCE OF NURSING CARE

Study Guide to Accompany

# FUNDAMENTALS OF
# NURSING

THE ART AND SCIENCE OF NURSING CARE

Second Edition

**Carol Taylor, CSFN, RN, MSN, PhD** (candidate)
Assistant Professor, Nursing
Georgetown University
Washington, DC
Holy Family College
Philadelphia, Pennsylvania

**Carol Lillis, RN, MSN**
Associate Professor
Delaware County Community College
Media, Pennsylvania

**Priscilla LeMone, RNC, DSN**
Assistant Professor
University of Missouri–Columbia
Columbia, Missouri

**Marilee LeBon**
Mountaintop, Pennsylvania

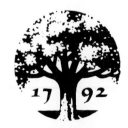

**J. B. Lippincott**
Philadelphia

*Sponsoring Editor:* Donna L. Hilton, RN, BSN
*Coordinating Editorial Assistant:* Susan Perry
*Production Manager:* Lori Bainbridge
*Production:* NB Enterprises
*Printer/Binder:* Courier Kendallville
*Cover Printer:* Lehigh Press

2nd Edition

6  5  4  3  2

ISBN 0-397-54948-2

Any procedure or practice described in this book should be applied by the health care practitioner under appropriate supervision in accordance with professional standards of care used with regard to the unique circumstances that apply in each practice situation. Care has been taken to confirm the accuracy of information presented and to describe generally accepted practices. However, the authors, editors, and publisher cannot accept any responsibility for errors or omissions or for any consequences from application of the information in this book and make no warranty, express or implied, with respect to the contents of the book.

Every effort has been made to ensure drug selections and dosages are in accordance with current recommendations and practice. Because of ongoing research, changes in government regulations, and the constant flow of information on drug therapy, reactions, and interactions, the reader is cautioned to check the package insert for each drug for the indications, dosages, warnings, and precautions, particularly if the drug is new or infrequently used.

# PREFACE

The authors of the second edition of *Fundamentals of Nursing: The Art and Science of Nursing Care,* together with Marilee LeBon, have carefully developed these student learning guides. We recognize that beginning students in nursing must learn an enormous amount of information and skills in a short period of time. The questions in the learning guides, arranged by chapter, are structured to help you integrate and begin to apply the knowledge in the practice of nursing. Each chapter includes the following sections:

- *Introduction:* This section, placed at the beginning of the study guide, summarizes the material in the corresponding textbook chapter.
- *Chapter Objectives:* The chapter objectives are identical to those listed at the beginning of each textbook chapter. The objectives are written so that you can focus your study time on the critical elements of each chapter and structure your learning to gain essential information.
- *Exercises:* The exercises in each chapter group similar types of questions together to help you in learning the information in a variety of different formats. The types of questions included will fol-

low the same format in each learning guide chapter. Please note that not all of these types of questions will be found in each learning guide chapter. The format is:

> Matching Questions
> Multiple Choice Questions
> Correct the False Questions
> Completion Questions
> Sequencing Questions
> Case Study Questions

The case studies in the clinical nursing care chapters provide a unique opportunity for you to "encounter" an actual client and to use the nursing process to assess and diagnose the client's need for nursing and to meet these needs.

The answers to the questions are included in the back of the book so that you can immediately assess your own learning as you complete each study guide.

We hope you find this study guide to be helpful and enjoyable and we wish you every success as you begin the exciting journey toward becoming a nurse.

*Carol Taylor*
*Carol Lillis*
*Priscilla LeMone*

# Contents

## Unit I: The Nurse: Foundations for Nursing Practice

| | | |
|---|---|---|
| 1. | Introduction to Nursing | 1 |
| 2. | Promoting Wellness in Health and Illness | 4 |
| 3. | The Health-Care System | 7 |
| 4. | Theoretical Base for Nursing Practice | 10 |
| 5. | Values and Ethics in Nursing | 12 |
| 6. | Legal Implications of Nursing | 16 |

## Unit II: The Client: Concepts for Holistic Care

| | | |
|---|---|---|
| 7. | Basic Human Needs: Individual, Family, and Community | 20 |
| 8. | Culture and Ethnicity | 23 |
| 9. | Stress and Adaptation | 26 |

## Unit III: Promoting Wellness Across the Lifespan

| | | |
|---|---|---|
| 10. | Developmental Concepts | 30 |
| 11. | Conception Through Midlife | 33 |
| 12. | The Older Adult | 37 |
| 13. | Loss, Grief, and Death | 40 |

## Unit IV: The Nursing Process

| | | |
|---|---|---|
| 14. | Introduction to Nursing Process | 43 |
| 15. | Assessing | 46 |
| 16. | Diagnosing | 50 |
| 17. | Planning | 54 |
| 18. | Implementing and Documenting | 57 |
| 19. | Evaluating | 61 |

## Unit V: Roles Basic to Nursing Care

| | | |
|---|---|---|
| 20. | Communicator | 64 |
| 21. | Teacher and Counselor | 67 |
| 22. | Leader, Researcher, and Advocate | 71 |

## Unit VI: Actions Basic to Nursing Care

| | | |
|---|---|---|
| 23. | Vital Signs | 75 |
| 24. | Nursing Assessment | 80 |
| 25. | Safety | 86 |
| 26. | Asepsis | 93 |
| 27. | Diagnostic Procedures | 99 |
| 28. | Continuity of Care | 104 |

## Unit VII: Promoting Healthy Physiologic Responses

| | | |
|---|---|---|
| 29. | Hygiene | 107 |
| 30. | Activity | 114 |
| 31. | Rest and Sleep | 124 |
| 32. | Comfort | 132 |
| 33. | Nutrition | 140 |
| 34. | Urinary Elimination | 150 |
| 35. | Bowel Elimination | 158 |
| 36. | Oxygenation | 166 |
| 37. | Fluid, Electrolyte, and Acid-Base Balance | 176 |

## Unit VIII: Promoting Healthy Psychosocial Responses

| | | |
|---|---|---|
| 38. | Self-Concept | 188 |
| 39. | Sensory Stimulation | 194 |
| 40. | Sexuality | 198 |
| 41. | Spirituality | 206 |

## Unit IX: Promoting Optimal Health in Special Situations

| | | |
|---|---|---|
| 42. | Medications | 212 |
| 43. | Care of Wounds | 224 |
| 44. | Perioperative Nursing | 229 |

| | |
|---|---|
| **Answers** | **237** |

Study Guide to Accompany

# FUNDAMENTALS OF
# NURSING

## THE ART AND SCIENCE OF NURSING CARE

# 1

# Introduction to Nursing

Chapter 1 introduces the historical context and aims of nursing as an emerging profession and discipline. The major aims of nursing are discussed: promoting wellness, preventing illness, restoring health, and facilitating coping with disability and death. Educational preparation, professional organizations, and guidelines for nursing practice are presented; and nursing trends and issues are discussed in terms of nursing in transition.

## OBJECTIVES

After studying this chapter the learner will be able to:

Define key terms used in the chapter.

Describe the historical background, the definitions of nursing, and the status of nursing as a profession and a discipline.

Identify the aims of nursing as they interrelate to facilitate maximum function and quality of life for clients.

Describe the various levels of educational preparation in nursing.

Discuss the effect of nursing organizations, standards of nursing practice, nurse practice acts, and the nursing process on the practice of nursing.

Identify current trends in nursing.

## EXERCISES

## Matching

Match the term in Part A with the correct definition in Part B.

Part A

a. dependent nursing actions

b. nursing

c. in-service education

d. licensure

e. interdependent nursing actions

f. nursing education

g. independent nursing actions

h. holistic health care

i. continuing education

j. nurse practice act

k. professional standards

Part B

1. _____ The education of R.N.s and L.P.N.s.

2. _____ The foundation for the practice of professional nursing.

3. _____ A law that regulates nursing practice.

4. _____ Collaborating with other health team members.

5. _____ Institutional education and training for employees.

6. _____ Nursing actions based on physician orders.

7. _____ Planned learning experiences beyond basic professional education.

8. _____ Nursing actions based on assessments, knowledge, and judgment.

9. _____ Most basically, the care of others.

10. _____ Integrates physical, psychosocial, and spiritual dimensions.

11. _____ Legal right to practice nursing.

Match the definitions in Part A with the correct terms in Part B.

Part A

a. Conducted the first organized visiting of the sick.

b. Criteria include having a code of ethics and standards set by a professional organization.

c. Based on research in the late 1950s by Dr. Montag.

d. Has a specific and unique body of knowledge.

e. A major guideline for nursing practice.

f. A theory used by early civilizations to explain illness.

g. The diagnosis and treatment of human responses to actual or potential health problems.

h. The professional organization of RNs in the United States.

i. The freedom to regulate one's work behavior.

j. Recommended by professional nursing organizations as the entry level for professional nursing practice.

Part B

12. _____ animism

13. _____ ANA definition of nursing practice

14. _____ discipline

15. _____ Associate degree in nursing

16. _____ American Nurses' Association

17. _____ deaconesses

18. _____ nursing process

19. _____ profession

20. _____ Baccalaureate in nursing

21. _____ autonomy

## Completion

1. List six of the nine contributions (discussed in the chapter) made to nursing by Florence Nightingale.

a. _____

_____

b. _____

_____

c. _____

_____

d. _____

_____

e. _____

_____

f. _____

_____

Nursing has been defined in many ways, but there are essential elements present in most thoughtful perspectives. Use your own words to expand the following short definitions of nursing.

2. Nursing is caring. _____

_____

_____

3. Nursing is sharing. _____

_____

_____

4. Nursing is touching. _____

_____

_____

5. Nursing is feeling. _____

_____

_____

6. Nursing is listening. _____

_____

_____

7. Nursing is accepting. _____

_____

_____

8. Nursing is respecting. _____

_____

_____

Write the names of the organizations associated with the initials.

9. ANA _____

10. ICN _____

11. NLN _____

12. NSNA _____

13. CNA _____

14. List the four broad aims of nursing.

a. _____

b. _____

c. _____

d. _____

Identify in the space provided the role of the nurse described by nursing functions.

15. _____ The provision of care to clients that combines both the art and science of nursing in meeting physical, emotional, intellectual, sociocultural, and spiritual needs.

16. _____ The use of communication skills to assess, implement, and evaluate individualized teaching plans.

17. _____ The use of therapeutic interpersonal communication skills to provide information, make referrals, and facilitate the client's problem-solving and decision-making skills.

18. _____ The protection of human or legal rights and the securing of care for all clients, based on the belief that clients have the right to make informed decisions about their own health and life.

19. _____ The assertive, self-confident practice of nursing when providing care, effecting change, and functioning with groups.

20. _____ The participation in or conduct of research to increase knowledge in nursing and improve client care.

21. _____ The use of effective interpersonal and therapeutic communication skills to establish and maintain helping relationships with clients.

Complete the table with the correct word or phrase to differentiate among the nursing roles that are listed.

| Title | Education/Preparation | Role Description |
|---|---|---|
| *Example:* | | |
| *Nurse Reasearcher* | *Advanced degree* | *Conducts research relevant to nursing practice and education* |
| 22. Nurse Midwife | a. | b. |
| 23. Nurse Practioner | a. | b. |
| 24. Nurse Anesthetist | a. | b. |

# 2

# Promoting Wellness in Health and Illness

Chapter 2 discusses the way in which the practice of nursing is influenced by the client—the person receiving care. Definitions of wellness are provided. Models of health and illness and factors affecting health and illness are presented. Wellness promotion and illness prevention are described, incorporating risk factors, acute and chronic illness, and effects of illness on the family. Levels of preventive care and the nurse as role model in promoting wellness are identified.

O B J E C T I V E S

After studying this chapter the learner will be able to:

Define key terms used in the chapter.

Describe wellness, health, and illness.

Identify the factors influencing health and illness, including the human dimensions, basic human needs, and self-concept.

Compare and contrast acute illness and chronic illness.

Summarize the role of the nurse in promoting wellness based on knowledge of risk factors for illness, illness behaviors, and the effects of illness on the family.

Describe the levels of preventive care.

## E X E R C I S E S

## Matching

Match the term in Part A with the correct definition in Part B.

Part A

a. acute illness
b. agent-host-environment model
c. basic human needs
d. chronic illness
e. health
f. health-belief model
g. health-illness continuum
h. health-risk appraisal
i. high-level wellness
j. illness
k. primary preventive care
l. risk factor
m. self-concept
n. tertiary preventive care
o. secondary preventive care

Part B

1. _____ A model based on what individuals perceive to be true about their own health.

2. _____ Functioning to one's maximum potential.

3. _____ Essential and common to all people.

4. _____ A factor that increases possible injury or illness.

5. _____ Often described in terms of feeling state, symptoms, or ability to carry out activities of daily living.

6. _____ An abnormal process in which one's level of function is changed in comparison to a previous level.

7. _____ In this model, a combination of factors increases the possibility of illness.

8. _____ A model that describes health as a constantly changing state.

9. _____ Has both physical and emotional aspects and can be altered by illness.

10. _____ A permanent change in normal anatomy or physiology.

11. _____ Care aimed at restoring clients to maximum function following an illness.

12. _____ Care that focuses on health maintenance for clients with health problems.

13. _____ Has a rapid onset of symptoms that last for a limited period of time.

14. _____ Care that is directed toward health promotion activities.

## Multiple Choice

Circle the letter that corresponds to the best answer for each question.

1. What is a risk factor?
   a. An appraisal that indicates areas of health and areas for illness.
   b. A factor in the human dimensions that increases the chance for illness.
   c. A pathologic change in human functioning that results in disease.
   d. Something that is essential to emotional and psychologic health.

2. Which of the following statements best describes an acute illness?
   a. An acute illness is a pathophysiologic change in physical function that rarely requires treatment.
   b. An acute illness and a chronic illness can occur at the same time in an individual.
   c. An acute illness has a rapid onset of symptoms but lasts a limited and short period of time.
   d. An acute illness is caused by an irreversible and permanent pathophysiologic change.

3. A chronic illness commonly has periods of remission and exacerbation. What is indicated by the term *remission?*
   a. Symptoms of the illness reappear.
   b. A time during which most symptoms occur.
   c. A time during which new symptoms occur.
   d. Symptoms are not experienced.

4. During the recovery and rehabilitation stage of illness, the person who has been ill is expected to do which of the following?
   a. Give up the dependent role.
   b. Assume a dependent role.
   c. Seek medical attention.
   d. Recognize symptoms of illness.

5. The major cause of injury and death in the older adult is:
   a. automobile accidents
   b. falls
   c. burns
   d. increasing age

## Completion

1. Write the World Health Organization definition of health. _____
   _____
   _____

2. Compare and contrast *disease* and *illness.* _____
   _____
   _____
   _____
   _____
   _____
   _____

3. List the six human dimensions that influence behaviors of persons receiving health care.
   a. _____
   b. _____
   c. _____
   d. _____
   e. _____
   f. _____

4. In the space below, draw and label the health–illness continuum.

   _____

   _____

5. Where do you fit on the health–illness continuum and why? _____
   _____
   _____

6. Name six common causes of disease.
   a. _____
   b. _____
   c. _____
   d. _____
   e. _____
   f. _____

Relate each level of preventive care with the corresponding nursing actions by writing the number of each action in the space provided.

**Level of Preventive Care**

PRIMARY: _____

SECONDARY: _____

TERTIARY: _____

**Nursing Actions**

7. Giving medications.

8. Facilitating a support group.

9. Giving decubitus care.

10. Teaching self-breast exam.

11. Giving immunizations.

12. Providing accident prevention lectures.

13. Providing dental care teaching.

14. Providing physical therapy.

15. Doing range-of-motion exercises.

16. Doing diabetic teaching.

# 3

## The Health Care System

Chapter 3 provides information about the components of the health care system. Types of health care settings are discussed: in-patient settings, out-patient settings, community health settings, government agencies, voluntary agencies, and home care. Members of the health care team are discussed in terms of education and responsibilities. The economics of health care delivery includes information about private insurance, group plans, and federal health care support in the United States and Canada. Trends and issues in the health care system include a focus on wellness, consumerism, cost containment, fragmentation of care, increasing numbers of older and chronically ill adults, and health care as a right or a privilege.

### O B J E C T I V E S

After studying this chapter the learner will be able to:

Define key terms used in the chapter.

Compare and contrast in-patient and out-patient health care settings.

Discuss the services provided by community health care agencies and in community settings.

Describe government health care agencies and services.

Describe the roles of members of the health care team.

Discuss various private insurance, group plans, and Federal support in the United States and Canada.

Discuss trends and issues affecting the health care delivery system.

## E X E R C I S E S

### Matching

Match the term in Part A with the correct definition in Part B.

Part A

a. hospital

b. extended care facility

c. out-patient settings

d. ambulatory care centers

e. community health settings

Part B

1. _____ Usually offer walk-in services and are open longer than traditional office hours.

2. _____ Care is focused on acute care needs of the client.

3. _____ Provide care in agencies, homes, day-care centers, crisis intervention centers, and drug/alcohol programs.

4. _____ Includes skilled care facilities, nursing homes, retirement centers, and residential institutions.

5. _____ Services are provided in hospitals, physicians' offices, ambulatory care centers, and clinics.

Match the term in Part A with the correct definition in Part B.

Part A

a. health maintenance organizations

b. preferred provider organizations

c. long-term care insurance

d. Medicare

e. Medicaid

Part B

6. _____ A United States federal health insurance program for persons 65 years of age or older.

7. _____ Insurance plan that covers a variety of services, including adult day-care centers and respite care.

8. _____ The subscriber pays premiums, and then receives all health care free, as long as it is received through this plan.

9. _____ Any arrangement where clients are channeled to specific health providers.

10. _____ The federally funded health insurance program (United States) for very low income persons.

## Multiple Choice

Circle the letter that corresponds to the best answer for each question.

1. Public hospitals in the United States are classified as:
   a. for-profit institutions
   b. not-for-profit institutions
   c. tertiary care institutions
   d. extended care facilities

2. Canadian hospitals receive funding from what sources?
   a. they do not have a source of funding
   b. business and industry
   c. federal and provincial sources
   d. private citizens

3. Almost all extended care facilities require 24-hour coverage of skilled nursing care. What does the phrase *skilled nursing care* mean?
   a. Technicians must have completed a basic patient care course.
   b. Nurses must pass an examination to validate skills.
   c. The agency can only employ registered nurses.
   d. The care given to clients can only be done by or under the direction of a licensed nurse.

4. Nurses who work in crisis intervention centers must have what abilities?
   a. strong communication and counseling skills
   b. well-developed technical skills
   c. low tolerance for frustration
   d. dependence on others

5. Special services that are available to terminally ill persons and their families are called:
   a. public health services
   b. rehabilitation centers
   c. hospices
   d. hospitals

6. Which of the following members of the health care team would most likely be trained to help a stroke victim learn how to verbally communicate?
   a. occupational therapist
   b. physical therapist
   c. respiratory therapist
   d. speech therapist

7. Diagnosis-related groups were implemented by the federal government to meet what health care problem?
   a. increasing health care costs
   b. increasing numbers of ill elderly
   c. increasing fragmentation of care
   d. increasing consumer complaints

8. Which of the following programs illustrates a focus on wellness in our society?
   a. research on the treatment of AIDS
   b. incarceration of drug addicts
   c. anti-smoking ads on television
   d. aggressive therapy for cancer

9. What does the phrase *fragmentation of care* mean?
   a. Care is given by many different providers.
   b. Care is provided only on certain days.
   c. The health care provider does not have time.
   d. The health care provider does total care.

10. The most rapidly growing segment of our population is what age group?

    a. infants under the age of one year

    b. females under the age of 18

    c. adolescent males

    d. older adults (over 70 years)

## Completion

1. How are government health care agencies financed? _____

_____

_____

2. Describe the services provided by each of the following:

a. Public Health Service _____

_____

b. Centers for Disease Control _____

_____

c. National Institutes of Health _____

_____

_____

3. What four types of home health services are provided to clients?

a. _____

b. _____

c. _____

d. _____

Complete the following information: (a) role, (b) education, and (c) license/title.

4. Pharmacist

a. _____

b. _____

c. _____

5. Physical Therapist

a. _____

b. _____

c. _____

6. Physician's Assistant

a. _____

b. _____

c. _____

7. Occupational Therapist

a. _____

b. _____

c. _____

8. Dietician

a. _____

b. _____

c. _____

9. Respiratory Therapist

a. _____

b. _____

c. _____

10. What are diagnostic related groups (DRGs)? _____

_____

_____

_____

11. Describe the Canada Health Act. _____

_____

_____

_____

_____

12. List six of the eight ways (described in the box *Computer Applications in Nursing*) that computers are used to reduce health care costs.

a. _____

b. _____

c. _____

d. _____

e. _____

f. _____

# 4

# Theoretical Base for Nursing Practice

Chapter 4 provides an introduction to the theoretical base for nursing practice. Nursing theory is discussed in relation to underlying theories, and the basic characteristics and common components of nursing theory are examined. Historical perspectives and the evolution of nursing theory provide a framework for appreciation of nursing theory today. Selected models and theories of nursing are described; these models and theories are applied to the care of one client to illustrate application in clinical practice.

O B J E C T I V E S

After studying this chapter the learner will be able to:

Define key terms used in the chapter.

Describe the underlying processes and characteristics of nursing theory.

Define the four common components of nursing theory.

Summarize the historical background, cultural influences, and value of nursing theory.

Discuss selected nursing theories, including definitions, assumptions, beliefs, and applications to nursing practice.

## Matching

Match the term in Part A with the correct definition in Part B.

Part A

a. philosophy          d. theory

b. concept             e. process

c. conceptual

   framework (model)

Part B

1. _____ Abstract impressions, organized into symbols of reality that describe objects, properties, and events.

2. _____ A series of actions, changes, or functions that brings about a desired result.

3. _____ The study of wisdom, fundamental knowledge, and the processes used to develop our perceptions.

4. _____ A group of concepts that follow an understandable pattern.

5. _____ A statement that explains a process, an occurrence, or an event; derived through inductive and deductive reasoning.

Match the nursing theorist in Part A with the central theme of the model or theory listed in Part B.

Part A

a. Dorothy Johnson

b. Imogene King

c. Madeline Leininger

d. Dorthea Orem

e. Martha Rogers

f. Sr. Calista Roy

g. Jean Watson

Part B

6. _____ human science and human care

7. _____ self-care

8. _____ open systems

9. _____ transcultural care

10. _____ behavioral systems

11. _____ a science of unitary man

12. _____ adaptation model

## Completion

Fill in the blank with the correct word or phrase.

1. General systems theory explains the breaking of whole things into (a) _____.
Adaptation theory explains human adaptation as occurring on three levels: the internal or
(b) _____, the social or
(c) _____, and the physical or
(d) _____.

2. Developmental theory states that the process of growth and development in humans is
(a) _____ and
(b) _____.

3. List the five basic characteristics of nursing theory.

a. _____

b. _____

c. _____

d. _____

e. _____

4. List the four concepts common to nursing theory.

a. _____

b. _____

c. _____

d. _____

For each nursing theorist listed, define that theorist's belief about nursing.

5. *Dorothy Johnson:* Nursing is _____

_____

_____

_____

_____

6. *Imogene King:* Nursing is _____

_____

_____

_____

_____

_____

7. *Madeline Leininger:* Nursing is _____

_____

_____

_____

_____

_____

8. *Dorthea Orem:* Nursing is _____

_____

_____

_____

_____

_____

9. *Sr. Calista Roy:* Nursing is _____

_____

_____

_____

_____

_____

10. *Jean Watson:* Nursing is _____

_____

_____

_____

_____

# 5

# Values and Ethics in Nursing

Chapter 5 introduces the learner to the process of values clarification and identifies the values essential to the professional nurse. Codes of professional ethical conduct for nursing are explored and a process of ethical decision making is highlighted. Common ethical problems encountered by practicing nurses are presented.

O B J E C T I V E S

After studying this chapter the learner will be able to:

Define key terms used in the chapter.

List five common modes of value transmission.

Identify the seven basic values essential in the practice of nursing.

Describe seven steps in the valuing process.

Utilize values clarification strategies in clinical practice.

Identify three sources of standards for professional ethical conduct.

Describe nursing practice that is consistent with the code of ethics for nursing.

Describe three typical concerns of the nurse advocate.

Recognize ethical issues as they arise in nursing practice.

Utilize an ethical framework and decision-making process to resolve ethical problems.

Identify four functions of institutional ethics committees.

## Matching

Match the term in Part A with the correct definition in Part B.

Part A

a. value system

b. value neutrality

c. value

d. attitude

e. beliefs

f. values clarification

Part B

1. _____ Nonjudgmental commitment to clients whether or not the nurse and clients hold the same values.

2. _____ A special class of intellectual attitudes based primarily on faith as opposed to fact.

3. _____ Feeling or emotion generally including positive or negative judgment toward persons, objects, or ideas.

4. _____ Process by which persons come to understand their own values and value system.

5. _____ Personal belief about worth that acts as a standard to guide one's behavior.

6. _____ An organization of values in which each value is ranked along a continuum of importance.

Match Part B, the nurses' responses to the situation related below, with Part A, the six basic types of values underlying a person's interests and motives (Feldman, 1969).

*Situation:* The nursing supervisor on a cardiac unit has been suffering from emotional distress for a prolonged period of time, due to a difficult divorce. Her attention is diverted from her job, resulting in sporadic client record-keeping, nurse scheduling problems, and diminished quality of client care.

Part A

a. economical

b. religious

c. theoretical

d. social

e. aesthetic

f. political

Part B

7. _____ This nurse is distressed with the diminishing quality of client care and attempts to correct the problem by working harder to cover for her charge nurse. She encourages other nurses to work with her to resolve the problem.

8. _____ This nurse unites all the nurses in an effort to confront their supervisor and encourage her to seek professional help.

9. _____ This nurse keeps an accurate record of all problems experienced by the staff that are directly related to her charge nurse's situation in order to document the need for intervention.

0. _____ This nurse meets with the other nurses assigned to the unit to establish a united effort to report their charge nurse to a higher authority.

1. _____ This nurse doesn't want to "rock the boat" and accepts the working conditions as they are, because finding a solution to the problem isn't worth losing a good job.

2. _____ This nurse believes the charge nurse will eventually work out her problems on her own and deals with each problem as it arises. She takes comfort in a pleasant working environment.

Match the universal moral principles reflected in the Nursing Codes of Ethics (ICN, ANA, CNA), listed in Part A, with their definitions in Part B.

Part A

a. beneficence          e. respect for persons

b. nonmaleficence       f. autonomy

c. confidentiality       g. fidelity

d. justice              h. veracity

Part B

13. _____ Self-determination.

14. _____ Truth telling.

15. _____ Doing good.

16. _____ Treating people fairly.

17. _____ Keeping promises.

18. _____ Avoiding harm.

19. _____ Patient dignity.

20. _____ Respecting privileged information.

## Multiple Choice

Circle the letter that corresponds to the best answer for each question.

1. Which of the following was developed by the American Hospital Association to enumerate the rights and responsibilities of clients while receiving hospital care?
   a. Code of Ethics
   b. Patient Bill of Rights
   c. Biomedical Ethics
   d. Hospital Patient Advocacy

2. Of the following, which is the system of reflection that attempts to explain how we ought to live and why?
   a. Biomedical Ethics
   b. Institutional Ethics Committees
   c. Ethical Theory
   d. Values Clarification

3. In which of the following ethical theories is an action right or wrong independent of the consequences it produces?

   a. utilitarian
   b. deontological
   c. nonmaleficence

4. Which of the following offers the nurse a means to look at and evaluate alternative courses of right action using basic moral concepts and principles?

   a. values
   b. Bill of Rights
   c. modeling
   d. ethics

## Correct the False Statements

Circle the word *true* or *false* that follows the statement. If the word *false* has been circled, change the underlined word/words to make the statement true. Place your answer in the space provided.

1. Personal standards of right or wrong are called <u>morals</u>.

   True    False    _____

2. An action guide that determines the rightness or wrongness of an action depending on the consequences the action produces is <u>deontological</u>.

   True    False    _____

3. Keeping patients in restraints against their wishes to keep them from hurting themselves is an example of <u>paternalism</u>.

   True    False    _____

4. <u>Advocacy</u> is the protection and support of another's rights.

   True    False    _____

5. <u>Altruism</u> is the inherent worth and uniqueness of an individual.

   True    False    _____

6. Some areas of medicine in which <u>biomedical ethics</u> may apply are gene therapy, physician-assisted suicide, and treatment withdrawal.

   True    False    _____

## Completion

1. Give two examples of moral issues that can arise between nurse/client, nurse/physician, and nurse/nurse.

   a. Nurse/client: _____

   _____

   _____

   _____

   b. Nurse/physician: _____

   _____

   _____

   _____

   c. Nurse/nurse: _____

   _____

   _____

   _____

2. List and describe the six-step procedure for ethical decision making according to Jameton, 1984.

   Step 1. _____

   Step 2. _____

   Step 3. _____

   Step 4. _____

   Step 5. _____

   Step 6. _____

3. List the four chief functions of institutional ethics committees.

   a. _____

   b. _____

   c. _____

   d. _____

4. Identify the common modes of value transmission illustrated below.

   a. _____: A child learns that family unity is important by observing his mother's attempts to have everyone together for family meals.

   b. _____: A child is grounded for fighting with his sister and is later praised for sharing his candy with her.

   c. _____: A child of nine is allowed to stay up as late as he desires, although he is expected to be up at 7:30 for school.

_____: A child is reprimanded by his teacher for failing to turn in his homework on time.

_____: A 13-year-old child is allowed to go to the movies with her friends, but guidelines are set down as to what behavior should accompany this freedom.

List five of the seven values the American Association of Colleges for Nursing identified as essential for the practicing nurse.

_____

_____

_____

_____

_____

## Sequencing

Items 1–7 illustrate the steps in the valuing process as related to the situation described below. Place each step in the correct sequence by numbering the items.

*Situation:* A 45-year-old male client with a history of heart disease decides to give up smoking because he values his health.

1. _____ The client realizes that if he stops smoking his blood pressure will stabilize and his chances of survival will increase dramatically; if he does not stop smoking his condition could worsen. He chooses to stop.

2. _____ Although his wife has been begging him to stop smoking for years, it was the client's own decision to stop based on his desire to be healthy.

3. _____ The client tells his wife she was right about his need to quit smoking and asks for her help and understanding in his attempt to break his habit.

4. _____ The client knows he could improve his health by not smoking or he could wait and see if his condition worsens with no action.

5. _____ The client stops smoking and chews gum or takes a walk when he feels the urge to smoke.

6. _____ A feeling of satisfaction and pride in his ability to order his life encompasses the client.

7. _____ The client has not had a cigarette for three months and his desire for nicotine has decreased dramatically.

# 6

# Legal Implications of Nursing

Chapter 6 introduces the learner to basic legal concepts and describes the professional and legal regulation of nursing practice. Crimes and torts related to nursing practice are explained. The chapter highlights legal safeguards for the nurse and explores nursing roles in malpractice litigation. Student liability, laws affecting nursing practice, and legal issues related to death and dying are all briefly addressed.

## OBJECTIVES

After studying this chapter the learner will be able to:

Define key terms used in the chapter.

Define law, describing its four sources.

Describe the professional and legal regulation of nursing practice.

Identify the purpose of credentialing; using as examples accreditation, licensure/registration, and certification.

Differentiate intentional torts (assault and battery, defamation, invasion of privacy, false imprisonment, fraud) and unintentional torts (negligence).

Evaluate personal areas of potential liability in nursing.

Describe the legal procedure once a plaintiff files a complaint against a nurse for negligence.

Describe the roles of the nurse as defendent, fact witness, and expert witness.

Utilize appropriate legal safeguards in nursing practice.

Explain the purpose of incident reports.

Describe laws affecting nursing practice.

## EXERCISES

### Matching

Match the intentional torts listed in Part A with their correct examples, listed in Part B.

Part A

a. assault

b. battery

c. slander

d. false imprisonment

e. fraud

f. libel

g. invasion of privacy

Part B

1. _____ An HIV-negative sports celebrity is admitted to the hospital for viral pneumonia. The charge nurse on his floor speculates to her co workers that the case may be AIDS related.

2. _____ A nurse seeking a middle management position in long-term care claims to be certified in gerontological nursing when this is not the case.

3. _____ A client recovering from a stroke refuses to eat her lunch because she has difficulty swallowing. The nurse takes the client's spoon and forces the food into her mouth, causing her to choke.

4. _____ A nurse threatens to use restraints on a 70-year-old client who has had hip surgery, if he continues to attempt to get out of bed on his own.

5. _____ A Down's syndrome client is placed in restraints after minor surgery to prevent him from harming himself or others, even though he has shown no violent tendencies.

6. _____ A nurse is responsible for supplying the information for a newspaper article describing a local politician's struggle against cancer.

7. _____ A nurse circulates a petition among her co-workers to remove a nurse from her unit who has engaged in inappropriate behavior with a client. The nurse's alleged inappropriate behavior is described in detail at the top of the petition.

Match the terms in Part A with their definitions in Part B.

Part A

a. litigation       f. appellate court

b. laws            g. trial court

c. tort            h. felony

d. crimes          i. misdemeanor

e. precedent

Part B

8. _____ A wrong against a person or his property considered to be against the public as well.

9. _____ The process of a lawsuit.

10. _____ A case that first sets down a rule by decision.

11. _____ Crimes punishable by imprisonment in state or federal penetentiaries for more than one year.

12. _____ Crimes punishable by fine or imprisonment for less than one year or both.

13. _____ Only hears cases questioning a point of law decided by trial court.

14. _____ A wrong committed by a person against another person or his property generally resulting in a civil trial.

15. _____ A standard or rule of conduct established and enforced by the government of a society.

16. _____ The first level of court which hears evidence and makes decisions according to the facts, usually involving a jury.

Match the legal safeguards for nurses in Part A with their examples in Part B.

Part A

a. client education

b. contract

c. professional liability insurance

d. competent practice

e. documentation

f. executing physician orders

g. risk management program

Part B

17. _____ A nurse administers the exact dosage of antibiotics prescribed by the client's physician.

18. _____ A hospital committee of doctors, nurses, and hospital managers meets every Wednesday to discuss safety and quality assurance.

19. _____ A nurse executes a legal agreement with a hospital to work as a licensed nurse for a specific salary.

20. _____ A nurse notices a client is having an adverse reaction to a drug and calls the client's physician. She carefully writes down the client's symptoms on his chart and records all directions given over the phone.

21. _____ A nurse refuses to perform a procedure on a client for which she feels unprepared. She later signs up for a class detailing that procedure.

22. _____ A nurse seeks legal advice to find out if she is covered by her hospital in case of negligence.

23. _____ A nurse describes a procedure for cleansing sutures to a woman who delivered a baby.

## Multiple Choice

Circle the letter that corresponds to the best answer for each question.

1. What is the process by which a person who has met certain criteria established by a non-governmental association is granted recognition?

   a. accreditation
   b. litigation
   c. licensure

2. What legal protection is available to health practitioners when they give aid to persons in emergency situations?

   a. informed consent
   b. Good Samaritan Laws
   c. licensure
   d. Negligence Liability Act

3. What is a tool used by health care institutions to document the occurrence of anything out of the ordinary that results in or has potential to harm a client, employee, or visitor?

   a. incident reports
   b. risk management programs
   c. precedents
   d. witness document

4. What is the process by which an educational program is evaluated and recognized as having met certain predetermined criteria?

   a. licensure
   b. registration
   c. accreditation

## Correct the False Statements

Circle the word *true* or *false* that follows the statement. If the word *false* has been circled, change the underlined word/words to make the statement true. Place your answer in the space provided.

1. The two persons involved in a lawsuit are the <u>plaintiff</u>, the person or government bringing suit against another; and the defendant, the person being accused of a crime or tort.

   True    False    _____

2. The American Nurses Association Standards of Practice and the Canadian Nurses Association Standards of Practice are examples of <u>legal</u> standards of nursing practice.

   True    False    _____

3. <u>The State Board of Nurses Examiners</u> may revoke or suspend a nurse's license for drug/alcohol abuse, fraud, or negligence.

   True    False    _____

4. A signed consent form is needed <u>only for experimental procedures</u>.

   True    False    _____

5. <u>Living Wills</u> appoint an agent that a person trusts to make decisions in the event of the appointing person's subsequent incapacity.

   True    False    _____

6. "Do not recussitate" or "no code" prevent the improper use of <u>CPR</u>.

   True    False    _____

7. The <u>U.S. Occupational Safety and Health Act of 1970</u> states that nurses must inform clients of advance directives.

   True    False    _____

8. Student nurses <u>are responsible</u> for their own acts of negligence.

   True    False    _____

## Completion

Name the four elements that must be established to prove liability as described below.

a. _____ Obligation to use due care.

b. _____ Failure to meet standard of care.

c. _____ Failure to meet standard of care, which actually causes the injury.

d. _____ Actual harm or injury resulting to client.

. Define the four sources of law existing at both the federal and state (provincial) level.

. Constitutions: _____
_____
_____
_____

. Statutes: _____
_____
_____
_____

. Administrative: _____
_____
_____
_____

. Common Law: _____
_____
_____
_____

3. Give and define examples of two kinds of advance directives.

a. _____
_____
_____

b. _____
_____
_____

4. Name six of the eight elements of competent nursing practice described in this chapter.

a. _____

b. _____

c. _____

d. _____

e. _____

f. _____

5. Place a check next to each of the recommendations below which would serve the best interests of a "nurse defendant."

a. _____ Discuss the case only with the key people (client, doctor) involved.

b._____ Be available for questions from the plaintiff's lawyer.

c. _____ Do not discuss the case with reporters.

d. _____ Change the client's records to correspond to each action you performed.

e. _____ Go to the witness stand prepared.

f. _____ Volunteer any information on the witness stand that you feel is pertinent to the case.

g. _____ Be courteous on the witness stand.

h. _____ Do not hide any information from your lawyer.

# 7

# Basic Human Needs: Individual, Family, and Community

Chapter 7 discusses the levels of basic human needs in each person. Definitions, structures, functions, and developmental tasks of families are described, as are family risk factors in health and illness. The community is defined, and community risk factors and nursing in the community are broadly addressed.

O B J E C T I V E S

After studying this chapter, the learner will be able to:

Define the terms used in the chapter.

Describe each level of Maslow's hierarchy of basic human needs.

Discuss nursing actions necessary to meet needs for each level of Maslow's hierarchy.

Discuss family concepts, including family roles, structures, functions, developmental stages, tasks, and health risk factors.

Identify aspects of the community that affect individual and family health.

Describe nursing interventions to promote and maintain wellness in the individual as a member of a family and as a member of the community.

## E X E R C I S E S

### Matching

Match the correct risk factor category (L, S, E, or B) with the appropriate family risk factor.

**Risk Factor Categories**

Life-style (L)

Social/Psychological (S)

Environmental (E)

Biologic (B)

**Family Risk Factors**

1. _____ birth defects

2. _____ chemical dependence

3. _____ inadequate child-care resources

4. _____ crowded living conditions

5. _____ conflict between family members

6. _____ lack of knowledge about sexual roles

7. _____ inadequate nutrition

8. _____ mental retardation

9. _____ genetic predisposition to sickle cell anemia

10. _____ child abuse

11. _____ water pollution

Match the family stage in Part A with the appropriate family task in Part B.

Part A

a. beginning family

b. childbearing family

c. preschool family

d. schoolage family

e. adolescent/young adult family

f. postparental family

g. aging family

Part B

12. _____ Adjusting to retirement.

13. _____ Establishing a mutually satisfying marriage.

14. _____ Preparing for retirement.

15. _____ Having and adjusting to infant.

16. _____ Maintaining open communication among members.

17. _____ Promoting joint decision-making between children and parents.

18. _____ Coping with parental loss of energy and privacy.

6. List six of the ten community risk factors described in the chapter.

a. _____

b. _____

c. _____

d. _____

e. _____

f. _____

In the space provided, write the type of family described.

7. The _____ family is composed of a father, a mother, and their children.

8. The _____ family is made up of family units who join together to form new family structures.

9. Children in a _____ family live most often with one birth parent and with one non-birth parent.

10. In the traditional _____ family, the father works outside the home and the mother cares for home and children.

11. Aunts, uncles, and grandparents are part of the _____ family.

## Completion

List the five levels of needs as defined by Maslow in hierarchial order in the diagram below (with number 5 being the first or most basic need).

1 _____

2 _____

3 _____

4 _____

5 _____

Complete the table below by providing an examples of how the family functions listed could be met within the family.

| Family Functions | Examples |
| --- | --- |
| 12. Physical | |
| 13. Economic | |
| 14. Reproductive | |
| 15. Affective/coping | |
| 16. Socialization | |

# 8

# Culture and Ethnicity

Chapter 8 presents concepts of culture and ethnicity. Included in the chapter is a discussion of cultural and ethnic influences on health care, and a discussion of folk medicine. The chapter concludes with concepts of transcultural nursing, including the culture of health care, cultural imposition, and providing transcultural care.

O B J E C T I V E S

After studying this chapter the learner will be able to:

Define key terms used in the chapter.

Discuss the concepts of culture, ethnicity, race, and stereotyping.

Describe cultural and ethnic characteristics that influence health care, including gender roles, language and communication, orientation to space and time, food and nutrition, socioeconomic factors, importance of family, physical and mental characteristics, spiritual characteristics, and perceptions of illness and health.

Compare and contrast the culture of the health care system with the broad concept of culture.

Identify the factors that affect the interaction of the nurse and the client in terms of health care values.

Discuss the guidelines that are useful in practicing transcultural nursing.

Use knowledge of specific cultural and ethnic factors in providing holistic, individualized nursing care to clients.

E X E R C I S E S

## Matching

Match the term in Part A with the correct definition in Part B.

Part A

a. culture

b. subculture

c. dominant group

d. minority group

e. cultural assimilation

f. ethnicity

g. race

h. stereotyping

Part B

1. _____ Categorizing persons into subgroups according to some specific physical characteristic.

2. _____ Subgroups of people with a distinct identity but having certain characteristics common to a larger culture.

3. _____ A group with some physical or cultural characteristic that identifies the people within it as different.

4. _____ The set of values, beliefs, and traditions held by a specific social group.

5. _____ A group within a culture that has the authority to control the value system and determine rewards.

6. _____ When one assumes that all members of a culture or ethnic group will act alike.

7. _____ The sense of identification held collectively by a cultural group.

8. _____ A minority group living within a dominant group lose cultural characteristics that make them different.

## Multiple Choice

Circle the letter that corresponds to the best answer for each question.

1. What is the primary means of transmitting culture from one generation to the next?
   a. written documents
   b. formal education
   c. language
   d. touch

2. Nursing is a subculture of a larger culture in our society. What is the larger culture?
   a. health care providers
   b. organizations of nurses
   c. institutions
   d. health care system

3. Which of the following statements is an example of negative stereotyping?
   a. Women are just as smart as men.
   b. A woman could never do that job; it takes a man.
   d. Jewish people have good business sense.
   e. All nurses are caring people.

4. Your client, Mr. Samz, draws back when you touch his arm. This may mean you have entered the area of:
   a. personal space
   b. no touching
   c. cultural sensitivity
   d. ethnic consideration

5. Your neighbor is of Native American heritage, and tells you she has "awful gas" after drinking milk. You recognize this as being:
   a. a keloid formation
   b. lactase deficiency
   c. a symptom of thalassemia
   d. G-6-PD deficiency

6. The feelings a person experiences when placed in a different and often strange culture is describe by the phrase:
   a. covert hostility
   b. Yin and Yang
   c. hot and cold
   d. culture shock

7. Mrs. Sanchez tells the nurse that the folk healer gave her some herb tea for her diarrhea. The nurse tells Mrs. Sanchez that this is totally wrong and will not be tolerated. The nurse is practicing:
   a. cultural sensitivity
   b. transcultural care
   c. cultural imposition
   d. cultural diversity

8. The folk medicine system classifies illness as natural or unnatural. An unnatural illness would be the result of which of the following?
   a. Punishment for failing to follow God's rules.
   b. Being exposed to smog in the environment.
   c. Not dressing warmly enough.
   d. Eating contaminated food.

9. Why is it important to assess the family for the dominant member when a client enters the hospital?
   a. The dominant member is the financial provider.
   b. The dominant member often makes decisions about health care.
   c. The dominant member rarely makes decisions.
   d. The dominant member must remain at the hospital.

10. In what population would you expect to find keloid formation?
    a. Asian-American
    b. African-American
    c. Hispanic
    d. White American

## Correct the False Statements

Circle the word *true* or *false* that follows the statement. If the word *false* has been circled, change the underlined word/words to make the statement true. Place your answer in the space provided.

1. Mrs. Quiet has been admitted to the hospital. Her husband answers the nurse's questions during the health history. Mr. Quiet is the <u>dominant</u> member of the family.

   True    False    _____

2. An increasing number of families living in poverty are headed by <u>males</u>.

   True    False    _____

3. Sickle cell anemia is a disease that occurs most commonly in <u>white middle-class</u> persons.

   True    False    _____

4. Reactions to culture shock are most often expressed as <u>anger</u>.

   True    False    _____

5. A major theme of transcultural nursing care is to focus on the <u>caring practices</u> of various cultures.

   True    False    _____

## Completion

List the common and unique cultural and social beliefs and behavior patterns shared by people within an ethnic group.

1. _____

2. _____

3. _____

4. _____

5. _____

6. _____

7. _____

8. _____

Provide definitions for the following terms.

9. Yin and Yang _____

_____

_____

10. Ataques _____

_____

_____

11. Acupunture _____

_____

12. Compadrazgo _____

_____

_____

13. Curanderas (os) _____

_____

_____

14. Write the word or phrase to complete the definition of transcultural nursing by Leininger (1990) that is provided in the chapter.

Transcultural nursing is a formal area of study and practice focused on a comparative study of

(a) _____ with respect to discovering (b) _____ and

(c) _____ as related to nursing phenomena of (d) _____,

(e) _____, or illness patterns within a cultural context.

15. What three groups of people are most at risk for living in poverty?

   a. _____

   b. _____

   c. _____

16. List the four factors that affect an interaction of the nurse with the client specific to *culture*.

   a. _____

   _____

   _____

   _____

   b. _____

   _____

   _____

   _____

   c. _____

   _____

   _____

   _____

   d. _____

   _____

   _____

# 9

# Stress and Adaptation

Chapter 9 discusses basic concepts of homeostasis, stress, and adaptation. Physiologic and psychologic responses to stress are described, including the mind-body interaction, local adaptation syndrome, general adaptation syndrome, and coping mechanisms. The effects of stress on the person and the family are addressed. Nursing actions to promote stress reduction, with specific activities, are presented. The chapter concludes with a discussion of stress management for nurses.

## O B J E C T I V E S

After studying this chapter the learner will be able to:

Define key terms used in the chapter.

Describe the mechanisms involved in maintaining physiologic homeostasis.

Explain the interdependent nature of stressors, stress, and adaptation.

Compare and contrast developmental and situational stress, incorporating the concepts of physiologic and psychosocial stressors.

Describe the physical and emotional responses to stress, including mind-body interaction, local adaptation syndrome, general adaptation syndrome, and coping/defense mechanisms.

Discuss the effects of short- and long-term stress on basic human needs, health and illness, and the family.

Integrate knowledge of healthy life-style, support systems, stress management techniques, and crisis intervention into nursing care plans.

Recognize and effectively cope with stress unique to the nursing profession.

## E X E R C I S E S

### Matching

Match the term in Part A with the correct definition in Part B.

Part A

a. homeostasis          f. anxiety

b. stress               g. defense mechanisms

c. stressor             h. caregiver burden

d. adaptation           i. crisis

e. developmental crisis j. situational stress

Part B

1. _____ Occurs when coping and defense mechanism are no longer effective, producing high level of anxiety.

2. _____ A vague sense of impending doom or apprehension.

3. _____ The change that takes place as a result of the response to a stressor.

4. _____ The return to a normal state of balance through physiologic and psychologic mechanisms.

5. _____ Anything that causes a person to experience stress.

6. _____ A condition in which the human system responds to changes in its normal balance state.

7. _____ Stress that occurs as the individual progresses through normal growth and development stages.

8. _____ Reactions used to protect one's self-esteem are useful in mild to moderate anxiety.

9. _____ Reactions to home care of family member for long periods of time.

10. _____ Stress that does not occur in predictable patterns; can occur at any time.

Match the homeostatic effect in Part A with the correct body system in Part B.

Part A

a. parasympathetic nervous system

b. sympathetic nervous system

c. pituitary

d. adrenals

e. thyroid

f. cardiovascular

g. renal

h. respiratory

i. gastrointestinal

Part B

11. _____ Regulates metabolic rate and growth.

12. _____ Slows heart rate.

13. _____ Provides oxygen and nutrients to cells.

14. _____ Stimulates the adrenal cortex and thyroid.

15. _____ Maintains fluid and electrolyte balance.

16. _____ Increases heart rate and cardiac output.

17. _____ Energy sources.

18. _____ Prepares the person for emergencies.

19. _____ Helps maintain acid-base balance.

## Multiple Choice

Circle the letter that corresponds to the best answer for each question.

1. When physiologic mechanisms within the body respond to internal changes to maintain an essential balance, the process is named:
   a. stress
   b. self-regulation
   c. homeostasis
   d. fight-or-flight response

2. Which of the following is an example of an external stressor?
   a. Having the flu.
   b. Hearing a loud noise.
   c. Experiencing menopause.
   d. Being afraid of flying.

3. Which of the following is an example of developmental stress?
   a. Starting a new job.
   b. The 2-year old is toilet trained.
   c. Being promoted to a head nurse.
   d. Having a car accident.

4. You respond to an approaching examination with a rapidly beating heart and shaking hands. This is the result of what type of response?
   a. coping mechanism
   b. stress adaptation
   c. defense mechanism
   d. mind-body interaction

5. While preparing to wash dishes, you fill the sink with hot water. When you put your hands in the water, you immediately take them out again. This illustrates what response?
   a. local adaptation syndrome
   b. inflammatory response
   c. reflex pain response
   d. general adaptation syndrome

6. Which of the following phrases best illustrates the panic level of anxiety?
   a. Loss of control and rational thought.
   b. Increases alertness and motivates learning.
   c. Narrow focus on specific detail.
   d. Narrows the perceptual field.

7. Following a clinical experience in which everything seemed to go wrong, the student nurse said, "That's it. I quit." This is an example of what type of task-oriented reaction?
   a. attack behavior
   b. compromise behavior
   c. constructive behavior
   d. withdrawal behavior

8. Which of the following statements would demonstrate habits that help in stress reduction and health?
   a. "I eat breakfast on the run; usually have a soda."
   b. "I get plenty of exercise cleaning the house."
   c. "I never get to bed before 1 AM and get up at 5 AM."
   d. "I walk for half an hour, four days a week."

9. The nurse teaches the client about the procedures and activities that will be experienced before, during, and after surgery. What type of stress reduction method is this?

   a. anticipatory guidance
   b. meditation
   c. biofeedback
   d. crisis intervention

10. When nurses become overwhelmed in their jobs and develop symptoms of anxiety and stress, they are said to be experiencing:

    a. culture shock
    b. adaptation
    c. burnout
    d. ineffective coping

## Completion

1. List the four results of adaptation.

   a. _____
   b. _____
   c. _____
   d. _____

2. You have a cut on your finger. Describe the phases of the inflammatory response that allow healing.

   Phase 1: _____
   _____
   _____
   _____

   Phase 2: _____
   _____
   _____
   _____

   Phase 3: _____
   _____
   _____
   _____
   _____

Write the names of the stages of the general adaptation syndrome described.

3. _____ Having perceived a threat and responded by mobilizing resources, the body now attempts to adapt to the stressor.

4. _____ A specific stressor is perceived and various defense mechanisms are activated.

5. _____ The adaptive mechanisms are ineffective; death may occur.

Define the defense mechanisms.

6. Compensation _____
   _____
   _____
   _____

7. Denial _____
   _____
   _____
   _____

8. Projection _____
   _____
   _____

9. Regression _____
   _____
   _____
   _____

10. Sublimation _____
    _____
    _____
    _____

## Sequencing

Items 1–5 illustrate the steps in the problem-solving technique used in crisis intervention. Place each step in the correct sequence by numbering the items from 1 to 5 (1 = the first step).

*Situation:* A senior nursing student is half-way through the last nursing course in the program. He realizes he is failing the course and may not graduate as planned. He realizes this is a crisis situation.

1. _____ The student makes a list of activities that could be eliminated or decreased, including nights out with friends, movies, and a part-time job.

2. _____ The student looks at each activity, saying to himself, "What would happen if I didn't do this?"

3. _____ The student acknowledges that he is not spending enough time reading the textbook and preparing for clinical experiences.

4. _____ The student chooses to eliminate every activity on the list until the course is completed.

5. _____ The student's plan is successful; he passes the course.

# 10

# Developmental Concepts

Chapter 10 describes growth and development from a theoretical perspective. Principles of growth and development are presented, and theories are described for psychoanalytic theory, psychosocial theory, developmental tasks, moral development, and faith development. The application of these concepts in nursing is discussed in terms of the family and implications for nursing.

O B J E C T I V E S

After studying this chapter the learner will be able to:

Define key terms used in the chapter.

Summarize basic principles of growth and development.

Discuss the theories of Freud, Erikson, Havighurst, Piaget, Kohlberg, Gilligan, and Fowler.

Describe the importance of incorporating multiple theories of growth and development in assessing and planning nursing care for individuals and families.

Describe the dynamics of family in providing nursing care.

List implications for nursing practice that uses a knowledge base of growth and development.

## E X E R C I S E S

### Matching

Match the term in Part A with the appropriate theorist in Part B.

Part A

a. id

b. intimacy versus isolation

c. sensorimotor stage

d. "good boy–good girl" stage

e. selfishness

Part B

1. _b_ Erikson

2. _a_ Freud

3. _e_ Gilligan

4. _c_ Piaget

5. _d_ Kohlberg

Match the term in Part A with the correct definition in Part B.

Part A

a. libido          d. accommodation

b. ego             e. assimilation

c. oral stage

Part B

6. _e_ The process of integrating new experiences into existing schemata.

7. _d_ An alteration of thought processes to correlate more complex information.

8. _b_ The conscious part of the psyche that serves as a mediator.

9. _a_ General pleasure-seeking instincts.

10. _c_ Pleasures center around gratification by sucking and satisfying hunger.

## Multiple Choice

Circle the letter that corresponds to the best answer for each question.

1. The development of the fetus proceeds from head to tail. This pattern of growth and development is called:

   a. proximodistal
   b. symmetrical
   c. cephalocaudal
   d. central/peripheral

2. Freud believed the underlying stimulus for human behavior was:

   a. sexuality
   b. faith
   c. crisis
   d. morality

3. A mother notices her 5-year-old masturbating during his bath. Based on Freud's theory, she should do which of the following?

   a. Punish the child by restricting television viewing.
   b. Ask her husband to give the child his bath.
   c. Explain why the child should not do this.
   d. Accept the behavior as normal.

4. Erikson believed that providing an infant with inconsistent, inadequate, or unsafe care would result in:

   a. shame
   b. mistrust
   c. inferiority
   d. guilt

5. Based on Piaget's theory of cognitive development, which of the following school activities would be most difficult for a third-grader?

   a. Reading from a third-grade reader.
   b. Writing in cursive style.
   c. Measuring body height and weight.
   d. Working with fractions in math.

6. Fowler's universalizing faith stage corresponds with which of Erikson's psychosocial stages?

   a. integrity vs despair
   b. trust vs mistrust
   c. identity vs role confusion
   d. intimacy vs isolation

7. According to Havighurst, a developmental task of later maturity is to:

   a. Take on a civic responsibility.
   b. Learn to get along with age-mates.
   c. Adjust to declining physical strength.
   d. Acquire a set of values and an ethical system.

## Correct the False Statements

Circle the word *true* or *false* that follows the statement. If the word *false* has been circled, change the underlined word/words to make the statement true. Place your answer in the space provided.

1. Upper limits that can be achieved in growth and development are imposed primarily by one's <u>environment</u>.

   True    False    _____

2. The <u>id</u> is the part of the psyche concerned with self-gratification.

   True    False    _____

3. When parents encourage toddlers to put on their own clothes, the parents are encouraging <u>autonomy</u>.

   True    False    _____

4. The young adult who fears commitment to others may have <u>stagnation</u>.

   True    False    _____

5. Gilligan defines the female morality as being an orientation of <u>"the ethic of law and order."</u>

   True    False    _____

## Completion

List the five broad principles of growth and development discussed in the chapter.

1. _____

_____

_____

2. _____

_____

_____

3. _____

_____

_____

4. _____

_____

_____

5. _____

_____

_____

6. List the four major organizing concepts for psychosocial theory:

a. _____

b. _____

c. _____

d. _____

List the levels of Gilligan's theory of moral development.

7. Level 1: _____

8. Level 2: _____

9. Level 3: _____

10. List the functions of the family as described by Friedman.

a. _____

b. _____

c. _____

d. _____

e. _____

f. _____

Use the space provided to identify the stages of faith described by Fowler.

11. _____ Prestage when trust, courage, hope, and love compete with threats of abandonment.

12. _____ Typical of ages 3–7, when children imitate religious gestures and behaviors of caregivers.

13. _____ Found in the school-age child; includes concept of reciprocal fairness.

14. _____ The adolescent begins to question values and religious practices to stabilize own identity.

15. _____ The young adult accepts responsibility for commitments, beliefs, and attitudes.

16. _____ Others' viewpoints about faith are integrated into one's understanding of truth.

17. _____ Characterized by total trust in the principle of being and the existence of the future.

Identify the stage of the theorist noted that can be used by the nurse in responding to statements made by the client in the following situation.

*Situation:* A 15-year-old boy, Toby, has been admitted to the hospital following a three-wheeler accident. Toby has multiple fractures and several deep cuts in his face that require stitches.

18. *Freud:* _____ "My dad told me not to ride that thing. I should have listened to him and this never would have happened."

19. *Erikson:* _____ "I am going to be so ugly with these scars on my face. I won't ever be able to have a girl look at me again."

20. *Piaget:* _____ "Tell me the best way to be sure I don't lose strength in my muscles. If I do those exercises you taught me, I will be able to go back to school and play basketball next year."

21. *Fowler:* _____ "I don't believe in God. If there is a God he would never have let this happen to me."

# 11

# Conception Through Midlife

Chapter 11 discusses the person from conception through midlife: conception, the neonate, infancy, toddlerhood, preschooler, school-age, adolescence, young adult, and middle adult. Included in the discussion of each stage of life in this chapter are physiologic development, cognitive development, psychosocial development, common health problems, and the role of the nurse in health care. Adult developmental theories are presented in the section about young and adult development, as are adaptations and needs during pregnancy.

## OBJECTIVES

After studying this chapter the learner will be able to:

Define key terms used in the chapter.

Summarize major physiologic, cognitive, psychosocial, moral, and spiritual development for each age period from conception through the middle years.

List common health problems of each age period from the newborn through middle adulthood.

Describe nursing actions to promote wellness at each developmental level.

Discuss the adult developmental theories of Gould, Levinson, and Erikson.

## EXERCISES

### Matching

Match the term in Part A with the correct definition in Part B.

Part A

a. prelinguistic

b. attachment

c. play

d. temperament

e. separation anxiety

f. negativism

g. regression

h. puberty

i. menopause

j. andropause

Part B

1. _____ The stage in which secondary sex characteristics develop and reproductive organs function.

2. _____ Behavior that is more characteristic of a younger age.

3. _____ The beginning stage of language development.

4. _____ An active, affectionate, reciprocal relationship between two people.

5. _____ Primarily inborn, influenced by environment, allows labeling the baby as "easy" or "difficult."

6. _____ Allows the infant/child to discover the environment and to begin to learn to control it.

7. _____ A normal, gradual decrease in ovarian function in the middle-adult woman.

8. _____ Occurs when a child is afraid of being sent away from those persons who are loved and represent security.

9. _____ The result of the toddler's effort to have some control over his or her environment.

10. _____ Decreased androgen levels that normally occur in the middle-adult man.

Match the specific age group in Part A with the appropriate behaviors in Part B according to Gould's theory of adult development.

Part A

a. 18–22 years

b. 23–28 years

c. 29–34 years

d. 35–43 years

e. 44–50 years

f. 51–60 years

Part B

11. _____ Establishes control of self.

12. _____ Demonstrates competence as an independent adult.

13. _____ Questions self and values; sees time as having an end.

14. _____ Realization of mortality.

15. _____ Increased self-confidence; no longer has need to prove self.

16. _____ Set personalities/special interests.

## Multiple Choice

Circle the letter that corresponds to the best answer for each question.

1. Many different factors influence the development of the zygote. A neonate born with defects in the bones of the lower legs may have had interference with what cell layer in the pre-embryonic stage?

   a. ectoderm
   b. mesoderm
   c. endoderm
   d. ovum

2. The test administered to the neonate immediately after birth is named the:

   a. Denver Developmental Screening
   b. Neonatal Test
   c. Apgar Rating Scale
   d. Infant Scoring Mode

3. The process that occurs during a sensitive period in the first few hours of life and that is necessary to attachment is called:

   a. bonding
   b. binding
   c. borning
   d. attaching

4. Which of the following toys would be most age-appropriate for the toddler?

   a. stuffed animal
   b. building blocks
   c. basketball
   c. tricycle

5. Which of the following words, if repeated frequently, is considered normal for the preschooler?

   a. no!
   b. why?
   c. bye-bye
   d. potty

6. Andee, age 4, often cries out at night and wants a night light on in her room. When her mother asks you about this, your reply is based on the knowledge that this is:

   a. normal for Andee's age
   b. abnormal behavior for a preschooler
   c. the result of a severe trauma
   d. something that must be stopped

7. The influential group in stabilizing self-concept in the adolescent are his or her:

   a. parents
   b. siblings
   c. peers
   d. teachers

8. The leading cause of death in adolescents is:

   a. infectious diseases
   b. cancer
   c. smoking
   d. accidents

9. Midlife transition is a phenomenon that seems to occur in both men and women during their late 30s and 40s. What area of life is *not* usually affected by this transition?

   a. physiology
   b. economics
   c. work
   d. relationships

10. You have been asked to implement a sex education program in the public schools. With which
grade level would you begin the program?

    a. kindergarten
    b. elementary
    c. junior high
    d. high school

## Correct the False Statements

Circle the word *true* or *false* that follows the statement. If the word *false* has been circled, change the
underlined word/words to make the statement true.
Place your answer in the space provided.

1. A developmental task of <u>infancy</u> is learning to control elimination.

    True     False     _____

2. "Playing doctor" is normal behavior for the
<u>preschooler</u>.

    True     False     _____

3. Suicide is more prevalent in <u>middle adults</u> than in
any other age group.

    True     False     _____

4. The most common STD among adolescents of both
sexes is <u>syphilis</u>.

    True     False     _____

5. During the <u>second</u> trimester of pregnancy, body
changes and fetal movements make the baby real
to the pregnant woman.

    True     False     _____

## Completion

1. You have completed an Apgar on a newborn, and
the score is 10. What does this number represent?

    _____

    _____

    _____

    _____

2. Describe the risks for the infant born to the mother
who:

    a. smokes cigarettes _____

    _____

    _____

    b. drinks alcohol _____

    _____

    _____

    _____

    c. uses cocaine, crack, and/or heroin _____

    _____

    _____

    _____

    _____

3. List the areas of development assessed with the
DDST.

    a. _____

    b. _____

    c. _____

    d. _____

4. List five of the six psychosocial needs of the
prospective father described in the chapter.

    a. _____

    _____

    b. _____

    _____

    c. _____

    _____

    d. _____

    _____

    e. _____

    _____

5. Define the term "child abuse."

_____

_____

_____

_____

6. Describe five teaching activities nurses can use to promote wellness in the infant in the area of accident prevention and safety.

a. _____

_____

b. _____

_____

c. _____

_____

d. _____

_____

e. _____

_____

7. Describe four teaching activities nurses can use to promote wellness in the school-age child in the area of sexuality.

a. _____

_____

b. _____

_____

c. _____

_____

d. _____

_____

8. Describe normal physiologic changes that take place in the middle adult years

a. Body structure: _____

_____

_____

_____

b. Skin and hair: _____

_____

_____

_____

c. Musculoskeletal: _____

_____

_____

_____

d. Sensory: _____

_____

_____

_____

e. Reproductive: _____

_____

_____

_____

# 12

## The Older Adult

Chapter 12 focuses on the older adult. Information presented includes theories of aging, with discussion of physiologic and functional status, cognitive development, and developmental tasks specific to those over 65 years. Meeting health care needs of the older adult includes the implications of chronic illness, injuries, and acute care needs. Nursing implications for the care of the elderly are included.

O B J E C T I V E S

After studying this chapter the learner will be able to:

Define key terms used in the chapter.

Describe common myths and stereotypes that perpetuate ageism.

Gain awareness of own feelings and attitudes toward the aging process and the older adult.

Compare physiologic and functional changes that occur with normal aging.

Discuss developmental tasks of the older adult, as described by Erikson and Havighurst.

Identify socioenvironmental factors in our society that may inhibit the older adult from meeting needs and realizing potentials.

Discuss nursing implications concerning the continued growth and development of the elderly client.

List family and community resources that can be utilized to maintain the health and independence of the elderly client.

Describe the health care needs of the older adult in terms of chronic illness, accidental injuries, and acute care needs.

## E X E R C I S E S

### Matching

Match the term in Part A with the correct definition in Part B.

Part A

a. ageism

b. dementia

c. sundowning syndrome

d. reminiscence

e. gerontology

Part B

1. _____ A form of prejudice about older adults.

2. _____ The scientific and behavioral study of all aspects of aging and its consequences.

3. _____ The older adult habitually becomes confused in darkness.

4. _____ A variety of organically caused disorders that progressively affect cognitive functioning.

5. _____ A way for the older adult to relive and restructure life experiences.

## Multiple Choice

Circle the letter that corresponds to the best answer for each question.

1. After what age is one considered an older adult?

   a. 45
   b. 55
   c. 65
   d. 75

2. Which of these organizations is a strong social and political force for older adults?

   a. Medicare
   b. AARP
   c. White Panthers
   d. WKRP

3. In general, where do most older adults live?

   a. in their own homes
   b. in nursing homes
   c. in retirement communities
   d. with their children

4. Based on an understanding of the cognitive changes that normally occur with aging, what would you expect a newly hospitalized older adult to do?

   a. Talk rapidly, but be confused.
   b. Withdraw from strangers.
   c. Interrupt with frequent questions.
   d. Take longer to respond and react.

5. Which of the following nursing actions would help maintain safety in the older adult?

   a. Treat each client as a unique individual.
   b. Orient the client to new surroundings.
   c. Encourage independence.
   d. Provide planned rest and activity times.

6. As defined by Erikson, in what stage of human development is the older adult?

   a. intimacy versus isolation
   b. identity versus role diffusion
   c. ego-integrity versus despair
   d. generativity versus stagnation

7. According to Havighurst, which of the following is a developmental task of later maturity?

   a. Adjusting to declining physical strength and health.
   b. Moving from one's own home to the home of others.
   c. Learning to live by oneself after losing spouse.
   d. Establishing oneself in the community.

8. Which of the following questions might you expect your elderly client to have difficulty answering?

   a. When were your children born?
   b. Where did you live when you got married?
   c. How old were you when you started school?
   d. What did you have for breakfast?

9. Reduced muscle tone and decreased peristalsis cause a common problem in the older adult. What is the problem?

   a. loss of appetite
   b. wrinkling of skin
   c. constipation
   d. visual deficits

10. Your 85-year-old neighbor, Mrs. Panoose, tells you she notices that she has to "get up and go to the toilet two or three a times a night." Your answer to her is based on the knowledge that this is:

    a. abnormal; she must have a bladder infection
    b. abnormal; having six children ruined her kidneys
    c. normal; she drinks a lot of liquids during the day
    d. normal; bladder capacity is decreased with age

## Completion

. What is meant by the term "old-old"? _____

_____

_____

. List the six developmental tasks of later maturity
escribed by Havighurst:

. _____

_____

. _____

_____

. _____

_____

. _____

_____

. _____

_____

. _____

_____

. What are the most commonly occurring chronic
llnesses in the older adult?

. _____

. _____

. _____

. _____

. _____

. What is the most common surgery in persons over
5? _____

_____

5. Describe five normal physiologic changes in the
neurologic system that occur in older adulthood.

a. _____

_____

b. _____

_____

c. _____

_____

d. _____

_____

e. _____

_____

6. Describe the questions you would ask to collect the
necessary information to meet the needs of the hospitalized older adult in the area of sleep and rest.

a. _____

b. _____

c. _____

d. _____

e. _____

# 13

## Loss, Grief, and Death

Chapter 13 provides an overview of loss, grief, and death. Loss and grief are defined and described. Factors affecting grief and death are discussed. The dying client is addressed in terms of the needs of the dying, the impact of terminal illness, stages of dying, and meeting needs of the client and the family. Ethical and legal dimensions as well as nursing responsibilities are described.

O B J E C T I V E S

After studying this chapter the learner will be able to:

Define key terms used in the chapter.

Differentiate the types of loss.

Describe the grief process and the stages of grief.

Outline physiologic and psychologic care of a dying client.

Identify ethical/legal issues concerning death.

List the clinical signs of approaching death.

Outline nursing responsibilities following death.

Discuss the role of the nurse in caring for a client's family.

## Matching

Match the term in Part A with the correct definition in Part B.

Part A

a. loss

b. actual loss

c. perceived loss

d. anticipatory loss

e. grieving

f. bereavement

g. mourning

h. grief

i. dysfunctional grief

j. restitution

Part B

1. _____ Involves the rituals surrounding loss (Engel, 1964).

2. _____ Occurs when a valued person, object, or situation is changed or made inaccessible.

3. _____ Abnormal or distorted grief; may be unresolved or inhibited.

4. _____ Loss that can be recognized by others as well as by the person sustaining the loss.

5. _____ The emotional pain caused by loss.

6. _____ Loss perceived by the individual, but intangible to others.

7. _____ The period of acceptance of loss and grief.

8. _____ The individual displays loss and grief behaviors for a loss that has yet to take place.

9. _____ The state of grieving during which an individual goes through grief reaction.

10. _____ The emotional reaction to loss; occurs with loss due to separations as well as loss due to death.

Match the stages of grief, as defined by Kübler-Ross and listed in Part A, with the appropriate statements for each stage listed in Part B.

**Part A**

a. denial and isolation

b. anger

c. bargaining

d. depression

e. acceptance

**Part B**

11. _____ "Why me . . . I did everything I was supposed to do!"

12. _____ "They made a mistake. I don't have cancer."

13. _____ "I can't stand the thought of never seeing my children grow up. . . ."

14. _____ "If I can just live long enough to go to my daughter's wedding, I will be happy."

15. _____ "I can die with peace. I've done all I can."

## Multiple Choice

Circle the letter that corresponds to the best answer for each question.

1. The nurse provides care for the grieving family primarily within which role?
   a. caretaker
   b. communicator
   c. researcher
   d. teacher

2. An examination of the organs and tissues of a human body following death is called a/an:
   a. euthanasia
   b. homicide
   c. autopsy
   d. bereavement

3. According to Engel (1964), the exaggeration of the good qualities of the person or object lost, followed by acceptance of the loss is:
   a. idealization
   b. restitution
   c. awareness
   d. outcome

4. Following the death of her husband, Sardi complained of frequent headaches and loss of appetite. No medical cause was found. Sardi probably had what type of grief?
   a. abbreviated grief
   b. anticipatory grief
   c. unresolved grief
   d. inhibited grief

5. When a client dies, the nurse's first nursing action should be to:
   a. Place proper identification on the body.
   b. Ask the family for permission to donate organs.
   c. Allow the family to spend time with the body.
   d. Call the funeral home or mortician.

## Completion

1. List the clinical symptoms of grief described by Schultz:
   a. _____
   b. _____
   c. _____
   d. _____
   e. _____
   f. _____
   g. _____

2. Describe three of the five personal questions a nurse may ask to help clarify feelings about death.
   a. _____
   _____
   b. _____
   _____
   c. _____
   _____

3. What is the last sense believed to leave the body in the dying person? _____

4. What physical needs of the dying client should be met by the nurse?

a. _____

b. _____

c. _____

d. _____

e. _____

f. _____

5. In what circumstances of death must a coroner be legally notified?

a. _____

b. _____

c. _____

d. _____

6. Complete the following definition of death by filling in the blank spaces:

Death is present when an (a) _____

has sustained either irreversible cessation of

(b) _____ and

(c) _____ functions, or irreversible

cessation of all functions of the entire

(d) _____, including the

(e) _____.

7. List the needs of grieving families for *participating*.

a. _____

b. _____

c. _____

d. _____

# 14

# Introduction to Nursing Process

As the practice of nursing became more complex, nurses began to study the process of nursing to both understand and improve the means nurses use to accomplish their aims. Chapter 14 discusses the five major steps in the nursing process: assessing, diagnosing, planning, implementing, and evaluating. Five key descriptors of the nursing process highlighted in this chapter are: systematic, dynamic, interpersonal, goal-oriented, and universally applicable. Problem solving as it relates to the nursing process is also discussed and several benefits of the nursing process are described.

## OBJECTIVES

After studying this chapter the learner will be able to:

Define key terms used in the chapter.

Describe the historical evolution of the nursing process.

Describe the nursing process and each of its five steps.

List five characteristics of the nursing process.

List three client and three nursing benefits of using the nursing process correctly.

## EXERCISES

## Matching

Match the actions listed in Part B with the nursing process steps listed in Part A.

Part A

a. assessing

b. diagnosing

c. planning

d. implementing

e. evaluating

Part B

1. _____ The nurse sits down with the client and determines what nursing measures will be used to assist the client in achieving his goals for recovery.

2. _____ The nurse and client together measure the extent to which client goals have been met.

3. _____ The nurse collects all data pertinent to the case, evaluates the data, and communicates this to the client.

4. _____ Actions are performed by the nurse to carry out the plan.

5. _____ The nurse analyzes client data in order to identify actual or potential health problems and coping patterns or strengths of the client.

## Multiple Choice

Circle the letter that corresponds to the best answer for each question.

1. The initial determination of whether or not the client needs nursing care is made during which step of the nursing process?
   a. assessing
   b. diagnosing
   c. planning
   d. implementing
   e. evaluating

2. The fact that each nursing task is part of an ordered sequence of activities, and that each activity is dependent on the accuracy of the activity that precedes it, is indicative of which characteristic of the nursing process?
   a. dynamic
   b. goal-oriented
   c. interpersonal
   d. systematic
   e. universally applicable

3. The nursing process is applicable:
   a. When nurses work with clients who are able to participate in their care.
   b. When families are clearly supportive and wish to participate in care.
   c. Whenever patients are totally dependent on the nurse for care.
   d. In all nursing situations.

4. As students struggle to master nursing process skills, it would be most helpful to remember that:
   a. Nurses in the "real world" no longer need to worry about the nursing process.
   b. When used well, the nursing process achieves for clients scientifically based, holistic, individualized care.
   c. Although the nursing process offers nurses no benefits, there are important client benefits achieved through its use.

5. Which method of problem solving is "a direct apprehension of a situation based upon a background of similar and dissimilar situations and embodied intelligence and skill" (Benner, 1984)?
   a. intuitive problem solving
   b. scientific method
   c. trial and error method
   d. nursing process

## Correct the False Statements

Circle the word *true* or *false* that follows the statement. If the word *false* has been circled, change the underlined word/words to make the statement true. Place your answer in the space provided.

1. The Joint Commission on Accreditation of Health Care Organizations requires that care be documented according to the <u>nursing plan.</u>

   True    False    _____

2. In addition to roles as caregivers, nurses also fill roles as <u>care managers/coordinators,</u> teachers, counselors, advocates and researchers.

   True    False    _____

3. In l967, <u>Hall and Hammond</u> published the first comprehensive book on nursing process, which described the four steps of assessment, planning, intervention, and evaluation.

   True    False    _____

4. The steps of the nursing process were legitimized in l973, when the American Nurses Association Congress for Nursing Practices developed <u>Standards of Practice</u> to guide nursing performance.

   True    False    _____

5. The <u>scientific method</u> is a systematic method that directs the nurse and client as they determine the need for nursing care, plan and implement the care and evaluate the results.

   True    False    _____

6. The <u>trial and error</u> method of problem solving involves testing any number of solutions until one is found that works for that particular problem.

   True    False    _____

7. The <u>intuitive problem solving</u> method is a systematic, seven-step process that is closely related to the more general, six-step problem solving process used by health care professionals as they work with clients.

   True    False    _____

## Completion

. List and describe five characteristics of the nursing process.

. _____
_____

. _____
_____

. _____
_____

. _____
_____

. _____
_____

. List four benefits of the nursing process.

. _____

. _____

. _____

. _____

. List three key professional events in the evolution of nursing diagnosis as an integral component of nursing process.

. _____

. _____

. _____

## Sequencing

Items 1–5 below are steps in the nursing process. Place each step in the proper sequence by numbering the items.

1. _____ The nurse and the client develop a plan of care that details client goals and determines which nursing actions are likely to obtain these goals.

2. _____ The nurse determines if the nursing plan is effective in terms of client goal achievement.

3. _____ The nurse obtains all data pertinent to this case and reviews it systematically.

4. _____ The nurse carries out the predetermined plan of care.

5. _____ The nurse lists client strengths and health problems and determines if each health problem is best treated by nursing or by another health discipline.

# 15

# Assessing

Assessing, the systematic and continuous collection, validation and communication of client data, is the main focus of Chapter 15. The learner is provided with concepts essential to obtaining a data base, enabling an effective plan of care to be designed and implemented for the client. Interviewing the client to obtain a nursing history and performing a nursing examination to collect data are discussed, and other sources of client information, including support persons, client records, client's health care professionals, and nursing and health care literature, are detailed. Methods for verifying and recording data are also presented in this chapter.

## OBJECTIVES

After studying this chapter the learner will be able to:

Define key terms used in the chapter.

Describe the purposes of the initial nursing assessment and of ongoing nursing assessments.

Differentiate a nursing assessment from a medical assessment.

Differentiate objective and subjective data.

Describe the purposes of nursing observation, interview, and physical assessment.

Obtain a nursing history using effective interviewing techniques.

Identify five sources of client data useful to the nurse.

Differentiate comprehensive admission assessments from focused assessments.

Plan client assessments by identifying assessment priorities and structuring the data to be collected systematically.

Identify common problems encountered in data collection, noting their possible cause and etiology.

Explain when data need to be validated and several ways to accomplish this.

Describe the importance of knowing when to report significant client data and the importance of proper documentation.

Obtain complete, accurate, relevant, and factual client data.

## EXERCISES

### Matching

Match the term in Part A with the definition in Part B.

Part A

a. data base

b. observation

c. subjective data

d. physical assessment

e. validation

f. objective data

Part B

1. _____ Information perceived only by the affected person, which cannot be perceived or verified by another person.

2. _____ Includes all the pertinent client information collected by the nurses and other health care professionals.

3. _____ The conscious and deliberate use of the five physical senses to gather data.

4. _____ Information perceived by the senses; can be verified by another person.

5. _____ The act of confirming or verifying; helps keep data free from error, bias, and misinterpretation.

6. _____ The examination of the client for objective data that may help the nurse in planning care.

Match the examples of data in Part B with the type of data (a or b) in Part A.

**Part A**

a. objective data

b. subjective data

**Part B**

7. _____ Redness and swelling are noticed at the site of an incision.

8. _____ Client complains of pain in his left arm.

9. _____ Client has a violent spell of coughing.

0. _____ A client recovering from knee surgery favors his impaired leg while walking.

1. _____ Client is nauseated at the sight of food.

2. _____ Client worries about what will happen to her children during her hospital stay.

Match the characteristics of data listed in Part A with the related nursing measure in Part B.

**Part A**

a. relevant

b. accurate and factual

c. complete

**Part B**

3. _____ Verifying what is heard with what is observed using other senses, and validating questionable data.

4. _____ Determining what type of data to collect for each client.

5. _____ Identifying all client data necessary to understand a client health problem.

## Multiple Choice

Circle the letter that corresponds to the best answer for each question.

1. The primary purpose of the nursing assessment is which of the following?
   a. To help define underlying pathology.
   b. To assist in identifying the client's medical problem.
   c. To help identify the causes of the client's physical symptoms.
   d. To explore client responses to health problems.

2. Mrs. Smith is admitted to the hospital with c/o left sided weakness and difficulty speaking. Which of the following assessments contains the data that best represents a nursing assessment?
   a. Neurological exam reveals partial paralysis and aphasic speech.
   b. Brain scan shows evidence of a clot in the middle cerebral artery.
   c. Unable to communicate basic needs and perform hygiene measures with left hand.
   d. Left-sided weakness and speech deficit indicate probable stroke.

3. Mr. Martin is an energetic 80-year-old admitted to the hospital with c/o difficulty urinating, bloody urine, and burning on urination. In assessing Mr. Martin, which of the following data collection priorities should be included?
   a. Focusing on altered patterns of elimination common in the elderly.
   b. Only assessing the urinary system.
   c. A detailed assessment of the client's sexual history.
   d. A thorough systems review to validate data on the client's record.

4. Mrs. Jones is a 48-year-old woman admitted to your unit with diabetes mellitus. Which of the following would be important for the nurse to remember during the nursing interview?
   a. Focus on the client during the interview.
   b. Be sure to get all your questions answered regardless of importance.
   c. Use questions that require a "yes" or "no" answer to speed up the interview.
   d. Assure the client that everything is going to be all right.

5. During the nursing examination Mrs. Jones becomes very tired. There are still questions the nurse practitioner would have liked to address in order to have data for planning Mrs. Jones' care. Which of the following actions would be most appropriate in this situation?
   a. Ask Mrs. Jones to wake up and try to answer your questions.
   b. Ask Mrs. Jones' husband to come in and answer your questions.
   c. Wait until the next day to obtain the answers to your questions.
   d. Ask Mrs. Jones if she objects to your interviewing her husband to obtain the needed data.

6. Actual and factual recording of client data is an important aspect of the nursing process. Which statement below would meet the criteria for factual?
   a. "Mrs. Jay is depressed today."
   b. "Jerry refused lunch today, would not engage in conversation, and was frequently observed staring out the window."
   c. "Client's behavior is weird."
   d. "Sara selected her lunch, deliberately avoiding high salt and fat content foods."

7. Mrs. Anderson is a 50-year-old female admitted to your unit with the diagnosis of scleroderma. You are unfamiliar with this condition. Which of the following would be your best source of information?
   a. Consult with the client.
   b. Consult with the client's doctor.
   c. Read the client's chart.
   d. Consult nursing and medical literature.

## Correct the False Statements

Circle the word *true* or *false* that follows the statement. If the word *false* has been circled, change the underlined word/words to make the statement true. Place your answer in the space provided.

1. Focused assessment is usually performed during the nurse's initial contact with the client, whereby the nurse collects data concerning all aspects of the client's health.

   True    False    _____

2. A general guideline when assessing clients is to gather as much data as possible, including information not directly related to the planned health care of the client.

   True    False    _____

3. Whenever possible, it is best to communicate with clients at eye level.

   True    False    _____

4. The purpose of validating data is to keep data as free from error, bias, and misrepresentation as possible.

   True    False    _____

5. Nurses are responsible for alerting appropriate health care professionals whenever assessment data differs significantly from the client baseline, indicating a potentially serious problem.

   True    False    _____

6. The focus of the nursing history is getting to know the data.

   True    False    _____

7. During the assessment step of the nursing process, the nurse interviews the client to obtain a nursing history.

   True    False    _____

8. Physical assessment is the examination of the client for subjective data that may be helpful to better define the client's condition.

   True    False    _____

9. Nursing physical assessments focus on the identification of the pathology and its etiology.

   True    False    _____

## Completion

Read each statement carefully and supply the information requested.

1. Name the phase of interview described below.

   a. _____ The nurse initiates the interview by stating his or her name and status, identifying the purpose of the interview and clarifying the roles of nurse and client.

   b. _____ The interview is carefully concluded; interview is recapitulated and key points are highlighted.

   c. _____ The nurse reads present and past records of the client and ensures the atmosphere for the interview is private and relaxed.

   d. _____ The nurse gathers all the information needed to form the subjective data base.

2. Name four methods commonly used to collect data during a physical assessment.

   a. _____

   b. _____

   c. _____

   d. _____

3. Name five sources of data for nurses.

   a. _____

   b. _____

   c. _____

   d. _____

   e. _____

4. Name three factors influencing assessment priorities.

   a. _____

   b. _____

   c. _____

5. List a remedy for the following problems of data collection:

   a. Pertinent data is omitted. _____

   _____

   _____

   b. Irrelevant or duplicate data is collected. _____

   _____

   _____

   c. Too little data is acquired from client._____

   _____

   _____

   d. Failure to update the data base._____

   _____

   _____

   e. Erroneous or misinterpreted data collected._____

   _____

   _____

# 16

# Diagnosing

The identification of actual and potential problems in the way the client responds to health or illness and the identification of etiologies and client strengths are the purposes of diagnosing discussed in Chapter 16. The distinction between nursing diagnosis versus collaborative problems is highlighted, as well as the interpretation and analysis of data. The learner is also presented with guidelines for writing a nursing diagnosis.

O B J E C T I V E S

After studying this chapter the learner will be able to:

Define key terms used in the chapter.

Describe the term "nursing diagnosis," distinguishing it from a collaborative problem and a medical diagnosis.

Describe the four steps involved in data interpretation and analysis.

Use the guidelines for writing nursing diagnoses when developing diagnostic statements.

List four advantages of using the NANDA-approved list of nursing diagnoses.

Develop a prioritized list of nursing diagnoses using identifiable criteria.

Describe the benefits and limitations of nursing diagnoses.

E X E R C I S E S

## Matching

Match the definitions in Part B with the terms in Part A. Each term may be used only once.

Part A

a. health problem

e. cue

b. nursing diagnosis

f. data cluster

c. medical diagnosis

g. problem statement

d. collaborative problem

h. wellness diagnosis

Part B

1. _____ A clinical judgment about an individual, family, or community in transition from a specific level of wellness to a higher level of wellness.

2. _____ Describes the health state or health problem of the client as clearly and concisely as possible.

3. _____ A condition related to health that requires intervention if disease or illness is to be prevented or resolved, and if coping and wellness are to be promoted.

4. _____ Describes problems for which the physician directs the primary treatment.

5. _____ Physiologic complications nurses monitor to detect onset or changes in status.

6. _____ Actual or potential health problems that can be prevented or resolved by independent nursing intervention.

7. _____ A grouping of client data that points to the existence of client health problems.

8. _____ Significant data, or data that influences decisions.

Match the examples in Part B with the four steps involved in the interpretation and analysis of data listed in Part A.

Part A

a. recognizing significant data.

b. recognizing patterns or clusters.

c. identifying strengths and problems.

d. reaching conclusions.

Part B

9. _____ A nurse notes that a client's refusal to stop smoking will adversely affect his recovery from cardiac surgery.

10. _____ A nurse compares a 15-month-old child's motor abilities with the norm for that age group.

11. _____ A nurse recognizes an unhealthy situation developing around a woman recovering from a mastectomy who cries at night, refuses to eat meals, and sleeps all day.

12. _____ A nurse decides no futher nursing response is indicated for a woman who recovered from gall bladder surgery according to schedule.

13. _____ A maternity nurse notices a newborn's skin tone is noticeably different than that of the other babies and checks for jaundice.

14. _____ A nurse determines that a man with a history of diabetes is highly motivated to develop a healthy pattern of nutrition in response to his problem.

15. _____ A nurse notices that a client with AIDS has an adverse reaction to a drug and consults the prescribing physician.

## Multiple Choice

Circle the letter that corresponds to the best answer for each question.

1. Which of the following factors is least significant when using Atkinson and Murray's (1990) guide for prioritizing client problems?
   a. client preference
   b. Maslow's hierarchy of human needs
   c. family needs
   d. anticipation of future problems

2. What is the primary benefit nursing diagnosis offers the client?
   a. Patient comprehension of medical problem.
   b. Individualization of client care.
   c. Relationship established between client and support persons.

3. Which of the following nursing diagnoses is correct when the health problem is likely to occur *unless* the nurse intervenes in a particular way?
   a. actual
   b. high risk
   c. possible

4. Which of the following identifies the physiologic, psychologic, sociologic, spiritual, and environmental factors believed to be related to the problem as either a cause or contributing factor?
   a. etiology
   b. nursing diagnosis
   c. problem statement
   d. cognitive abilities

5. Which of the following nursing diagnoses is correct when a health problem exists but more data is needed to confirm the diagnosis?
   a. actual
   b. high risk
   c. possible

## Completion

Place a check next to the nursing diagnoses that are written correctly, and identify the errors in the incorrect diagnoses on the lines that follow.

1. _____ High risk for injury related to absence of restraints and side rails. _____

_____

2. _____ Impaired skin integrity related to mobility deficit. _____

3. _____ Grieving related to loss of breast. _____

_____

4. _____ Self-care deficit: bathing related to immobility. _____

5. _____ Sleep pattern disturbance related to insomnia. _____

6. _____ Nutrition: alteration in: less than body requirements related to loss of appetite. _____

_____

7. _____ Powerlessness related to poor family support system. _____

_____

8. _____ Anxiety: mild related to changing life style/diet. _____

_____

9. _____ Ineffective airway clearance related to 20-year smoking habit. _____

_____

10. _____ Alteration in bowel elimination: constipation related to cancer of bowel. _____

_____

11. _____ Nausea and vomiting related to medication side effects _____

_____

12. _____ Knowledge deficit related to noncompliance with diet. _____

13. _____ Alteration in parenting related to knowledge deficit: child growth and development, discipline. _____

_____

14. _____ Pain related to discomfort in abdomen. ___

_____

15. _____ Impaired physical mobility: amputation of left leg related to gangrene. _____

_____

16. _____ Alteration in nutrition: more than body requirements related to obesity. _____

_____

17. _____ Noncompliance related to unresolved hostility. _____

_____

Read the three mini-cases that follow and in each, underline the cues that form a data cluster signifying a nursing diagnosis, and then write the appropriate nursing diagnosis as a three-part statement.

8. Mr. Klinetob, aged 86, has been seriously depressed since the death of his wife of 52 years, 6 months ago. While he suffers from degenerative joint disease and has talked for years about having "just a touch of arthritis," this never kept him from being up and about. Recently, however, he spends all day sitting in a chair and seems to have no desire to engage in self-care activities. He tells the visiting nurse that he doesn't get washed up anymore because he's "too stiff" in the morning to bathe and "just doesn't seem to have the energy." The visiting nurse notices that his hair is matted and uncombed, his face has traces of previous meals, and he has a strong body odor. His adult children have complained that their normally fastidious father seems not to care about personal hygiene any longer.

Nursing Diagnosis: _____

_____

_____

_____

_____

9. Miss Ebenezer sustained a right-sided cerebral infarct that resulted in left hemiparesis (paralysis on left side of body) and left "neglect." She ignores the left side of her body and actually denies its existence. When asked about her left leg, she stated that it belonged to the woman in the next bed—this while she was in a private room. This patient was previously quite active; she walked for 45–60 minutes four or five times a week and was an avid swimmer. At present she cannot move either her left arm or leg.

Nursing Diagnosis: _____

_____

_____

_____

_____

20. Ted and Rosemary Hines tried to conceive a child, unsuccessfully, for a period of 11 years. At this time, they sought the assistance of a fertility specialist who was highly recommended by a friend. It was determined that Ted's sperm was inadequate and Rosemary was inseminated with sperm from an anonymous donor. The Hines were told that the donor was healthy and that he was selected because he resembled Ted. Rosemary became pregnant after the second in vitro fertilization attempt and delivered a healthy baby girl named Sarah.

At the time they present for counseling, their child is seven and Ted and Rosemary have learned from blood tests that their fertility specialist is the biological father of their child. It seems that he lied to some couples about using sperm from anonymous donors, and deceived others into thinking the wives had become pregnant when he had simply injected them with hormones. Ted and Rosemary have joined other couples in pressing charges against this physician.

Rosemary informs the nurse in her pediatrician's office that she is concerned about how all this is affecting her family. "Ted and I both love Sarah and would do nothing to hurt her, but I am so angry about this whole situation that I am afraid I may be taking it out on her." Questioning reveals that Rosemary has found herself yelling at Sarah for minor disobediences and spanking her—something she rarely did before. Both Ted and Rosemary had commented before about Sarah's striking physical resemblance to the fertility specialist but attributed this to coincidence. "Whenever I see her now I can't help but see Dr. Clowser and everything inside me clenches up and I want to scream." Both Ted and Rosemary express great remorse that Sarah, who is innocent, is bearing the brunt of something that is in no way her fault.

Nursing Diagnosis: _____

_____

_____

_____

_____

# 17

## Planning

Chapter 17 introduces the learner to the planning stage of the nursing process. During this stage, the nurse works with the client and family to develop client goals and identify the nursing interventions that are most likely to assist the client in achieving these goals. The elements of planning are discussed, including writing goals and developing evaluative strategies, selecting nursing measures, and writing the nursing care plan.

### OBJECTIVES

After studying this chapter the learner will be able to:

Define key terms used in the chapter.

Describe the purpose and benefits of planning.

Identify three elements of comprehensive planning.

Prioritize client health problems and nursing responses.

Describe how client goals and nursing orders are derived from nursing diagnoses.

Develop a plan of nursing care with properly constructed goals and related nursing orders.

Use criteria to evaluate planning skills.

Describe five common problems related to planning, their possible causes, and remedies.

### EXERCISES

## Matching

Match the definition in Part B with the type of goal listed in Part A. Items in Part A may be used only once.

Part A

a. client goal

b. cognitive goals

c. psychomotor goals

d. long-term goals

e. affective goals

f. short-term goals

Part B

1. _____ Describes increases in client knowledge or intellectual behavior.

2. _____ Expected client outcome.

3. _____ Requires a longer period of time to be achieved, for example, discharge goals.

4. _____ Describes the client's achievement of new skills.

5. _____ Describes the goals that can be accomplished in most cases in less than a week.

6. _____ Describes changes in client values, beliefs, and attitudes.

## Multiple Choice

Circle the letter that corresponds to the best answer for each question.

1. Which of the following is *not* a basic type of planning critical to comprehensive nursing care?
   a. ongoing problem-oriented planning
   b. discharge planning
   c. standardized planning
   d. initial planning

2. Which of the following comprehensive plans is developed by a nurse who performs the admission nursing history and nursing examination?
   a. initial plan
   b. discharge plan
   c. ongoing plan

3. Which of the following comprehensive plans is carried out by the nurse who interacts with the patient and keeps the nursing plan up to date?
   a. initial
   b. ongoing
   c. discharge

4. Which of the following is *not* part of a well-written client goal?
   a. verb or action client will perform
   b. subject
   c. resolution
   d. criteria

## Completion

1. List four steps the nurse takes when preparing nursing orders for a client.
   a. _____
   b. _____
   c. _____
   d. _____

2. List five characteristics of well-written nursing orders.
   a. _____
   _____
   b. _____
   _____
   c. _____
   _____
   d. _____
   _____
   e. _____
   _____

3. Name the three types of information generally found on a Kardex care plan.
   a. _____
   b. _____
   c. _____

4. List five common problems student nurses encounter while developing nursing care plans.
   a. _____
   b. _____
   c. _____
   d. _____
   e. _____

Place a check mark next to the client goals that are written correctly, and on the line below, rewrite those that are written incorrectly.

5. _____ Teach Mrs. Myer one lesson per day on nutritional value of foods. _____

_____

6. _____ Mrs. Gray will know the dangers of smoking after viewing a film on smoking._____

_____

7. _____ By end of shift, client ambulates in hallway using crutches. _____

_____

8. _____ By 2/7, client correctly demonstrates sub Q injections using normal saline. _____

_____

9. _____ By next visit, client will understand benefits of psychotherapy. _____

_____

10. _____ By 6/12, client correctly demonstrates application of wet to dry dressing on leg ulcer. _____

_____

Identify a client goal that shows a direct resolution of the health problem expressed in the nursing diagnoses below.

11. Nursing Diagnosis: Fluid Volume Deficit, related to decreased fluid intake during fever.

Client Goal: _____

_____

_____

_____

12. Nursing Diagnosis: Altered Sexual Patterns: Loss of desire related to change in body image and feelings of unattractiveness following mastectomy.

Client Goal:_____

_____

_____

_____

13. Nursing Diagnosis: Stress Incontinence, related to age-related degenerative changes and weak pelvic muscles and structural supports.

Client Goal:_____

_____

_____

_____

14. Nursing Diagnosis: Activity Intolerance, related to decreased amount of oxygenated blood available to tissues.

Client Goal:_____

_____

_____

_____

15. Nursing Diagnosis: Acute Postoperative Pain, related to fear of taking prescribed analgesics.

Client Goal:_____

_____

_____

_____

## Sequencing

Place each step in the correct sequence by numbering the following steps in developing a comprehensive plan of care for a client.

1. _____ The nurse writes goals for each nursing diagnosis that, if achieved, demonstrate a direct resolution of the problem.

2. _____ The nurse writes nursing orders that communicate to the entire staff specific nursing measures that are to be implemented for the client.

3. _____ The nurse reviews the list of nursing diagnoses and ranks them as high priority, medium priority, or low priority.

4. _____ The nurse selects nursing measures that specifically address all the factors causing or contributing to the client's problem.

# 18

# Implementing and Documenting

Chapter 18 describes the implementing step of the nursing process, in which all the nursing actions developed during the planning step are carried out. The purposes of implementation—to assist the client in achieving desired health goals, to promote wellness, to prevent disease/illness, to restore health, and to facilitate coping with altered functioning—are discussed. The learner is also introduced to documentation guidelines.

## OBJECTIVES

After studying this chapter the learner will be able to:

Define key terms used in the chapter.

Distinguish independent, interdependent or collaborative, and dependent nursing interventions.

Use intellectual, interpersonal, and technical skills to implement a plan of nursing care.

Describe six variables that influence the way a plan of care is implemented.

Use seven guidelines for implementation.

Compare and contrast different documentation systems: source-oriented record, problem-oriented record, and computer record.

Document nursing interventions completely, accurately, concisely, and factually.

Describe nursing's role in communicating with other health-care professionals by reporting, conferring, and referring.

## EXERCISES

### Matching

Match the examples in Part B with the types of nursing interventions listed in Part A.

Part A

a. independent intervention (nurse-initiated)

b. dependent intervention (physician-initiated)

c. interdependent intervention (collaborative)

Part B

1. _____ A nurse notices her client is extremely anxious prior to surgery and recommends psychiatric evaluation.

2. _____ A nurse administers the prescribed dosage of pain medication for his client recovering from knee surgery.

3. _____ A nurse teaches the daughter of a client with leg ulcers how to apply the dressings.

4. _____ A nurse meets with a client's physician to describe what she feels is the client's lack of response to prescsribed therapy.

5. _____ A nurse prepares a client for surgery by performing a bowel cleansing.

6. _____ A nurse meets in conference with a client's physician, social worker, and phychiatrist to discuss client's failure to progress.

Match the examples in Part B with the prerequisite nursing skills listed in Part A.

Part A

a. intellectual skills

b. interpersonal skills

c. technical skills

Part B

7. _____ Obtaining vital signs on a newborn.

8. _____ Designing a plan of care for a client with TMI that reflects client's strengths and resolves problems.

9. _____ Communicating the nursing care plan to a young client with cystic fibrosis.

10. _____ Using nursing resources to better understand a client with developmental problems.

11. _____ Performing a heplock procedure for a patient with CHF.

12. _____ Holding the hand of a client who is dying.

Match the statements in Part B with the purposes for which the client record may be used, listed in Part A.

Part A

a. communication

b. care planning

c. audit

d. research

e. education

f. legal documentation

g. historic documentation

Part B

13. _____ Client records may be entered into court proceedings as evidence.

14. _____ Client records may be studied to learn how to treat similar cases.

15. _____ Years later, information concerning a client's past health care may become pertinent.

16. _____ Client records help health care professionals from different disciplines to speak to each other.

17. _____ Charts may be reviewed to evaluate retrospectively the quality of care received and the competence of nurses providing that care.

18. _____ Health-care professionals reading a client's chart learn much about clinical manifestations of health problems, effective treatment modalities, and factors affecting client goal achievement.

19. _____ Each professional working with the client has access to the client's baseline and ongoing data, and can see client's response to treatment.

## Multiple Choice

Circle the letter that corresponds to the best answer for each question.

1. As the nurse bathes a client, she notes his skin color and integrity, his ability to respond to simple directions, and his muscle tone. Which of the following statements explains why such continuing data collection is so important?
   a. It is difficult to collect complete data in the initial assessment.
   b. It is the most efficient use of the nurse's time.
   c. It enables the nurse to revise the care plan appropriately.
   d. It meets current standards of care.

2. If the nurse telephones the physician with a client problem that the physician either fails to treat, or about which the physician gives a questionable order, the nurse should take which of the following actions?
   a. Have a second nurse listen to the conversation and co-sign the documentation.
   b. Call the physician back after talking to the nursing supervisor.
   c. Tell the physician she/he cannot carry out the order.
   d. Carry out the order, since the physician is responsible for it and has more medical knowledge.

3. Which of the following is *not* typical information shared among nurses during a change-of-shift report?
   a. Basic identifying information about each client.
   b. Current appraisal of each client's health status.
   c. Current orders, especially any recently changed.
   d. Past history of illness for client and family.

4. You are finding it difficult to plan and implement care for Mr. Rivers. You decide to have a nursing case conference. Which of the following best defines this action?
   a. Consult with someone in order to exchange ideas or to seek information, advice, or instructions.
   b. A meeting of nurses to discuss some aspect of client care; other health practitioners may be invited.
   c. A procedure in which a group of nurses visit selected clients individually at each client's bedside.
   d. Send or direct someone for action or help in a specific nursing care problem.

5. Which of the following is a significant disadvantage of audiotaped change-of-shift reports?
   a. There is no permanent record of the message.
   b. The message usually cannot be validated with the sender.
   c. The senders do not like to talk into recorders.
   d. The recorders are too expensive.

## Correct the False Statements

Circle the word *true* or *false* that follows the statement. If the word *false* has been circled, change the underlined word/words to make the statement true. Place your answer in the space provided.

1. A <u>source oriented</u> client record is one in which each health care group keeps data on its own separate form.

   True    False    _____

2. <u>Charting by exception</u> is a type of client record that is organized around a client's problems rather than around sources of information.

   True    False    _____

3. <u>Standing orders</u> are written plans that detail the nursing activities to be executed in specific situations commonly encountered in a unit.

   True    False    _____

4. Admission protocals for OB/GYN and protocals for bowel programs that allow nurses to select and administer certain bowel interventions are examples of <u>standing orders.</u>

   True    False    _____

5. During the <u>implementing</u> step of the nursing process, all the nursing actions developed during the planning step are carried out.

   True    False    _____

6. <u>Validating</u> is the written, legal record of all pertinent interventions with the client; assessing, diagnosis, planning, implementing, and evaluating.

   True    False    _____

7. JCAHO specifies that nursing care data related to patient assessments, the nursing diagnosis and/or client needs, nursing interventions, and patient outcomes are permanently integrated into the clinical information system.

True    False    _____

## Completion

1. List three areas in which nurses use specialized skills to carry out the plan of care.

a. _____

b. _____

c. _____

2. List five variables influencing the way a plan of care is implemented.

a. _____

b. _____

c. _____

d. _____

e. _____

3. List seven documentations that must be included to fully implement the nursing process.

a. _____

b. _____

c. _____

d. _____

e. _____

f. _____

g. _____

4. List three specific communication strategies frequently used by nurses.

a. _____

b. _____

c. _____

# 19

## Evaluating

The last step of the nursing process—evaluating—is the main topic discussed in chapter 19. When evaluating, the nurse and client together measure how well the client has achieved the goals specified in the plan of care. The three options the nurse may take based on the client's response to the plan of care are: terminate, modify, or continue the plan of care. Evaluation criteria and standards, as well as factors influencing goal achievement, are also highlighted in this chapter.

### OBJECTIVES

After studying this chapter the learner will be able to:

Define key terms used in the chapter.

Describe evaluation, its purpose, and its relationship to other steps in the nursing process.

Evaluate the client's achievement of goals specified in the plan of care.

Manipulate factors contributing to the client's success or failure in goal achievement.

Use the client's responses to the plan of care to modify the plan as needed.

Explain the relationship between quality assurance programs and excellence in health care.

Value self-evaluation as a critical element in developing the ability to deliver quality nursing care.

## EXERCISES

### Matching

Match the examples in Part B with the measurement tool listed in Part A.

Part A

a. criteria

b. standard

Part B

1. _____ Client will be able to walk length of hall by 5/15.

2. _____ The admission data base will be completed on all patients within 24 hours of admission to the unit.

3. _____ All patients in active labor will have continuous external fetal heart monitoring.

4. _____ Upon completion of EKG course, the nurse will be able to recognize common arrhythmias when they appear on a heart monitor.

5. _____ The student will be able to name and describe steps of nursing procedure by end of semester.

Match the examples of goals in Part B with the type of goal listed in Part A.

Part A

a. cognitive goals

b. psychomotor goals

c. affective goals

Part B

6. _____ By 10/2, client will demonstrate the proper method of bathing an infant.

7. _____ By 10/6, client will be able to list three foods high in saturated fats.

8. _____ By 2/14, client will plan a weekly menu low in fat.

9. _____ By 2/16, client will demonstrate willingness to try a coping strategy that worked in the past.

10. _____ After viewing a movie on smoking, client will value his health enough to participate in a program to stop smoking.

11. _____ By 10/3, client will perform three exercises to facilitate leg flexibility.

## Multiple Choice

Circle the letter that corresponds to the best answer for each question.

1. The nurse collects data in the evaluative step to determine which of the following?
   a. The identification of client health problems.
   b. The resolution of health problems through goal achievement.
   c. The ability of client to cope with health problems.
   d. The existence of support systems to assist client.

2. Which of the following is written by the nurse, once data have been collected, to determine client goal achievement?
   a. goal planning statement
   b. assessment sheet
   c. evaluative statement
   d. goal assessment

3. Which of the following is a specially designed program that has as its aim the promotion of excellence in nursing?
   a. quality assurance program
   b. case review program
   c. nursing care assessment program
   d. standards of nursing care program

4. Which of the following is a method of evaluating nursing care that involves a review of client records to assess the outcome of nursing care or process by which these outcomes were achieved?
   a. nursing care assessment
   b. nursing review
   c. nursing audit
   d. nursing care appraisal

5. Which of the following is the evaluation of nursing care conducted while the patient is receiving the care?
   a. retrospective evaluation
   b. nursing audit
   c. ongoing evaluation
   d. concurrent evaluation

6. Which of the following actions should the nurse take when client data indicates that the stated goals have not been achieved?
   a. Collect more data for the data base.
   b. Review each preceding step of the nursing process.
   c. Implement a standardized plan of care.
   d. Change the nursing orders.

7. The nurse observes that a new mother holds her infant closely, makes eye contact, calls the baby by name, smiles and coos at the baby. The nurse is probably collecting data to evaluate whether the client has achieved which type of goal?
   a. cognitive
   b. psychomotor
   c. affective
   d. physical change

8. For a client with a self-care deficit, the long-term goal is that the client will be able to dress himself by the end of the six-week therapy. For best results, the nurse should evaluate the client's progress toward this goal at which of the following times?
   a. When the client is discharged.
   b. At the end of the six-week therapy.
   c. Only when the client shows some progress.
   d. As soon as possible.

9. The quality assurance model of the ANA identifies three essestial components of quality care. Which one of these components does the nurse use when determining whether or not a client has met the goals stated on the care plan?

   a. structure

   b. process

   c. retrospective

   d. outcome

10. Which of the following are common problems encountered during the evaluation phase of the nursing process?

   a. Vague or missing nursing diagnoses.

   b. Properly developed nursing goals.

   c. Nursing care plans kept up to date.

   d. Positive communication between nurses.

## Completion

1. List three options the nurse can employ when evaluating client goal achievement to direct future nurse-client interactions.

a. _____

b. _____

c. _____

2. List two integral parts of an evaluative statement.

a. _____

b. _____

3. List and describe the three essential components of quality nursing care according to the ANA quality assurance program.

a. _____

_____

_____

b. _____

_____

_____

c. _____

_____

4. List five steps in the evaluating component of the nursing process.

a. _____

b. _____

c. _____

d. _____

e. _____

# 20

# Communicator

Communication—the process of sharing information and generating and transmitting meanings, is the focus of Chapter 20. The learner is introduced to the basic characteristics of communication, as well as to the various forms of communication that take place in the health care setting. Communication as a component of therapy, the documentation of communication, and developing skills in communication are also presented in Chapter 20.

OBJECTIVES

After studying this chapter the learner will be able to:

Define key terms used in the chapter.

Describe the communication process.

List at least eight ways in which people communicate nonverbally.

Describe the interrelationship between communication and the nursing process.

Identify client goals for each phase of the helping relationship.

Utilize each of the effective communication techniques when interacting with clients.

Evaluate self in terms of the interpersonal skills needed in nursing.

Describe how each of the ineffective communication techniques hinders communication.

Explain how to facilitate nurse-client interactions in special circumstances.

Establish therapeutic relationships with clients assigned to your care.

## EXERCISES

## Matching

Match the examples of client goals in Part B with the appropriate phase of a helping relationship listed in Part A.

Part A

a. orientation phase

b. working phase

c. termination

Part B

1. _____ The client will demonstrate ability to maneuver on crutches.

2. _____ The client will acknowledge goals he has accomplished in physical therapy.

3. _____ The client will learn the name of physical therapist and address him by his name.

4. _____ An anorexic client will establish an agreement with her health care professional to gradually return to a normal eating pattern.

5. _____ The client will express his desire to go home despite the excellent care he received at the agency.

6. _____ The client will attend a counseling session dealing with smoking.

Match the definition in Part B with the appropriate communication term listed in Part A.

Part A

a. communication          e. decoder

b. encoder                f. feedback

c. message                g. noise

d. channel                h. body language

Part B

7. _____ Verbal and nonverbal evidence that the message is received and understood.

8. _____ A term used in communication theory to denote the actual physical product of the source.

9. _____ A term used in communication theory that specifies the person or object to which the message is directed.

10. _____ Nonverbal communication.

11. _____ A term used in communication theory to specify the one who prepares and sends the message to the receiver.

12. _____ A term used in communication theory to denote the medium selected to convey the message.

13. _____ The process of sharing information.

14. _____ Factors that distort the quality of a message.

Match the interviewing questions in Part B with the interviewing techniques useful in nurse-client interactions listed in Part A.

Part A

a. validating question/comment

b. clarifying question/comment

c. reflective question/comment

d. sequencing question/comment

e. directing question/comment

Part B

15. _b_ "You say you've always been healthy and active; is this the first time you've ever been hospitalized?"

16. _c_ "You expressed concern about your children at home..."

17. _a_ "At home you've been treating your ulcer with antacid. Did you take any today?"

18. _e_ "You've been on your present medication for three years. Did you experience any side-effects?"

19. _d_ "Your chest pain began after exercising on a life cycle?"

## Multiple Choice

Circle the letter that corresponds to the best answer for each question.

1. During the preoperative teaching, the client laughs and says, "I know two other guys who've had this done, it's a piece of cake." The nurse notices that the client is sitting rigidly in the bed, clenching his jaws and twisting his ring on his finger. The nurse should conclude that the client is which of the following?

   a. being deceptive
   b. giving unimportant nonverbal cues
   c. probably anxious
   d. probably not anxious

2. When changing linens for an incontinent patient, the nurse may feel repulsed by odors and appearances. In trying to gain control and proceed with the care, it is important to realize that the nurse's facial expression will do which of the following?

   a. It is not likely to be noticed by the client.
   b. It will convey a message to the client.
   c. It is less important than what is said.
   d. It will probably not reflect her/his feelings.

3. Which phase of the therapeutic (helping relationship) is usually the longest?

   a. orientation
   b. working
   c. termination
   d. evaluation

4. A client consistently replies instantly, saying the first thing that comes to mind. The nurse writes a goal: "By the end of therapy, the client will begin to take a moment to think before speaking in nurse-patient interaction." This goal is aimed at improving which of the following client skills?

   a. conversational skills
   b. interviewing skills
   c. interpersonal skills
   d. listening skills

5. In evaluating a conversation with a client, which of the following would indicate that the client is listening attentively?

   a. The client makes frequent eye contact.
   b. The client sits with crossed legs.
   c. The client stares for long periods of time.
   d. The client has little facial expression.

6. A 36-year-old client who is four days post hysterectomy says to the nurse, "I wonder if after all this surgery, I will still feel like a woman." Which of the following responses would most likely encourage the client to expand on this and express her concerns in more specific terms?

a. "When did you begin to wonder about this?"
b. "Do you want more children?"
c. "Feel like a woman. . . ."
d. To remain silent.

## True or False

Place a "T" for *True* or an "F" for *False* in the space provided.

1. _____ Communication is continuous and reciprocal.

2. _____ Nonverbal communication is more likely to be voluntary.

3. _____ Verbal and nonverbal communication occurs simultaneously.

4. _____ One person may be involved in the communication process.

5. _____ Communication is not influenced by the way people feel about themselves and others.

6. _____ Communicating persons respond to the messages they receive.

7. _____ The person sending the message must have knowledge to send and the person receiving the message must have knowledge to understand.

8. _____ Past experiences of the encoder and decoder do not affect the message.

9. _____ A person's position within a sociocultural system may influence the process of communication.

10. _____ Three forms in which communication occur are one-to-one, small groups, and large groups.

## Completion

1. List five of the ten forms of nonverbal communication.

a. _____

b. _____

c. _____

d. _____

e. _____

2. List three characteristics of the helping relationship.

a. _____

b. _____

c. _____

3. List five interpersonal skills essential to the promotion of a nurse-client relationship that will be therapeutic for the client.

a. _____

b. _____

c. _____

d. _____

e. _____

4. List examples of ways in which the nurse uses communication in each phase of the nursing process.

a. Data collection: _____

_____

_____

b. Diagnosis: _____

_____

_____

c. Planning:_____

_____

_____

d. Implementation: _____

_____

_____

e. Evaluation: _____

_____

_____

# 21

## Teacher and Counselor

The professional nursing role of teacher/counselor is explored in Chapter 21. The chief aims of teaching and counseling—promoting wellness, preventing illness, restoring health, and facilitating coping—are presented in this chapter, as well as examples of teaching strategies. The learner is also introduced to the three types of counseling needed to assist clients through crises or motivate them to work toward health promotion.

OBJECTIVES

After studying this chapter the learner will be able to:

Define key terms used in the chapter.

Describe the teaching-learning process, including domains, developmental concerns, and specific principles.

Describe what factors should be assessed for the learning process.

Compose diagnoses for identified learning needs.

Explain how to create a teaching plan for a client.

Describe what is involved in implementing a teaching plan.

Name three methods for the evaluation of learning.

Explain what should be included in the documentation of the teaching-learning process.

Discuss the nurse's role as a counselor.

Summarize how the nursing process is used to assist clients in problem solving.

Describe how to use the counseling role to motivate a client toward health promotion.

## EXERCISES

### Matching

Match the examples of teaching strategies in Part B with the aims of nursing listed in Part A.

Part A

a. promoting wellness

b. preventing illness

c. restoring health

d. facilitating coping

Part B

1. _____ A nurse demonstrates to a diabetic client the correct procedure for self-injection of insulin.

2. _____ A nurse explains to a new mother the importance and availability of immunizations for her baby.

3. _____ A nurse counsels a woman in her first trimester on proper nutrition.

4. _____ A nurse refers a recovering alcoholic to a local group meeting.

5. _____ A nurse presents a lecture on baby-proofing a home to a group of new parents.

6. _____ A nurse teaches a young athlete stretching exercises to be used before running track.

7. _____ A nurse refers a daughter of a terminally ill client to a counseling session on dealing with death and dying.

8. _____ A nurse introduces a client recovering from a broken hip to the physical therapy staff.

9. _____ A nurse refers a 42-year-old woman to a clinic providing free mammagrams.

10. _____ A nurse teaches relaxation techniques to a client recovering from heart by-pass surgery.

Match the definitions in Part B with the appropriate term listed in Part A.

Part A

a. teaching

b. learning

c. pedagogy

d. andragogy

e. teaching strategies

f. informal teaching

g. formal teaching

h. team teaching

Part B

11. _____ Unplanned teaching sessions dealing with client's immediate learning needs and concerns.

12. _____ The technique used by a teacher to promote learning.

13. _____ The study of teaching adults.

14. _____ A planned method or series of methods to help someone learn.

15. _____ The science of teaching.

16. _____ Planned teaching done to fulfill learner objectives.

17. _____ The process by which a person acquires or increases knowledge or changes behavior in a measurable way as a result of an experience.

18. _____ When two or more nurses plan and coordinate the implementation of a teaching plan.

Match the examples of teaching strategies in Part B with the appropriate teaching strategy listed in Part A.

Part A

a. role modeling        e. discussion

b. demonstration        f. role playing

c. discovery            g. audio-visual materials

d. lecture

Part B

19. _____ A nurse chooses a low-calorie diet for herself when eating with an obese client on a weight loss program.

20. _____ A nurse bathes a newborn while his mother watches.

21. _____ A nurse shows a film on relaxation techniques to a cardiac patient.

22. _____ A nurse exchanges information with a client about client's feelings of powerlessness following a TIA.

23. _____ A nurse presents information on the dangers of smoking to a group of forty smokers.

24. _____ A nurse describes the symptoms of an anxiety attack to a client with panic disorder and lets him choose which measures to take during and after the attack.

25. _____ One student pretends to be a patient while another student conducts a nursing interview.

## Multiple Choice

1. The chief purpose of teaching and counseling is:
   a. Giving clients all the information they need about their disease and treatment regimen.
   b. Aswering all the questions of the client and family.
   c. Developing the self-care abilities that enable clients and families to maximize their functioning and quality of life.
   d. Promoting high level wellness.

2. What type of goals should be written for a client who repeatedly presents with diabetes-related complications because she sees no value in the appropriate self-care measures?

   a. affective
   b. cognitive
   c. psychomotor
   d. physical behaviors

3. Which of the following assumptions ought to guide planning learning experiences for *adult* learners?

   a. As a person matures, his or her self-concept is likely to move from dependence to independence.
   b. Adult learners are generally motivated by a love for learning in and of itself.
   c. Most adults prefer learning that prepares them for future challenges.
   d. It is often true that you "can't teach an old dog new tricks."

4. The nurse who wishes to evaluate whether or not a new parent has mastered basic parenting skills should:

   a. Check to see if nurses have documented that they instructed the parent about feeding, bathing, and general parenting skills.
   b. Check the sign-out sheet on the parenting skills video to make sure that the parent has watched these educational aids.
   c. Ask the parent if she feels able to care for her newborn once she gets home.
   d. Observe the parent as she feeds, bathes, and interacts with her baby.

5. When a student appeals to the school nurse and confides that she is pregnant and needs to make a quick decision about whether or not to have an abortion (as her boyfriend is recommending) ,the nurse engages in what type of counseling?

   a. short-term
   b. long-term
   c. motivational
   d. compliance

6. When a client refuses to adhere to the diet which is part of his medical regimen, the nurse should first:

   a. Report this information promptly to the physician and document his refusal.
   b. Order a consultation with the dietician.
   c. Wite a nursing diagnosis that labels the client "noncompliant."
   d. Explore the reasons for the client's "noncompliance."

7. In which of the following examples has the client *not* reached the stage of learning that Piaget refers to as "formal operations"?

   a. A mother understands the need for her daughter to completely finish the course of the antibiotics prescribed for her infection, even though the symptoms have disappeared.
   b. A male client with heart problems recognizes the role stress plays in maintaining healthy blood pressure.
   c. A client in a nursing home takes medication as needed for pain, but is unaware of what triggers the pain.
   d. A sexually active teenager purchases contraceptives to prevent pregnancy and protect against AIDS.

## Correct the False Statements

Circle the word *true* or *false* that follows the statement. If the word *false* has been circled, change the underlined word/words to make the statement true. Place your answer in the space provided.

1. A return demonstration is an excellent evaluative method for the <u>cognitive domain.</u>

   True    False    _____

2. <u>Teaching</u> may be defined as the interpersonal process of assisting clients to make decisions that promote their overall well-being.

   True    False    _____

3. <u>Short-term</u> counseling focuses on the immediate problem or concern.

   True    False    _____

4. A <u>situational</u> crisis may occur when a woman going through menopause needs the assistance of a nurse when adjusting to the changes she experiences.

   True    False    _____

5. <u>Motivational counseling</u> involves discussing feelings and incentives with the client.

   True    False    _____

6. When the nurse's best counseling efforts fail to produce motivation in the client to adhere to a treatment regimen, the client may be described as <u>noncompliant.</u>

    True    False    _____

7. Ineffective individual coping, hopelessness, anxiety, and social isolation are examples of NANDA approved <u>nursing diagnoses</u> for which counseling is the appropriate intervention.

    True    False    _____

## Completion

1. List four elements that need to be considered in each assessment of client learning needs.

    a. _____

    b. _____

    c. _____

    d. _____

2. List four aims of teaching/counseling

    a. _____

    b. _____

    c. _____

    d. _____

3. When establishing learning objectives it is helpful to use verbs reflective of the learning domain. Place the verbs in the list below in the appropriate domain listed on the chart.

| Verbs | |
|---|---|
| arranges | explains |
| assembles | helps |
| categorizes | justifies |
| chooses | lists |
| constructs | shares |
| defends | shows |
| defines | states |

| a. Cognitive Domain | b. Affective Domain | c. Psychomotor Domain |
|---|---|---|
| | | |

4. List three types of counseling that nurses use to guide their client.

    a. _____

    b. _____

    c. _____

# 22

# Leader, Researcher, and Advocate

In Chapter 22, the learner is introduced to the professional nursing role of leader, researcher, and advocate. As a leader, the nurse directs or motivates others toward the achievement of predetermined goals. The role of researcher entails expanding nursing's body of knowledge in order to learn improved ways to promote and maintain health. As an advocate, it is the nurse's responsibililty to protect and support the client's rights. Chapter 22 explores how the roles of leader, researcher, and advocate enhance the basic caregiver role of the nurse.

OBJECTIVES

After studying this chapter the learner will be able to:

Define key terms used in the chapter.

Identify the qualities, four skills, and three styles of leaders.

List the four managerial functions.

Summarize the steps in the process of change.

Describe areas in which the beginning nurse can develop leadership skills that enhance the caregiver role.

Give an example of mentorship in nursing.

Compare the strengths and limitations of three sources of nursing knowledge.

Describe three ways the beginning nurse can utilize research to enhance the caregiver role.

Explain different ways nurse caregivers can be advocates for clients.

Describe the nurse advocate's role in situations requiring ethical decision making.

Explain how two types of advance directives promote client dignity and well-being.

## EXERCISES

## Matching

Match the examples of leadership in Part B with the leadership traits listed in Part A. Use each trait only once.

Part A

a. assertiveness

b. flexibility

c. political awareness

d. knowledge

e. role models

f. vision

Part B

1. _____ A nurse belongs to the local chapter of the ANA to keep abreast of local nursing legislation.

2. _____ A nurse motivates her colleagues to become the best nurses possible.

3. _____ A nurse is open to suggestions from colleagues about how best to meet the needs of a client who is not achieving his targeted outcomes.

4. _____ A nurse has a positive self-image, which is reflected in her work.

5. _____ A nurse empowers her clients to claim their right to knowledge and respectful treatment.

6. _____ A nurse implements a new technique for sterile procedure that she read about in a nursing manual.

Match the examples of leadership in Part B with the styles of leadership listed in Part A.

Part A

a. autocratic leadership

b. democratic leadership

c. laissez-faire leadership

Part B

7. _____ A head nurse works with her staff to come to an agreement about work schedules.

8. _____ A head nurse takes charge of a "code blue" situation and directs the other nurses to their tasks.

9. _____ A head nurse seeks input from staff members on procedures for dealing with contagious diseases.

10. _____ A head nurse makes schedules of meetings of the ANA available to any staff members who are interested.

11. _____ A head nurse directs the triage unit after several earthquake victims arrive at the emergency room.

## Multiple Choice

Circle the letter that corresponds to the best answer for each question.

1. Which of the following is *not* one of the four management functions listed by Hersey and Blanchard (1977)?
   a. evaluating
   b. controlling
   c. organizing
   d. planning

2. Which of the following concerning patient advocacy is true?
   a. Advocacy is necessary only for those who cannot defend themselves.
   b. Nurses can make ethical decisions for their patients as advocates.
   c. Nurses use assertiveness to ensure patient compliance with prescribed treatment regimens.
   d. Nurses give patients the information needed to manage their health care.

3. Which of the following characterizes an informal group?
   a. Membership requirements are stipulated.
   b. Group goals are outlined.
   c. There are few or no rules and regulations.

4. Which of the following is an example of a task role in a group?
   a. active listener
   b. information giver
   c. dominator
   d. supporter

5. Which of the following is an example of a self-serving role in a group?
   a. coordinator
   b. harmonizer
   c. evaluator
   d. blocker

6. Which of the following is an example of a maintenance role in a group?
   a. tension reliever
   b. withdrawer
   c. clarifier
   d. aggressor

## Correct the False Statements

Circle the word *true* or *false* that follows the statement. If the word *false* has been circled, change the underlined word/words to make the statement true. Place your answer in the space provided.

1. Preceptorship is a relationship in which an experienced individual advises and assists a less experienced individual.

   True    False    _____

2. Authoritative knowledge comes from an expert and is accepted as truth based on a perceived level of expertise.

   True    False    _____

3. Scientific knowledge is that part of nursing practice passed down generation after generation.

   True    False    _____

4. <u>Variables</u> are factors in the scientific method that might interfere with the outcome.

   True    False    _____

5. <u>Independent variables</u> are the consequences that vary as changes occur with other variables.

   True    False    _____

6. <u>Advocacy</u> involves combining the three roles of teacher, counselor and leader to form a new role to protect and support the client's rights.

   True    False    _____

7. A nurse who helps clients attain their rights is acting in an <u>assertive</u> manner.

   True    False    _____

## Completion

1. Give an example of how the following indicators of resistance to change can be overcome:

a. Threat to self: _____

_____

b. Lack of understanding: _____

_____

_____

c. Limited tolerance for change: _____

_____

_____

d. Disagreement about benefit of change:_____

_____

_____

e. Fear of increased responsibility: _____

_____

_____

2. List the three stages of change as proposed by Kurt Levin (1951).

a. _____

b. _____

c. _____

3. List the four basic types of skills needed for nursing leadership.

a. _____

b. _____

c. _____

d. _____

4. List and define two legal instruments a client may use to state how choices about their health care should be made if certain circumstances (such as terminal illness) develop in the future that leave them unable to communicate their wishes.

a. _____

_____

_____

b. _____

_____

_____

5. Give two specific examples for each of the nursing research skills listed below:

a. Using research findings to improve practice: _____

_____

_____

_____

b. Identifying researchable problems: _____

_____

_____

_____

c. Protecting the rights of research subjects: _____

_____

_____

_____

_____

6. Give examples of two types of patients who may require nursing advocacy and describe the advocacy role you would play.

| Patient Situation | Nursing Advocacy Response |
| --- | --- |
| a. | |
| b. | |

# 23

## Vital Signs

Chapter 23 provides a thorough discussion of vital signs: body temperature, pulse, respirations, and blood pressure. Physiologic factors, normal and abnormal findings, assessment methods, and assessment sites are described for each vital sign.

### O B J E C T I V E S

After studying this chapter the learner will be able to:

Define key terms used in the chapter.

Discuss nursing responsibilities in assessing temperature, pulse, respirations, and blood pressure.

Compare normal and abnormal vital sign assessments, including causes, effects, and implications of abnormal findings.

Describe the equipment necessary to assess vital signs.

Identify sites for assessing temperature, pulse, and blood pressure.

### E X E R C I S E S

## Matching

Match the term in Part A with the correct definition in Part B.

Part A

a. circadian rhythm

b. pyrexia

c. hyperpyrexia

d. antipyretic

e. hypothermia

Part B

1. _____ A body temperature below the lower limit of normal.

2. _____ Predictable fluctuations in measurement of body temperature.

3. _____ A high fever, usually above 41 degrees Centigrade.

4. _____ An elevation of normal body temperature.

5. _____ A fever-reducing drug.

Match the term in Part A with the correct definition in Part B.

Part A

a. tachycardia

b. bradycardia

c. arrhythmia

d. amplitude

e. radial pulse

f. apical pulse

g. pulse deficit

h. bigeminal

i. premature beat

Part B

6. _____ The difference between the apical and radial pulse.

7. _____ A normal pulse rhythm of two beats is followed by a pause.

8. _____ Pulse that is assessed by using a stethoscope.

9. _____ A rapid heart rate; over 100 beats per minute.

10. _____ A slow heart rate; below 60 beats per minute.

11. _____ A heartbeat occurs before the normal one.

12. _____ An irregular pattern of heartbeats.

13. _____ Pulse that is assessed by palpation.

14. _____ Fullness of the pulse; reflects the strength of the contraction of the left ventricle.

Match the term in Part A with the correct definition in Part B.

Part A

a. inspiration

b. expiration

c. apnea

d. dyspnea

e. orthopnea

f. stertorous breathing

g. stridor

h. eupnea

i. tachypnea

j. Cheyne-Stokes respirations

Part B

15. _____ A fast respiratory rate.

16. _____ A general term for noisy respirations.

17. _____ Difficult or labored breathing.

18. _____ The act of breathing in.

19. _____ The act of breathing out.

20. _____ A harsh, high-pitched sound on inspiration.

21. _____ A gradual increase, followed by a gradual decrease in the depth of respirations, and then a period of apnea.

22. _____ Normal respirations with equal rate and depth.

23. _____ Being able to breathe more easily in an upright position.

24. _____ Periods during which there is no breathing.

Match the term in Part A with the correct definition in Part B.

Part A

a. blood pressure

b. systolic pressure

c. diastolic pressure

d. pulse pressure

e. hypertension

f. hypotension

g. orthostatic hypotension

h. auscultation

i. Korotkoff sounds

j. Doppler apparatus

Part B

25. _____ The blood pressure is above normal for a sustained period.

26. _____ Low blood pressure associated with weakness when rising to an upright position.

27. _____ The force of the blood against arterial walls.

28. _____ The highest pressure present against arterial walls.

29. _____ The lowest pressure present against arterial walls.

30. _____ A blood pressure below normal.

31. _____ Listening for sounds within the body.

32. _____ The series of sounds for which the nurse listens when measuring the blood pressure.

33. _____ Amplifies sounds to obtain blood pressure.

34. _____ The difference between the systolic and diastolic pressures.

## Multiple Choice

Circle the letter that corresponds to the best answer for each question.

1. Mrs. Janski is recovering from surgery, which she had three days ago. Her temperature is 101.6 degrees Fahrenheit. In general, how often should her temperature be assessed?
   a. every 12 hours
   b. every 8 hours
   c. every 4 hours
   d. every hour

2. At what time of the day would you expect Mrs. Janski's oral temperature to be at its peak elevation?
   a. midnight
   b. 4 AM
   c. noon
   d. 4 PM

3. When an elevated temperature returns to normal gradually, it is said to have been resolved by:
   a. lysis
   b. crisis
   c. relapse
   d. remittence

4. What metal is contained in oral glass thermometers?
   a. lead
   b. silver
   c. lithium
   d. mercury

5. Which of the following patients would *not* have an oral temperature taken?
   a. A 16-year-old with an appendectomy.
   b. A 72-year-old with open-heart surgery.
   c. A 34-year-old with pneumonia.
   d. A 22-year-old who is unconscious.

6. Mrs. Marcum has severe heart disease. Which route would be contraindicated for taking her temperature?
   a. oral
   b. axillary
   c. rectal
   d. temperature patch

7. The pulse rate is the number of pulsations felt in what period of time?

    a. 1 minute
    b. 30 seconds
    c. 5 minutes
    d. 10 minutes

8. Mr. Ballot has an increased temperature and is also in severe pain. You would expect to find his pulse and respirations:

    a. decreased
    b. increased
    c. unchanged
    d. normal

9. The normal adult respiratory rate is:

    a. 2–4 respirations per minute
    b. 6–8 respirations per minute
    c. 16–20 respirations per minute
    d. 28–32 respirations per minute

10. You have just taken vital signs, and write down your findings: T = 98.6, P = 66, R = 18, BP = 124/82. Your instructor asks "which number is the systolic pressure?" You reply:

    a. 98.6
    b. 124
    c. 82
    d. 66

11. In which of the following situations would you expect to find a low blood pressure?

    a. A client who is overweight.
    b. A client who has just eaten.
    c. A client who is angry.
    d. A client who is dehydrated.

12. You are unable to obtain a blood pressure on your assigned client by using the brachial artery. Which artery would you use next?

    a. the popliteal artery
    b. the radial artery
    c. the dorsalis pedis
    d. the carotid artery

13. Your client, Mrs. Moe, is 84. What normal change in vital signs would you expect to assess?

    a. a higher than normal temperature
    b. a slower pulse
    c. a more rapid respiratory rate
    d. a lower blood pressure

14. When assessing the pulse on Mrs. Moe, you find that the pulsations are not easily felt, and slight pressure causes the pulse to disappear. You would describe this as what kind of pulse?

    a. bounding
    b. thready
    c. absent
    d. normal

15. Which of the following nursing actions when taking vital signs will be most helpful in encouraging client cooperation and reducing client apprehension?

    a. Wash your hands before and after the procedure.
    b. Gather all equipment before beginning.
    c. Wear disposable gloves for all procedures.
    d. Explain the procedure to the client.

## Correct the False Statements

Circle the word *true* or *false* that follows the statement. If the word *false* has been circled, change the underlined word/words to make the statement true. Place your answer in the space provided.

1. To take a rectal temperature on an adult, insert the thermometer 1/2 inch.

    True    False    _____

2. The first tapping sound heard when taking the blood pressure is the diastolic pressure.

    True    False    _____

3. The average adult blood pressure is 120/80.

    True    False    _____

4. The normal adult pulse rate is 80–130.

    True    False    _____

5. When pyrexia returns to normal suddenly, it is called resolution by crisis.

    True    False    _____

5. Taking vital signs is a <u>dependent</u> nursing action, requiring an order by a physician.

True   False   _____

## Completion

1. List the four physical processes by which heat is transferred.

a. _____

b. _____

c. _____

d. _____

2. Describe the symptoms that accompany fever.

a. _____

b. _____

c. _____

d. _____

e. _____

f. _____

3. Describe the appearance of the bulb of a glass thermometer for:

a. Oral route _____

b. Rectal route_____

4. List the types of clients for whom an oral temperature is contraindicated.

a. _____

b. _____

c. _____

d. _____

e. _____

f. _____

5. Describe the anatomical location used to take the apical pulse.

_____

_____

_____

_____

6. Why is the thumb *not* used to palpate an artery?

_____

_____

7. What is the normal ratio of respirations to the pulse rate? _____

8. What is the rationale for having dyspneic clients in an upright position?

_____

_____

_____

_____

_____

_____

_____

9. List the factors that are responsible for maintaining normal blood pressure.

a. _____

b. _____

c. _____

d. _____

e. _____

10. What two pieces of equipment are necessary to take a blood pressure?

a. _____

b. _____

11. For each of the following contributing causes to blood pressure errors, circle the correct word (high or low) for the assessment error that would result.

a. Noise in the background.          High     Low

b. Using too wide a cuff.            High     Low

c. Viewing the meniscus from         High     Low

   below eye level.

d. Releasing the valve too rapidly.  High     Low

e.  Releasing the valve too slowly.  High     Low

# 24

# Nursing Assessment

Chapter 24 presents the components of the nursing assessment. General guidelines provide information on instruments used, positions, draping, and preparing the environment and the client. Following a discussion of the techniques of assessment (inspection, palpation, percussion, and auscultation), the assessment of each body system is presented. A sample health history and physical assessment is included at the end of the chapter to illustrate documentation of data collected.

## OBJECTIVES

After studying this chapter the learner will be able to:

Define key terms used in the chapter.

Identify the purposes of the nursing assessment.

Describe the techniques used during a nursing examination.

Discuss the importance of client preparation for a nursing assessment.

Identify equipment used in performing a nursing assessment.

Describe positioning used for each body system examination.

Conduct a nursing assessment of each body system in a systematic manner, identifying normal and abnormal findings.

Document significant findings in a concise, descriptive manner.

## EXERCISES

### Matching

Match the term in Part A with the correct definition in Part B.

Part A

a. ophthalmoscope

b. otoscope

c. nasal speculum

d. vaginal speculum

e. tuning fork

f. percussion hammer

g. neurologic hammer

Part B

1. _____ Used to test reflexes and tissue density.

2. _____ Used to visualize the interior structures of the eye.

3. _____ Allows visualization of the lower and middle turbinates.

4. _____ Used to examine the vaginal canal and cervix.

5. _____ Used to test reflexes and sensory discrimination.

6. _____ Used for examining the external ear and tympanic membrane.

7. _____ Used for testing auditory function and vibratory perception.

Match the terms in Part A with the correct definitions for findings during skin assessment listed in Part B.

Part A

a. flushing          e. ecchymosis

b. cyanosis          f. petechiae

c. jaundice          g. lesion

d. pallor            h. turgor

Part B

8. _____ yellow color

9. _____ redness

10. _____ dusky bluish color

11. _____ purplish discoloration

12. _____ diseased or injured tissue

13. _____ paleness

14. _____ elasticity of the skin

15. _____ very small hemorrhagic spots

Match the terms in Part A with the correct description of findings during assessment of the thorax and lungs listed in Part B.

Part A

a. fremitus          d. rhonchi

b. crackles          e. pleural friction rub

c. wheezes

Part B

16. _____ High-pitched continuous sounds, may be inspiratory or expiratory.

17. _____ Vibrations palpated during respirations.

18. _____ Discrete, discontinuous, inspiratory sounds.

19. _____ A grating sound.

20. _____ Low-pitched continuous sounds; may be altered by coughing.

Match the terms in Part A with the correct definition for alterations in physical assessment with aging listed in Part B.

Part A

a. senile keratosis     f. cataract

b. senile lentigines    g. presbyopia

c. cherry angioma       h. presbycusis

d. alopecia             i. kyphosis

e. arcus senilis

Part B

21. _____ loss of hair

22. _____ raised dark spots on skin

23. _____ white ring around iris

24. _____ increase in dorsal spinal curve

25. _____ clouding of lens

26. _____ small, round, red spots

27. _____ flat brown age spots

28. _____ decrease in hearing acuity

29. _____ decrease in near vision

## Multiple Choice

Circle the letter that corresponds to the best answer for each question.

1. The client's height and weight are included in a general survey to assess:
   a. overall nutrition
   b. presence of obesity
   c. body shape
   d. muscle tone

2. An excess amount of perspiration, as when the entire skin surface of the body is moist, is called:
   a. ecchymosis
   b. diaphoresis
   c. turgor
   d. edema

3. A comparison of bilateral sides of a body part is an assessment for:

   a. tremor
   b. tic
   c. edema
   d. symmetry

4. When assessing a client's eyes for reaction to light, the normal response is that the pupil being examined will:

   a. remain the same
   b. dilate
   c. constrict
   d. retract

5. Mrs. Jones has a visual acuity of 20/100 in both eyes by the Snellen chart. This value means that Mrs. Jones:

   a. has better vision than normal.
   b. has poorer vision than normal.
   c. can see twice as well as normal.
   d. cannot see at all.

6. The structures of the internal eye are examined with what instrument?

   a. stethoscope
   b. otoscope
   c. Snellen chart
   d. ophthalmoscope

7. Where would you position yourself to assess a client's thyroid gland?

   a. Behind the client
   b. In front of the client
   c. To the right of the client
   d. To the left of the client

8. Mr. Rogers has been diagnosed as having a large tumor in his left lung. What percussion sound would you expect to hear over this tumor?

   a. tympany
   b. hyperresonance
   c. dullness
   d. flat tone

9. A normal assessment finding when examining the precordium is the apical impulse at the point of maximum impulse (PMI). Where is the PMI located?

   a. To the right of the sternum.
   b. At the 1st to 3rd intercostal space, right mid-clavicular line.
   c. Over the epigastric area.
   d. At the 4th or 5th intercostal space, left midclavicular line.

10. When assessing the abdomen, which technique should be used last?

    a. inspection
    b. auscultation
    c. percussion
    d. palpation

## Correct the False Statements

Circle the word *true* or *false* that follows the statement. If the word *false* has been circled, change the underlined word/words to make the statement true. Place your answer in the space provided.

1. <u>Palpation</u> is an assessment technique that uses visual, auditory, and olfactory senses as tools to gather data.

   True    False    _____

2. Excessive amounts of hair on the body is labeled <u>alopecia.</u>

   True    False    _____

3. A normal response to <u>convergence</u> during eye assessment is a crosseyed appearance.

   True    False    _____

4. If palpation of the precordium detects fine vibrations, they are documented as <u>thrills.</u>

   True    False    _____

5. When assessing the breasts, you may find normal tenderness one week <u>after</u> the menstrual period.

   True    False    _____

6. The rectum is assessed by the assessment technique of <u>inspection.</u>

   True    False    _____

7. When putting the joints of the arm through full range of motion, you hear a grating sound. This would be documented as <u>crepitus.</u>

   True    False    _____

8. A question to assess mental status for <u>time</u> is "what is today's date?"

   True    False    _____

9. A client who can not be aroused, even with painful stimuli, is described as being <u>comatose.</u>

True     False     _____

10. A client understands word, but can not respond verbally. This is <u>receptive</u> aphasia.

True     False     _____

## Completion

1. List the purposes of the nursing assessment.

a. _____

_____

_____

b. _____

_____

_____

c. _____

_____

_____

d. _____

_____

_____

e. _____

_____

_____

2. Fill in the blank with the position that is described in the accompanying sentence.

a. _____ Client lies flat on the back, with legs together, extended, and knees slightly flexed.

b. _____ Client lies on the abdomen, flat on the bed, head turned to one side.

c. _____ Client is in the standing position.

d. _____ Client sits upright in a chair, on the side of the bed or examining table, or is supine with head elevated.

e. _____ Client lies on the back, with legs separated, knees bent, and soles of the feet flat on the bed.

f. _____ Client lies either on the right or left side, with lower arm behind the body, upper arm flexed, and knees flexed.

g. _____ Client is in the dorsal recumbent position, with the buttocks at the end of the examining table and the feet supported in stirrups.

h. _____ Client kneels, using the knees and chest to bear the weight of the body.

3. There are seven characteristics of masses that are determined by palpation. List them below.

a. _____

b. _____

c. _____

d. _____

e. _____

f. _____

g. _____

4. For each of the following percussion tones, describe their relative intensity.

a. Flatness: _____

b. Dullness: _____

c. Resonance: _____

d. Hyperresonance: _____

e. Tympany: _____

5. List the arteries that are sites for palpation of peripheral pulses.

a. _____

b. _____

c. _____

d. _____

e. _____

f. _____

g. _____

6. List the four characteristics of sound that should be assessed by auscultation.

a. _____

b. _____

c. _____

d. _____

7. Complete the table below. For each cranial nerve, write the name below the number; identify it as sensory, motor, or both, and explain the function of the nerve.

| Cranial Nerve | Sensory/Motor | Function |
|---|---|---|
| a. I | | |
| b. II | | |
| c. III | | |
| d. IV | | |
| e. V | | |
| f. VI | | |
| g. VII | | |
| h. VIII | | |
| i. IX | | |
| j. X | | |
| k. XI | | |
| l. XII | | |

8. Complete the paragraph by filling in the blanks with the correct word.

During auscultation of the heart, the first heart sound heard is the (a) _____ of "lub-dub." This sound occurs when the (b) _____ and (c) _____ valves close and corresponds with the onset of (d) _____ contraction. This sound is called (e) _____, and heard best at the (f) _____ area. The second heart sound, (g) _____, occurs at the end of (h) _____ and represents the closure of the (i) _____ and (j) _____ valves. It is the (k) _____ of "lub-dub." These two sounds occur within (l) _____ second or less.

9. What risk factors should be considered when assessing the breasts?

a. _____

b. _____

c. _____

d. _____

e. _____

10. What three parameters are evaluated in the Glasgow Coma Scale?

a. _____

b. _____

c. _____

11. Provide one example for each of these basic types of skin lesions.

a. macule _____

b. papule _____

c. wheal _____

d. vesicle _____

e. pustule _____

f. fissure _____

g. comedo _____

h. nevus _____

12. List the organs underlying the right lower quadrant of the abdomen.

a. _____

b. _____

c. _____

d. _____

e. _____

# 25

## Safety

Chapter 25 provides the learner with the problem-solving tools needed to address safety issues—such as falls, fires, and poisoning—which occur with alarming regularity. The nursing process is discussed as a facilitator of the nurse's ability to recognize, assess, diagnose, and plan the nursing interventions that will effectively ensure safety for all ages in all environments.

O B J E C T I V E S

After studying this chapter the learner will be able to:

Define key terms used in the chapter.

Identify factors that may be safety hazards in the client's environment.

Describe ways in which the client's safety can be promoted in the home and health-care setting.

Identify clients at risk of falling.

Describe preventive strategies to decrease the incidence of client falls.

Identify alternatives to using restraints.

Identify nursing diagnoses associated with a client in an unsafe situation.

Describe nursing responsibilities for fire safety.

Identify teaching strategies that should be included in a safety program to prevent poisoning and suffocation.

## E X E R C I S E S

### Matching

Match the safety precaution listed in Part B with the appropriate age group listed in Part A. Use each answer only once.

Part A

a. fetus        e. adolescent

b. infant        f. adult

c. toddler and preschooler        g. elderly

d. school-age child

Part B

1. _____ This group needs assistance to evaluate activities that are potentially dangerous; needs to discuss specific interventions that provide for safety at home, at school, and in the neighborhood.

2. _____ Falls, fires and motor vehicle accidents are significant hazards for this group and safety measures should be directed toward preventing these injuries.

3. _____ Education for this group must focus on safe driving skills, drug and alcohol use, and formulation of a healthful life-style in response to the stress of daily living.

4. _____ A pregnant woman requires reinforcement about the risks associated with excess alcohol consumption, smoking, drug use and exposure to other dangers in the environment.

5. _____ This group needs reminders about the effect of stress on their life-style. Coping with the demands of raising a family and establishing and promoting a career may lead to development of unsafe health practices and reliance on drugs or alcohol.

6. _____ Vigilant supervision by parents and guardians should anticipate hazardous elements; protection with precautionary devices, such as child-proof locks, guard rails, and electric outlet covers is essential for this group.

7. _____ Safety care for this group entails never leaving the child unattended, using crib rails, and monitoring objects that may be placed in the mouth and swallowed.

Match the type of extinguisher in Part B with the class of fire it will extinguish listed in Part A. Answers may be used more than once.

Part A

a. Class "A" fire: wood, paper, rags

b. Class "B" fire: flammable liquids

c. Class "C" fire: energized electrical equipment

Part B

8. _____ Pressurized water

9. _____ Carbon dioxide

10. _____ Dry chemical

11. _____ All purpose

Match the definition in Part B with the term listed in Part A.

Part A

a. ground

b. macroshock

c. microshock

d. restraint

e. suffocation

Part B

12. _____ Results in a lack of air reaching the lungs and stoppage of breathing.

13. _____ A connection from an electricity source to the earth through which electric current leakage can be harmlessly conducted.

14. _____ A tingling sensation in the extremities and trunk resulting from an electric current passing through a relatively large area of the body.

15. _____ Devices used to limit a client's movement, which may be either physical or chemical/pharmacological.

16. _____ The transmission of an electric current through a relatively small area of the body, usually directly into the heart.

## Multiple Choice

Circle the letter that corresponds to the best answer for each question.

1. Which of the following is an accurate statistic regarding safety in the home or institution?
   a. Fire is the major safety problem in hospitals and the leading cause of accidental death for the elderly at home.
   b. The incidence of childhood poisoning has increased dramatically in the last ten years.
   c. Twenty percent of all homes are still not protected by smoke detectors and are involved in the majority of all house fires.
   d. The number of deaths related to cocaine abuse has decreased since 1988.

2. Which of the following statements concerning falls in the hospital is true?
   a. Mortality associated with a fall is not age-related.
   b. Older men fall more often than older women.
   c. The majority of hospital clients that fall are under the age of 65.
   d. More than one-third of falls in the elderly population are associated with the need to urinate.

3. Mrs. Nix is an 86-year-old woman admitted to the hospital with confusion and dehydration. Restraints were applied after Mrs. Nix got out of bed and fell. She began to fight and was rapidly becoming exhausted. She had black and blue marks on her wrists from the restraints. Which of the following would be the most appropriate nursing intervention?
   a. Sedate Mrs. Nix with sleeping pills and leave the restraints on.
   b. Take the restraints off and stay with Mrs. Nix and talk gently with her.
   c. Leave the restraints on and talk with Mrs. Nix. Tell her she must calm down.
   d. Talk with Mrs. Nix's family about taking her home since she is out of control.

4. Which of the following is emphasized in the hospital's procedure in case of a fire?
   a. Move anyone that is in immediate danger out of the area.
   b. Open the window in the area and close the door in the area.
   c. Take the elevator to the ground floor and get help.
   d. Stay upright if smoke is present and move out of the area.

5. Which of the following types of information are gathered according to Tideiksaar's use of the mnemonic SPLAT?
   a. severity of falls
   b. previous falls
   c. local environment
   d. age of client

6. Which of the following would be an appropriate automobile safety restraint for a toddler or preschool-age child?
   a. a rear-facing safety seat
   b. lap seat belts
   c. a booster seat with a shield or harness
   d. factory installed lap and shoulder belts

7. Which of the following statements regarding the use of restraints is accurate?
   a. Young clients and children are more likely to be restrained than elderly clients.
   b. In 1988, in the United States, over 50 percent of all nursing home residents were restrained, according to U.S. Health Care Financing Administration, 1988.
   c. According to Bock and Schilder (1988), heavy workloads and unquestioned or vague restraint policies foster the use of restraints for 10–15% of their clients.
   d. Physical and chemical restraints are never prescribed for the same client.

8. Which of the following would be an alternative to the use of restraints for ensuring client safety and preventing serious falls?
   a. Involve family in care.
   b. Allow client to use bathroom independently.
   c. Keep client sedated with tranquilizers.
   d. Maintain high bed position so client will not attempt to get out unassisted.

9. Which of the following would be the most important safety tip when counseling the parents of a toddler and preschool child?
   a. Remember that motor vehicle accidents are the leading cause of death.
   b. Safe care of the child includes never leaving the child alone.
   c. Drugs are the most common cause of death in this group.
   d. The focus for this group is childproofing the environment.

10. Mr. Kay is a 74-year-old man who lives alone since the death of his wife a year ago. Which of the following behaviors would be most dangerous to his safety?
    a. Driving a car in the immediate area of his home.
    b. Smoking in bed or in a stuffed arm chair.
    c. A floor with several small rugs in the room.
    d. Playing golf twice a week with friends.

11. You are visiting Mrs. King and her three children, age two, four, and five, in the home. You identify a safety problem and establish a nursing diagnosis of knowledge deficit concerning safety related to the danger of suffocation. Which of the following would be the most important action in the care plan?
    a. Remove old refrigerator from the neighborhood.
    b. Give sponge bath to children because of danger of suffocation in the bathtub.
    c. Remove all paper and plastic sacks from the home.
    d. Do not use seat belt in car because of the danger of suffocation.

12. Mrs. Ines tells you that she has a 3-year-old girl who is into everything. Which of the following would be the most common cause of poisoning death in children under 5?
    a. Cleaning agents, such as lysol, lye, and soap.
    b. Impure food, such as home canned items like green beans.
    c. Carbon monoxide poisoning from improperly vented space heater.
    d. Common household drugs, such as aspirin or laxatives.

13. Which of the following has been primarily responsible in reducing the number of child deaths from poisoning?
    a. childproof containers
    b. community education
    c. telephone hotlines
    d. identifying poisonous plants

## Correct the False Statements

Circle the word *true* or *false* that follows the statement. If the word *false* has been circled, change the underlined word/words to make the statement true. Place your answer in the space provided.

1. An accident in a health care agency requires the completion of a <u>problem report.</u>

   True    False _____

2. According to Stark and Flitcraft (1988), <u>domestic violence</u> may represent the single most common cause of injury to women.

   True    False _____

3. A <u>nursing history</u> should be done to determine if the client has a history of falls because that person is likely to fall again.

   True    False _____

4. Suffocation may occur in any age group but the incidence is greater in the <u>elderly.</u>

   True    False _____

5. A rear-facing safety seat is recommended for infants weighing less than <u>10 pounds.</u>

   True    False _____

6. Nurses consistently cite the risk of <u>injury from falls</u> as the primary reason for applying restraints.

   True    False _____

7. If your clothing catches fire, the appropriate safety measure would be to <u>run to the nearest person for help.</u>

   True    False _____

## Completion

1. Describe how the following factors affect safety.

a. Developmental considerations: _____

_____

_____

_____

b. Life style: _____

_____

_____

_____

c. Mobility: _____

_____

_____

_____

d. Sensory perception: _____

_____

_____

_____

e. Knowledge: _____

_____

_____

_____

f. Ability to communicate: _____

_____

_____

_____

g. Health state: _____

_____

_____

h. Psychosocial state: _____

_____

_____

2. List five factors that make a client high-risk for a fall.

a. _____

_____

b. _____

_____

c. _____

_____

d. _____

_____

e. _____

_____

3. Write a sample nursing diagnosis for each of the following situations:

a. A mother refuses to put her child in a car seat

when traveling by automobile: _____

_____

_____

b. An elderly client has poor vision and cannot read

the label on her medication: _____

_____

_____

c. A mother leaves her child unattended in the bath-

tub while she answers the phone: _____

_____

_____

d. A client admits she is "clumsy" and has fallen sev-

eral times in the past few years: _____

_____

_____

e. The windows and doors do not operate properly in

the home of an elderly couple living on a fixed

income. They state they do not have the finances

necessary to fix the problems: _____

_____

_____

4. List six safety measures recommended to reduce the number of falls in acute and extended care facilities.

a. _____

_____

b. _____

_____

c. _____

_____

d. _____

_____

e. _____

_____

f. _____

_____

5. Describe three situations in which safety restraints should be used to protect the client.

a. _____

_____

_____

b. _____

_____

_____

c. _____

_____

_____

6. List eight hazards associated with the immobility and restriction imposed by physically restraining a person.

a. _____

b. _____

c. _____

d. _____

e. _____

f. _____

g. _____

h. _____

7. Define the mnemonic "RACE" which is used by staff members in event of a hospital fire.

a. R: _____

b. A: _____

c. C: _____

d. E: _____

8. List six measures that should be taken when applying restraints to a client.

a. _____

_____

b. _____

_____

c. _____

_____

d. _____

_____

e. _____

_____

f. _____

_____

9. Many accidents occur at home. You are visiting the Jones family as part of your caseload in community health. Mrs. Jones wants help in making her home accident-free. The Jones have three children, age five, three, and one. What would be potential dangers specific to each room? What would you suggest to make each room/area accident free?

a. Kitchen: _____

_____

_____

_____

b. Living room: _____

_____

_____

c. Bedrooms: _____

_____

_____

d. Bathroom: _____

_____

_____

e. Porch and yard: _____

_____

_____

_____

10. List three poisonous products that may be found in each of the following rooms:

a. Kitchen: _____

b. Bedroom: _____

c. Laundry room: _____

d. Bathroom: _____

e. Garage/basement: _____

f. Living room: _____

11. List six guidelines for decreasing equipment-related accidents.

a. _____

_____

_____

b. _____

_____

_____

c. _____

_____

_____

d. _____

_____

_____

e. _____

_____

_____

f. _____

_____

## Sequencing

1. Place each step in the correct sequence by numbering the following steps in applying restraints.

a. _____ Explain reason for use to client and family. Clarify how care will be given and that use of restraints is a temporary measure.

b. _____ Determine the need for restraints

c. _____ Document reason for restraining client, type of restraint, times when removed, and result and frequency of nursing assessment for every shift.

d. _____ Reassure client at regular intervals and assess for signs of sensory deprivation, such as increased sleeping, day dreaming, anxiety, panic, and hallucinations.

e. _____ Remove restraint every two to four hours for at least 10 minutes according to agency policy and client need.

f. _____ Wash your hands.

g. _____ Apply restraints according to manufacturer's direction.

h. _____ Confirm agency policy for application of restraints. Secure physician's order if required.

i. _____ Wash your hands.

# 26

## Asepsis

Chapter 26 introduces the learner to aseptic techniques. The involvement of the nurse in identifying, preventing, controlling, and teaching the client about infection is discussed. The need for the consistent application of the nursing process to break the chain of infection is explained, along with techniques for achieving this goal. Controlling infectious agents by sterilization and disinfection, surgical asepsis and isolation, and barrier techniques are also presented in this chapter.

### OBJECTIVES

After studying this chapter the learner will be able to:

Define key terms used in the chapter.

Explain the infection cycle.

Describe nursing interventions used to break the chain of infection.

List the stages of an infection.

Identify clients at risk of developing an infection.

Identify factors that reduce the incidence of nosocomial infection.

Identify situations in which hand washing is indicated.

Identify nursing diagnoses associated with a client who has an infection or is at risk of developing an infection.

Differentiate between category-specific and disease-specific isolation systems.

Differentiate between universal precautions and the body substance isolation system.

## EXERCISES

### Matching

Match the definition in Part B with the term listed in Part A.

Part A

a. infection

b. pathogen

c. bacteria

d. aerobic bacteria

e. anerobic bacteria

f. virus

g. normal flora

h. opportunists

i. inflammatory response

j. immune response

k. antigen

l. antibody

Part B

1. _____ A protective mechanism that eliminates the invading pathogen and allows for tissue repair to occur.

2.. _____ Microorganisms that commonly inhabit various body sites and are part of the body's natural defense system.

3. _____ The most significant and most commonly observed agents causing infections in health care institutions.

4. _____ A disease state resulting from the presence of pathogens in or on the body.

5. _____ The body's response to an antigen.

6. _____ Bacteria that may potentially be harmful.

7. _____ The specific reactions in the body as it responds to an invading foreign protein such as bacteria, or in some cases, even the body's own proteins.

8. _____ Bacteria that require oxygen to live and grow.

9. _____ The smallest of all microorganisms.

10. _____ Bacteria that can live without oxygen.

11. _____ A disease producing microorganism.

12. _____ An invading foreign protein such as bacteria, or in some cases, the body's own proteins.

Match the stage of infection in Part B with its correct term listed in Part A.

Part A

a. incubation period

b. prodromal stage

c. full stage of illness

d. convalescent period

Part B

13. _____ The stage in which the presence of specific signs and symptoms are determined by the type of infection.

14. _____ The interval between the invasion of the body by the pathogen and the appearance of symptoms of infection.

15. _____ The stage that represents recovery from the infection; the signs and symptoms disappear.

16. _____ The stage in which a person is most infectious; early signs and symptoms of disease are present but are vague and nonspecific.

Match the type of infection in Part A with its definition listed in Part B.

Part A

a. nosocomial

b. exogenous

c. endogenous

d. iatrogenic

Part B

17. _____ An infection which occurs as a result of a treatment or diagnostic procedure.

18. _____ An infection that is hospital acquired.

19. _____ An infection in which the causative organism comes from microbial life the person himself harbors.

20. _____ An infection in which the causative organism is acquired from other persons.

Match the disease in Part B with the means of transmission listed in Part A. Answers may be used more than once.

Part A

a. direct contact

b. indirect contact

c. vehicles

d. airborne

e. vectors

Part B

21. _____ Malaria

22. _____ AIDS

23. _____ Staphylococcal infection

24. _____ Typhoid

25. _____ Hepatitis B

26. _____ Chicken pox

27. _____ Lyme disease

28. _____ Herpes simplex

29. _____ Salmonella

30. _____ Influenza

31. _____ Measles

## Multiple Choice

Circle the letter that corresponds to the best answer for each question.

1. Which of the following is a plant-like organism present in the air, soil, and water that can cause infection frequently resistant to treatment?
   a. bacteria
   b. virus
   c. fungi
   d. mold

2. Which of the following terms describes a nonhuman carrier that transmits organisms from one host to another?
   a. vehicle
   b. transmitter
   c. inducer
   d. vector

3. Which of the following laboratory test results indicates the presence of an infection?

   a. The presence of a pathogen in urine, blood, sputum, or other drainage cultures.
   b. A white blood cell count above 5,000 mm.
   c. A decrease in specific types of white blood cells.
   d. The presence of leukocytes in the blood.

4. Which of the following statements about nosocomial infections is accurate?

   a. At least 20 percent of all hospital admissions contract a nosocomial infection.
   b. Hospital-acquired infections are directly responsible for 20,000 deaths and contribute to another 60,000 deaths per year.
   c. Most hospital-acquired infections are caused by viruses.
   d. Gram-positive bacilli are responsible for more than 50 percent of hospital-acquired infections.

5. Which of the following nosocomial infections has the highest mortality rate?

   a. respiratory tract
   b. surgical wounds
   c. urinary tract
   d. intra-abdominal

6. John Smith is a 40-year-old man with systemic lupus erythematosus, an autoimmune disease in which the immune response involves specific reaction to the body's own tissue. Which of the following are two agents that interact to activate the immune response?

   a. antibiotic and antigen
   b. antibodies and infectious agent
   c. antigen and antibodies
   d. foreign protein and antigen

7. Which of the following is the most dependable and practical means for the destruction of microbial life?

   a. steam under pressure
   b. boiling water
   c. dry heat
   d. radiation

8. Susan, age 12, is in the hospital for chronic asthma. She has a history of frequent infections. Which of the following data would be most important in controlling infections for Susan?

   a. a diet history
   b. family history of disease
   c. evaluation of exercise program
   d. Susan's immunization status

9. Mrs. Teal is to have an indwelling urinary catheter inserted. Which of the following would be the precaution taken during this procedure?

   a. surgical asepsis technique
   b. medical asepsis technique
   c. good hand-washing technique
   d. strict reverse isolation

10. Which of the following statements about hand washing is accurate?

    a. Effective hand washing requires at least a 5-second scrub with plain soap or disinfectant and water.
    b. The frequency of hand washing and amount of soap used appear to positively influence the effectiveness of antiseptic products.
    c. Most studies on hand washing indicate that compliance is easily achieved.
    d. Wearing gloves is an acceptable substitute for proper hand washing.

## Correct the False Statements

Circle the word *true* or *false* that follows the statement. If the word *false* has been circled, change the underlined word/words to make the statement true. Place your answer in the space provided.

1. Disinfection is the process by which all microorganisms, including spores, are destroyed.

   True     False     _____

2. In surgical asepsis, areas are considered contaminated if they bear, or are suspected of bearing, pathogens.

   True     False     _____

3. Solutions generally are considered sterile for 24 hours once opened.

   True     False     _____

4. Isolation is a protective procedure that limits the spread of infectious diseases among hospitalized clients, hospital personnel, and visitors.

   True     False     _____

5. <u>Universal precautions</u> recommend that health care workers use gloves, gowns, and masks when exposure to blood or body fluids is likely, and to consider that all clients might be potentially infected.

True    False    _____

6. In the <u>body substance isolation system</u>, each infectious disease is listed separately along with the individual interventions and barriers that are necessary to prevent transmission of that specific pathogen.

True    False    _____

7. <u>Latex gloves</u> perform better in stressful care situations because they are more flexible, durable, and tiny glove punctures are able to reseal automatically.

True    False    _____

## Completion

1. List and define the six components in the infection cycle.

a. _____

_____

_____

_____

b. _____

_____

_____

_____

c. _____

_____

_____

_____

d. _____

_____

_____

_____

e. _____

_____

_____

_____

f. _____

_____

_____

_____

2. Define the following means of transmitting an organism.

a. Direct contact: _____

_____

_____

b. Indirect contact: _____

_____

_____

c. Vectors: _____

_____

_____

d. Airborne route: _____

_____

_____

e. Vehicles: _____

_____

_____

3. List six factors influencing the susceptibility of a host to infection.

a. _____

_____

_____

b. _____

_____

_____

c. _____

_____

_____

d. _____

_____

_____

e. _____

_____

_____

f. _____

_____

_____

4. Write four client goals that are appropriate to preventing infection. (Answers may vary.)

a. _____

_____

b. _____

_____

c. _____

_____

d. _____

_____

5. List two techniques for each of the following situations that clients should be taught to prevent the spread of infectious diseases.

a. In the home: _____

_____

b. Using public facilities: _____

_____

c. In the community: _____

_____

6. List five species of bacteria that are common causative organisms responsible for nosocomial infections.

a. _____

b. _____

c. _____

d. _____

e. _____

7. Describe three measures health agencies have found to be successful in reducing the incidence of nosocomial infections.

a. _____

b. _____

c. _____

8. List and describe the two types of bacterial flora normally found on the hands.

a. _____

_____

_____

_____

b. _____

_____

_____

_____

9. Explain why the following factors should determine the selection of sterilization and disinfectant methods.

a. Nature of organisms present: _____

_____

b. Number of organisms present: _____

_____

_____

c. Type of equipment: _____

_____

_____

d. Intended use of equipment: _____

_____

_____

e. Available means for sterilization and disinfection:

_____

_____

_____

f. Time: _____

_____

_____

10. List six precautions in the body substance isolation system that should be observed by everyone at all times regardless of the client's diagnosis.

a. _____

_____

_____

b. _____

_____

_____

c. _____

_____

_____

d. _____

_____

_____

e. _____

_____

_____

f. _____

_____

_____

## Sequencing

1. Place each step in the correct sequence by numbering the following steps in the hand washing procedure.

a. _____ Turn on water and adjust force.

b. _____ With firm rubbing and circular motion, wash the palms and backs of the hands, each finger, the areas between the fingers, the knuckles, wrists, and forearms.

c. _____ Use lotion on hands if desired.

d. _____ Continue the friction motion for 10–30 seconds.

e. _____ Rinse thoroughly.

f. _____ Stand in front of the sink. Do not allow your uniform to touch the sink during the hand-washing procedure.

g. _____ Wet the hands and wrist area. Keep hands lower than elbows to allow water to flow toward fingertips.

h. _____ Remove jewelry, if possible, and secure in a safe place or allow plain wedding band to remain in place.

i. _____ Dry hands and wrists with a paper towel. Use paper towel to turn off faucet.

j. _____ Use fingernails of the other hand or a clean orange-wood stick to clean under fingernails.

k. _____ Use about 1 teaspoon of liquid soap from dispenser or lather thoroughly with bar soap. Rinse bar and return to soap dish.

# 27

# Diagnostic Procedures

Chapter 27 introduces the learner to the basic responsibilities of the nurse assisting with all diagnostic tests. Major tests are summarized and procedures for obtaining laboratory specimens are provided.

OBJECTIVES

After studying this chapter the learner will be able to:

Define key terms used in this chapter.

Describe various diagnostic tests and their purposes.

Describe nursing responsibilities for a client prior to, during, and following a diagnostic test.

Discuss the importance of psychological preparation and support to clients having diagnostic tests.

Identify assessment data appropriate for specific diagnostic tests.

Evaluate the client's response following a diagnostic examination.

## Matching

Match the endoscopic study in Part A with its definition listed in Part B.

Part A

a. bronchoscopy

b. esophagogastroduodenoscopy

c. proctosigmoidoscopy

d. colonoscopy

e. cystoscopy

f. endoscopic retrograde cholangiopancreatography

Part B

1. _____ Visual examination of the entire large intestine.

2. _____ Visual examination of the trachea and bronchi.

3. _____ Visual examination of the bladder, urethra, and urethral orifices.

4. _____ Visual examination of the esophagus, stomach, and duodenum.

5. _____ Visual examination of the rectum, rectosigmoid junction, and lower sigmoid colon.

6. _____ Visual examination of the esophagus, stomach, and duodenum combined with x-ray visualization, by means of a contrast medium, of the pancreatic ducts and hepatobiliary tree.

Match the definition in Part B with the procedure listed in Part A.

Part A

a. liver biopsy

b. lumbar puncture

c. abdominal paracentesis

d. thoracentesis

e. electrocardiogram

f. electroencephalograph

g. endoscopic studies

h. radiography procedures

i. computed tomography

j. MRI

k. ultrasonography

l. laboratory tests

Part B

7. _____ Allows for direct visual examination of various body cavities and organs by means of a hollow, lighted tube.

8. _____ A noninvasive X-ray procedure in which a body part can be scanned from different angles with an x-ray beam and a computer calculates varying tissue densities and records a cross-sectional image on paper.

9. _____ The entering and aspirating of fluid from the pleural cavity.

10. _____ A noninvasive procedure that involves the use of ultrasound to produce an image or photograph of an organ or tissue.

11. _____ A needle aspiration of a sample of liver tissue.

12. _____ The withdrawal of fluid from the peritoneal cavity.

13. _____ An advanced scanning technique that uses magnetism and radio-frequency waves to produce cross-sectional images of body tissues on a computer screen.

14. _____ The use of X-rays to secure data about health status.

15. _____ An instrument that receives and records electrical currents in the brain.

16. _____ Studies done on blood, urine and bodily secretions.

17. _____ The insertion of a needle into the subarachnoid space in the spinal canal.

18. _____ A record of the electrical impulses of the heart.

## Multiple Choice

Circle the letter that corresponds to the best answer for each question.

1. When preparing a client for diagnostic tests, which of the following statements should be taken into consideration?

a. As a client advocate, the nurse must monitor all test preparations to ensure that the client is not in a prolonged fasting state.

b. An intravenous pyleogram must be scheduled after a barium study to properly visualize the kidneys.

c. A client who is given too much detailed information about a procedure is likely to be confused and ill prepared emotionally for the test.

d. The nurse is not responsible for gathering supplies and equipment for the test.

2. Mrs. Henry is scheduled for a liver biopsy. Which of the following statements are relative to this procedure?

a. Mrs. Henry will be emotionally prepared for a lengthy surgical procedure.

b. Mrs. Henry will receive general anesthesia prior to the test.

c. A prothrombin time and platelet count will be checked before the test is performed.

d. There are no dietary restrictions associated with this test.

3. When preparing a client for abdominal paracentesis, the nurse should be aware of which of the following?

a. The client should be placed in a supine position for the testing.

b. If the fluid is draining too rapidly, the container should be lowered to floor level.

c. No more than 2000 milliliters should be drained at one time.

d. After the procedure, the nurse should place a sterile, heavy dressing over the incision because leakage usually occurs.

4. Which of the following statements regarding elec-
trocardiograph findings is accurate?

 a. The electrical activity in the heart is received
through electrodes placed on the skin on various parts of the body.

 b. The placement patterns of electrodes are called
nodes.

 c. When cells are electrically stimulated they
polarize, or become charged, and contraction
occurs.

 d. The electrical activity that causes the heartbeat
originates in the atrioventricular node.

5. Computer tomography may cause nausea and
vomiting secondary to which of the following?

 a. The positioning necessary in the chamber.

 b. The idodine contrast media which may be given
IV.

 c. The length of time the X-ray beam is activated.

 d. The exposure to radiation.

6. Which of the following statements is correct to
teach a client who is scheduled to have a CT scan?

 a. The test usually lasts from one to two hours and
can be quite uncomfortable.

 b. Individuals allergic to other dyes need not
worry about this dye.

 c. Exposure to radiation from this test is approximately double that of conventional X-rays.

 d. The dye may cause a warm sensation and flushing of the face.

7. Prior to permitting a client to eat and drink who
has just returned from an endoscopy in which a
local anesthetic was used, the nurse must assess
which of the following?

 a. The client's ability to speak.

 b. The client's understanding of the procedure.

 c. The client's ability to cough or swallow.

 d. The client's understanding of the consent form.

8. A client undergoing a barium enema should be
aware of which of the following?

 a. The procedure should cause no discomfort.

 b. Fecal material may be black from the barium for
several days following the examination.

 c. There are no dietary restrictions prior to the
testing.

 d. Preparation generally includes cleansing of the
colon with laxatives and enemas.

## Completion

1. Explain the following nurse's responsibilities for
preparing a client for a diagnostic procedure prior to
the test.

a. Obtaining consent: _____

_____

_____

_____

_____

b. Scheduling tests: _____

_____

_____

_____

_____

c. Physical and psychologic preparation of the client:

_____

_____

_____

_____

d. Assembling equipment: _____

_____

_____

_____

_____

2. Explain the following nurse's responsibilities for
preparing a client for a diagnostic procedure during
the test.

a. Collecting baseline data: _____

_____

_____

_____

b. Evaluating the client: _____

_____

_____

_____

c. Supporting the client: _____

_____

_____

_____

d. Assisting the examiner: _____

_____

_____

_____

3. Explain the following nurse's responsibilities for client care after the test.

a. Assessing the client: _____

_____

_____

_____

b. Assisting the client: _____

_____

_____

c. Preparing specimens and caring for equipment: ___

_____

_____

_____

d. Documenting the procedure: _____

_____

_____

_____

4. Give a brief description of the following tests, listing the procedure and positioning of the client. Explain the nurse's responsibility for client care in each procedure.

a. Liver Biopsy

Procedure: _____

_____

_____

Nursing responsibilities: _____

_____

_____

_____

b. Lumbar Puncture

Procedure: _____

_____

_____

_____

Nursing responsibilities: _____

_____

_____

_____

c. Abdominal Paracentesis

Procedure: _____

_____

_____

Nursing responsibilities: _____

_____

_____

d. Thoracentesis

Procedure: _____

_____

_____

Nursing responsibilities: _____

_____

_____

e. Electrocardiography

Procedure: _____

_____

_____

_____

Nursing responsibilities: _____

_____

_____

_____

f. Radiography

Procedure: _____

_____

_____

_____

Nursing responsibilities: _____

_____

_____

_____

g. Magnetic Resonance Imaging

Procedure: _____

_____

_____

_____

Nursing responsibilities: _____

_____

_____

_____

h. Ultrasonography

Procedure: _____

_____

_____

_____

Nursing responsibilities: _____

_____

_____

_____

# 28

# Continuity of Care

Chapter 28 introduces the learner to the concept of continuity of care: the coordination of services provided to clients before they enter a health care setting, during the time they are in the setting, and after they leave the setting. Included in the discussion are the nursing roles and responsibilities in admission of clients to a health care setting, transferring client within and between settings, and discharge planning.

OBJECTIVES

After studying this chapter the learner will be able to:

Define key terms used in the chapter.

Describe the role of the nurse in ensuring continuity of care.

Discuss considerations for establishing an effective nurse-client relationship when admitting a client to a health-care setting.

Compare and contrast admission of a client to an ambulatory setting and a hospital setting.

Discuss transfer of clients within and among health-care settings.

Describe the components of discharge planning in providing continuity of care.

## Matching

Match the element of discharge teaching in Part A that would be implemented with the nursing actions in Part B.

Part A

a. medications

b. procedures and treatments

c. diet

d. referrals

e. health promotion

Part B

1._____ The nurse describes all aspects of the illness and the effects of treatment; the client is given verbal information and literature specific to learning needs.

2. _____ The nurse explains the purpose of the diet and provides examples of written diet plans and meals.

3. _____ The nurse demonstrates the dressing change, then has the client/family practice the procedure.

4. _____ The nurse discusses drug names, dosage, purposes, effects, times to be taken, and possible side effects.

5. _____ The nurse makes appointments with a local home health agency.

## Multiple Choice

Circle the letter that corresponds to the best answer for each question.

1. Which of the following is a normal response to admission to any type of health-care setting?
   a. anger
   b. fear
   c. happiness
   d. anxiety

2. There are many different types of ambulatory health care facilities. What does the word ambulatory describe when used in this context?
   a. The client must be able to walk upright.
   b. The client remains overnight, but is not bedfast.
   c. The client does not remain overnight.
   d. The client does not have surgery.

3. The identification band placed on a client's arm at the time of admission is essential to the client's:
   a. safety
   b. mobility
   c. care
   d. treatment

4. When clients are transferred within or among health-care settings, which of the following is most essential in ensuring continuity of care?
   a. Notification of all departments of room change.
   b. Accurate and complete communications.
   c. Careful moving of all personal items.
   d. Asking family members to take home jewelry.

5. Which of the following health-care providers is responsible for the comfort and well-being of the client on arrival to the unit?
   a. the admitting office clerk
   b. the nurse's aide
   c. the physician
   d. the nurse

## Correct the False Statements

Circle the word *true* or *false* that follows the statement. If the word *false* has been circled, change the underlined word/words to make the statement true. Place your answer in the space provided.

1. All persons who enter a health care setting take the role of <u>client.</u>

   True    False    _____

2. When admitting a client who will be arriving on a stretcher, the bed should be placed in the <u>lowest</u> position.

   True    False    _____

3. When transferring a client to a long-term facility for care, the original chart is <u>sent with the client.</u>

   True    False    _____

4. During admission, explaining the space and territory that will belong to the client gives the client a sense of <u>control</u> over the environment.

   True    False    _____

5. Your client says, "I'm going home today!" You verify this by checking the <u>nursing care plan.</u>

   True    False    _____

## Completion

1. In general, what must the nurse do to ensure continuity of care?

   a. _____
   _____
   _____

   b. _____
   _____
   _____

   c. _____
   _____
   _____

2. List the general guidelines that should be used to establish an effective nurse-client relationship, and in ensuring each client is considered as an individual during admission to a health-care setting.

a. _____

_____

_____

b. _____

_____

_____

c. _____

_____

_____

d. _____

_____

_____

e. _____

_____

_____

3. What is "discharge planning?"

_____

_____

_____

4. What should the nurse do if a client leaves the hospital against medical advice?

_____

_____

_____

_____

5. Describe the assessments that must be made about the environment as a part of discharge planning.

a. _____

b. _____

c. _____

d. _____

e. _____

f. _____

g. _____

# 29

## Hygiene

Chapter 29 provides the nurse with knowledge of the multiple factors that affect personal hygiene and of nursing measures that promote personal hygiene. A practical guide for assessing the adequacy of personal hygiene behaviors is presented. Client goals are provided, along with specific nursing strategies used when performing care of the skin, mouth, eyes, ears, and nose, feet, and perineal and vaginal areas.

### OBJECTIVES

After studying this chapter the learner will be able to:

List five functions of the skin, three factors influencing the skin's condition, and four basic principles that guide practices of skin care.

Identify factors affecting skin condition and personal hygiene.

Assess the integumentary system and the adequacy of hygiene self-care behaviors, using appropriate interview and physical assessment skills.

Develop nursing diagnoses related to deficient hygiene measures.

Describe the priorities of scheduled hygienic care, early morning care, morning care, afternoon care, and evening care.

Demonstrate the back massage, identifying at least four reasons for including the back massage in daily nursing care.

Demonstrate techniques used when assisting clients with hygiene measures, including those used when administering various types of baths and those used in cleaning each part of the body.

Describe agents commonly used on the skin and scalp and precautions to observe in their use.

Plan, implement, and evaluate nursing care for common problems of the skin and mucous membranes.

Describe the prevention and treatment of pressure ulcers.

## EXERCISES

### Matching

Match the definition in Part B with the term listed in Part A.

Part A

a. personal hygiene

b. integumentary system

c. epidermis

d. dermis

e. sebaceous glands

f. cerumen

g. dehydration

h. emollient

i. acne

j. rashes

k. pressure ulcers

l. dandruff

m. pediculosis

Part B

1. _____ Consists of the skin and its appendages, that is, the hair, glands in the skin, and the nails.

2. _____ Secretes an oily substance called sebum.

3. _____ Consists of smooth, muscular tissue, nerves, hair follicles, certain glands and their ducts, arteries, veins, and capillaries, and fibrous, elastic tissue.

4. _____ Infestation with lice.

5. _____ Condition characterized by itching and flaking of the scalp.

6. _____ Condition in which blackheads and pustules appear on the skin when secretions become dammed up in the sebaceous ducts, and inflammation with infection occurs.

7. _____ An agent used to soften, soothe, and protect dry skin after it is cleansed.

8. _____ Fluid loss through fever, vomiting, or diarrhea.

9. _____ Measures for personal cleanliness and grooming that promote physical and psychologic well-being.

*(Cont'd)*

10. _____  The superficial layer of skin, made up of layers of stratefied epithelial cells.

11. _____  Areas of cellular necrosis caused by the lack of blood circulation to the involved area.

12. _____  A heavy oil and brown pigment in the external ear canals.

13. _____  Eruptions or inflammations of the skin that may be found anywhere on the body.

Match the oral problem described in Part B with its medical term listed in Part A.

Part A

a. stomatitis

b. glossitis

c. cheilosis

d. dry oral mucosa

e. oral malignancies

Part B

14. _____  A condition related to dehydration, or caused by mouth breathing, an alteration in salivary functioning, or by certain medications.

15. _____  Lumps or ulcers in the mouth.

16. _____  An inflammation of the oral mucosa with numerous causes, such as bacteria, virus, mechanical trauma, irritants, nutritional deficiencies, and systemic infections.

17. _____  An ulceration of the lips most often caused by vitamin B deficiencies.

18. _____  An inflammation of the tongue.

Match the oral problem described in Part B with its medical term listed in Part A.

Part A

a. caries

b. plaque

c. gingivitis

d. pyorrhea

e. tartar

f. halitosis

Part B

19. _____  A strong mouth odor or persistent bad taste in the mouth.

20. _____  An invisible, destructive, bacterial film that builds up on everyone's teeth and eventually leads to the destruction of tooth enamal.

21. _____  The decay of teeth with the formation of cavities.

22. _____  Hard deposits on the gum lines of teeth, formed by unchecked plaque and dead bacteria.

23. _____  Periodontal disease.

24. _____  An inflammation of the tissue that surrounds the teeth.

## Multiple Choice

Circle the letter that corresponds to the best answer for each question.

1. When caring for the skin of clients of different age groups, which of the following should the nurse consider?

   a. An infant's skin and mucous membranes are protected from infection by a natural immunity

   b. An adolescent's skin ordinarily has enlarged sebaceous glands and increased glandular secretions caused by hormonal changes in the body.

   c. Secretions from skin glands are at their maximum from age three on.

   d. The skin becomes thicker and leathery with aging and is prone to wrinkles and dryness.

2. Illness affects the condition of the client's skin in which of the following ways?

   a. Very thin and very obese people tend to be less susceptible to skin irritation and injury.

   b. Fluid loss through fever, vomiting, or diarrhea reduces the fluid volume of the body and is called evaporation.

   c. Jaundice, a condition caused by excessisve bile pigments, results in a grayish skin color.

   d. Diseases of the skin are usually characterized by various lesions that require special care.

3. When caring for a client with dentures, which of the following should the nurse tell the client?

   a. Keeping dentures out for long periods of time permits the gum line to change, thus affecting their fit.

   b. Dentures should be wrapped in tissue or in a disposable wipe when they are out of the mouth, and stored in a disposable cup.

   c. Dentures should never be stored in water because the plastic material may warp.

   d. A brush and nonabrasive powder or paste should be used to clean the dentures, and hot water should be used to rinse them.

4. When caring for a client who is wearing contact lenses, the nurse should be aware of which of the following facts?

   a. It is recommended that extended-wear lenses be cleansed once a month.

   b. To allow the cornea to receive a maximal supply of oxygen, hard lenses should be removed before sleeping and should not be worn more than 24–30 hours.

   c. Extended-wear soft lenses can be left in place for 1 to 30 days, depending on the manufacturer.

   d. Nurses should try to remove the lenses from a client with an eye injury to facilitate healing.

5. Mrs. Green is a 55-year-old diabetic client. Which of the following precautions would apply when caring for her feet?

   a. Heating pads and hot water bottles should be applied to the feet to relieve soreness.

   b. The client should be encouraged to go barefoot whenever possible to allow the skin to breathe.

   c. The client's nails should be cut with scissors as files may put too much pressure on the nail.

   d. Preparations prescribed by a physician should be used to treat athlete's foot.

6. Mrs. Lucas has a pressure ulcer. The chart states that the ulcer is a stage-three classification. Which of the following best describes this finding?

   a. Redness persists, accompanied by edema and induration. The epidermis may blister and erode.

   b. Redness is the primary sign. The skin does not return to a normal color when pressure is relieved. There is no induration, the skin and underlying tissue remains soft.

   c. There is an open lesion and a crater exposing subcutaneous tissue. You may be able to see fascia at the base of the ulcer.

   d. Necrosis will extend through the fascia and may even involve the bone. Eschar is a common finding.

7. Mrs. Jensen has a pressure ulcer on her coccyx, which is about 1 1/2cm in size. Which of the following would be the most important nursing intervention to help heal the ulcer?

   a. Elevate the head to 45 degrees.

   b. Change position frequently, every one to two hours.

   c. Slide the client up in bed frequently.

   d. Use waterproof material on the client's bed.

8. Mrs. Jury is a 37-year-old woman admitted to the hospital. During her stay in the hospital, a vaginal douche is ordered. Which of the following would be the correct technique for this procedure?

   a. Hold the bag or hang it on a standard so that it is about 24–36 inches above the level of the hip.

   b. Fill a douche bag with a pint of douche solution; the solution may be warm soapy water.

   c. Use a bulb syringe because it is easier to inject the solution with force.

   d. Raise the level of the bag containing the douche for increased force of injection.

9. Which of the following is an ulceration of the lips most often caused by vitamin B deficiencies?

   a. satomatitis

   b. glossitis

   c. cheilosis

   d. caries

10. Which of the following responses would be appropriate when explaining to a client why antiembolism stockings are being applied?

    a. The stockings help force blood from the superficial veins to deeper veins and prevent stagnation.

    b. The stockings increase the arterial blood supply to the legs.

    c. The stockings are used so that the individual does not have to move.

    d. The stockings help by forcing blood out of the arteries and preventing blood clots.

## Correct the False Statements

Circle the word *true* or *false* that follows the statement. If the word *false* has been circled, change the underlined word/words to make the statement true. Place your answer in the space provided.

1. A <u>shearing force</u> results when layers of tissue move on each other.

   True      False      _____

2. Local anemia owing to poor circulation in the area is called <u>reactive hyperemia.</u>

   True    False    _____

3. The <u>clinitron bed</u> minimizes pressure and eliminates shear, friction and maceration by means of the fluidization principle.

   True    False    _____

4. Lice lay eggs called <u>nits</u> on the hair shafts.

   True    False    _____

5. The lateral angle of the eye where the upper and lower lids meet is known as the <u>inner canthus.</u>

   True    False    _____

6. The <u>esophagus</u> is the first part of the alimentary canal and is an adjunct of the respiratory system.

   True    False    _____

7. The odor of perspiration occurs when <u>bacteria</u> normally present on everyone's skin, act on the skin's normal secretions.

   True    False    _____

8. Deodorants and antiperspirants act as astringents and tend to <u>open</u> the exits of the sweat glands.

   True    False    _____

9. Problems concerning deficient hygiene are categorized as <u>self-care deficits.</u>

   True    False    _____

## Completion

1. Explain how the following functions of the skin operate.

a. The skin protects the body: _____

_____

_____

_____

_____

b. The skin helps regulate body temperature: _____

_____

_____

_____

_____

c. The skin is a sense organ: _____

_____

_____

_____

_____

d. The skin is an excretory organ: _____

_____

_____

_____

e. The skin helps maintain water and electrolyte balance: _____

_____

_____

_____

_____

f. The skin produces and absorbs vitamin D: _____

_____

_____

_____

_____

2. Summarize the hygienic care that should be performed during the following periods.

a. Early morning care: _____

_____

_____

_____

b. Morning care: _____

_____

_____

_____

_____

c. Afternoon care: _____

_____

_____

_____

d. Hour of sleep care: _____

_____

_____

_____

e. As needed care: _____

_____

_____

_____

3. Describe a safe bedside unit. What factors must be controlled to provide a comfortable bedside unit?

_____

_____

_____

_____

4. List five suggestions to alleviate dry skin.

a. _____

b. _____

c. _____

d. _____

e. _____

5. Write three nursing goals that will assist clients to develop or maintain oral hygiene practices to promote oral health and general well-being.

a. _____

_____

b. _____

_____

c. _____

_____

6. List the pertinent nursing measures that should be included in the plan of care for the following body parts.

a. Eyes: _____

_____

_____

_____

_____

b. Ears: _____

_____

_____

_____

c. Nose: _____

_____

_____

_____

_____

7. Describe the four stages of a pressure ulcer.

a. Stage 1: _____

_____

_____

b. Stage 2: _____

_____

_____

c. Stage 3: _____

_____

_____

d. Stage 4: _____

_____

_____

_____

## Case Study

Read the following case study and use your nursing process skills to answer the questions below.

Mrs. Chijioke, an 88-year-old woman who lived alone for years, was brought to the hospital after neighbors found her lying at the bottom of her cellar steps. She broke her hip and is now three days after hip repair surgery. The nurse assigned to care for Mrs. Chijioke noticed during the patient's bath that the skin of her coccyx, heels, and elbows was reddened. The skin did return to a normal color when pressure was relieved in these areas. There was no edema, nor was there induration or blistering. While Mrs. Chijioke was able to be lifted out of bed into a chair, she spent most of the day in bed, lying on her back with an abductor pillow between her legs. At 5', 89 pounds, Mrs. Chijioke looked lost in the big hospital bed. Her eyes were bright and she usually attempted a warm smile, but she had little physical strength and would lie seemingly motionless for hours. Her skin was wrinkled and paper thin and her arms were already bruised from unsuccessful attempts at initiating intravenous therapy. Dehydrated on admission, since she had spent almost 48 hours crumpled at the bottom of her steps before being found by her neighbors, Mrs. Chijioke was clearly in need of nutritional, fluid, and electrolyte support. A long-time diabetic, Mrs. Chijioke is now spiking a temperature (39.0°C/102.2°F), which concerns her nurse.

1. Identify pertinent client data by placing a single underline beneath the *objective* data in the case study and a double underline beneath the *subjective* data.

2. Complete the Nursing Process Worksheet on the opposite page to develop a three-part diagnostic statement and related plan of care for this client.

3. Write down the client and personal nursing strengths you hope to draw upon as you assist this client to better health.

Client strengths:_____

_____

_____

_____

_____

Personal strengths: _____

_____

_____

_____

_____

4. Pretend that you are performing a nursing assessment of this client after the plan of care is implemented. Document your findings below.

_____

_____

_____

_____

_____

_____

_____

_____

## Nursing Process Worksheet

**Health Problem (Title)**

Related to

↓

**Etiology (Related Factors)**

As Manifested by

↓

**Signs and Symptoms
(Defining Characteristics)**

**Client Goal***

**Nursing Interventions****

**Evaluative Statement:**

*More than one client goal may be appropriate. For the purposes of this exercise, develop the one client goal that demonstrates a direct resolution of the client problem identified in the nursing diagnosis.
**Be sure you are able to list the scientific rationale for each nursing intervention you ordered.

# 30

## Activity

Chapter 30 provides the learner with knowledge of the physiology of movement, the principles of body mechanics, and factors affecting body alignment and mobility. Types of exercises, the role of exercise in disease prevention and health promotion, risks related to exercise, and individualized exercise programs are presented. The effects of immobility of body systems are explored and a practical guide to assessing body alignment and mobility states is offered.

### OBJECTIVES

After studying this chapter the learner will be able to:

Define key terms used in this chapter.

Describe the role of the skeletal, muscular, and nervous systems in the physiology of movement.

Identify seven variables that influence body alignment and mobility.

Differentiate isotonic, isometric, and isokinetic exercise.

Describe the effects of exercise and immobility on major body systems.

Assess body alignment, mobility, and activity intolerance, utilize appropriate interview questions and physical assessment skills.

Develop nursing diagnoses that correctly identify mobility problems amenable to nursing therapy.

Utilize proper body mechanics when positioning, moving, lifting, and ambulating clients.

Design exercise programs.

Plan, implement, and evaluate nursing care related to select nursing diagnoses involving mobility problems.

### EXERCISES

## Matching

Match the definition in Part B with the term used to describe body positions and movements listed in Part A.

Part A

a. abduction

b. adduction

c. circumduction

d. flexion

e. extension

f. hyperextension

g. dorsiflexion

h. plantar flexion

i. rotation

j. internal rotation

k. external rotation

l. pronation

m. supination

n. inversion

o. eversion

Part B

1. _____ The assumption of a prone position.

2. _____ Lateral movement of a body part away from the midline of the body.

3. _____ Backward bending of the hand or foot.

4. _____ Movement of the sole of the foot outward.

5. _____ The state of being bent.

6. _____ A body part turning on its axis away from the midline of the body.

7. _____ Lateral movement of a body part toward the midline of the body.

8. _____ Movement of the sole of the foot inward.

9. _____ Movement of the distal part of the limb to trace a complete circle while the proximal end of the bone remains fixed.

10. _____ The assumption of the supine position.

11. _____ A body part turning on its axis toward the midline of the body.

12. _____ Flexion of the foot.

13. _____ The state of being in a straight line.

14. _____ The turning of a body part on the axis provided by its joint.

15. _____ The state of exaggerated extension.

Match the activity in Part B with the type of exercise listed in Part A. Answers may be used more than once.

Part A

a. aerobic exercise

b. stretching exercises

c. strength and endurance exercises

d. movement/daily life exercises

Part B

16. _____ House cleaning

17. _____ Hatha yoga

18. _____ Weight training

19. _____ Swimming

20. _____ Jogging

21. _____ Warm-up exercises

22. _____ Climbing stairs to an appointment

23. _____ Calisthenics

Match the definition in Part B with the type of joint listed in Part A. Give an example of the joint on the line provided after the definition.

Part A

a. ball and socket joint

b. condyloid joint

c. gliding joint

d. hinge joint

e. pivot joint

f. saddle joint

Part B

24. _____ Ring-like structure that turns on a pivot; movement is limited to rotation:

_____

25. _____ Rounded head of one bone fits into a cup-like cavity in the other:

_____

26. _____ Bone surfaces are convex on one side and concave on the other:

_____

27. _____ Oval head of one bone fits into shallow cavity of another bone:

_____

28. _____ Articular surfaces are flat, flexion-extension and abduction-adduction are permitted:

_____

29. _____ Spool-like surface fits into a concave surface:

_____

Match the definition in Part B with the term listed in Part A.

Part A

a. body mechanics

b. orthopedics

c. tonus

d. exercise

e. atelectasis

f. atrophy

g. contractures

h. ankylosis

i. osteoporosis

j. hypertrophy

k. muscle tone

l. flaccidity

m. spasticity

n. range of motion

o. paresis

Part B

30. _____ Impaired muscle strength or weakness.

31. _____ The complete extent of movement of which a joint is normally capable.

32. _____ The process of bone demineralization.

33. _____ Decreased muscle size.

34. _____ A consolidation and immobilization of a joint.

35. _____ The efficient use of the body as a machine and as a means of locomotion.

36. _____ The term used to describe the state of slight contraction in which we normally find skeletal muscles.

37. _____ Active exertion of muscles involving the contraction and relaxation of muscle groups.

38. _____ Increased muscle tone that interferes with movement.

39. _____ Increased muscle mass resulting from exercise or training

40. _____ The slight residual tension that remains in a resting normal muscle with an intact nerve supply.

41. _____ Decreased muscle tone.

42. _____ The correction or the prevention of disorders of the body's structures for locomotion.

43. _____ The incomplete expansion or collapse of lung tissue.

44. _____ Permanent contraction states of muscle.

Match the definitions in Part B with the type of involuntary body movements listed in Part A.

Part A

a. tremors

b. tics

c. chorea

d. athetosis

e. dystonia

f. fasciculations

g. myoclonus

h. oral-facial dyskinesias

Part B

45. _____ Sudden brief, rapid, unpredictable jerks, usually involving the limbs or trunk; may be single or repetitive.

46. _____ Movements that are slower, and more twisting and writhing than chorea movements, and that have a larger amplitude; commonly involve the face and distal extremities.

47. _____ Repetitive, bizarre movements that chiefly involve the face, mouth, jaw, and tongue.

48. _____ Relatively rhythmic oscillatory movements.

49. _____ Fine, rapid, flickering, or twitching movements originating in relatively small groups of muscle fibers; vary irregularly in frequency and extent, but rarely move a joint.

50. _____ Brief, repetitive, stereotyped, coordinated movements occurring at regular intervals.

51. _____ Movements similar to athetosis but that involve larger portions of the body, including the trunk; may result in grotesque, twisted postures.

52. _____ Brief, rapid, jerky, irregular, and unpredictable movements that occur at rest or interrupt normal, coordinated movements; seldom repeat themselves.

## Multiple Choice

Circle the letter that corresponds to the best answer for each question.

1. Which of the following is a type of muscle?
   a. skeletal
   b. disc
   c. vetebral
   d. rough

2. Which of the following stimulates muscles to contract?
   a. body mechanics
   b. diarthroses
   c. contractures
   d. nerve impulses

3. Which of the following statements about body balance and coordinated body movement should be incorporated into a nurse's practice?
   a. Nurses can increase body balance when working by decreasing the distance between their feet.
   b. Nurses can increase body balance by flexing their hips and knees, lowering the center of gravity.
   c. In order to move a client to the other side of the bed, a nurse should push the client, using the arm bones as levers and the elbows as fulcrums.
   d. Use the back muscles to help provide the power needed in strenuous activity.

4. Which of the following postural reflexes informs the brain of the location of a limb or body part as a result of joint movements stimulating special nerve endings in muscles, tendons, and fascia?
   a. extensor or stretch reflexes
   b. labyrinthine sense
   c. proprioceptor or kinesthetic sense
   d. visual or optic reflexes

5. Which of the following parts of the brain assumes the major role of controlling precise, discrete movements?
   a. basal ganglia
   b. pyramidal pathways
   c. cerebellum
   d. cerebral motor cortex

6. Mr. Bellas is a 40-year-old man with a sedentary job who is starting an exercise program. Which of the following statements about exercise should he be made aware of?
   a. The heart works harder when a person is exercising.
   b. Over time, regular exercise decreases the flow of blood to all body parts.
   c. High impact aerobic exercise predisposes a person to venous thrombosis, especially in the legs.
   d. Over time, regular exercise leads to improved pulmonary functioning.

7. Which of the following is an effect of immobility on the respiratory system?
   a. Decreased movement in the thoracic cage during respirations.
   b. Increased ventilatory effort.
   c. Increase in the depth and rate of respirations.
   d. Increase in the movement of secretions in the respiratory tract.

8. Mrs. Zachary has been admitted to your unit with severe rheumatoid arthritis. Which of the following nursing diagnoses would be most appropriate?
   a. Knowledge deficit related to surgery.
   b. Altered skin integrity related to chemotherapy.
   c. Impaired physical immobility related to disease process.
   d. Fluid volume excess related to increased appetite.

9. You are assessing an ambulatory client when you observe that both arms swing freely in alteration with leg swings. You are assessing which of the following?
   a. alignment
   b. gait
   c. joint function
   d. muscle tone

10. Your nursing diagnosis of Mr. Albert is "knowledge deficit related to crutch walking." Which of the following would be the best time to teach Mr. Albert about their correct use?
    a. prior to surgery on his knee
    b. the fourth day post-op
    c. prior to discharge
    d. when he is ready

11. The nursing diagnosis of "activity intolerance" has been given to Mr. Long. Which of the following observations indicates this problem has not been resolved?

    a. poor endurance
    b. orthostatic hypotension
    c. apathy
    d. diaphoresis, pallor, and weakness

12. Mr. Drennan will be ambulating for the first time since his cardiac surgery. Which of the following should the nurse know in order to assist Mr. Drennan?

    a. Clients who are fearful of walking should look at their feet to assure correct positioning.
    b. Clients who can lift their leg only one to two inches from the bed do not have sufficient power to permit walking.
    c. Nurses should never assist clients out of bed and help them to walk without a physical therapist present.
    d. If a client begins to fall, the nurse should slide the client down the nurse's own body to the floor, carefully protecting the client's head.

13. Mrs. Henry brings her 3-month-old baby to the doctor for a well-baby visit. When she questions her baby's motor abilities, which of the following should the nurse tell Mrs. Henry?

    a. By three months of age the infant in the prone position is generally able to raise the chest and head from the floor.
    b. By three months, head control is usually achieved in both the sitting position and when being held erect.
    c. The 3-month-old usually lies with extremeties flexed and hands closed.
    d. By 3 months of age, the infant should be able to roll over adeptly.

## Correct the False Statements

Circle the word *true* or *false* that follows the statement. If the word *false* has been circled, change the underlined word/words to make the statement true. Place your answer in the space provided.

l. The 206 bones in the human body are classified on the basis of their <u>size.</u>

   True    False    _____

2. <u>Synovial joints</u> are the freely movable joints in which there is a space between the articulating bones.

   True    False    _____

3. <u>Ligaments</u> are strong, flexible, inelastic fibrous bands that attach muscle to bone.

   True    False    _____

4. Attachment of a muscle to the more movable bone is the <u>point of origin</u>.

   True    False    _____

5. A <u>nerve impulse</u> stimulates muscles to contract.

   True    False    _____

6. The <u>center of gravity</u> of an object is the point at which its mass is centered.

   True    False    _____

7. A <u>dislocation</u> is the displacement of a bone from a joint with tearing of ligaments, tendons, and capsules.

   True    False    _____

8. <u>Isotonic exercise</u> involves muscle contraction without shortening.

   True    False    _____

9. <u>Hypostatic pneumonia</u> is a type of pneumonia that results from inactivity and immobility.

   True    False    _____

10. The acronym RICE stands for rest, ice, compression and <u>exercise.</u>

    True    False    _____

11. <u>Parapalegia</u> is paralysis of all four limbs.

    True    False    _____

12. <u>Footdrop</u> is a complication of plantar flexion in which the foot is unable to maintain itself in the perpendicular position, heel-toe gait is impossible, and client will experience difficulty walking.

    True    False    _____

## Completion

. Briefly explain the effects of exercise and immobility on the body systems listed on the chart below. Place our answers in the space provided on the chart.

| Body System | Effects of Exercise | Effects of Immobility |
|---|---|---|
| Cardiovascular | | |
| Respiratory | | |
| Gastrointestinal | | |
| Urinary | | |
| Musculoskeletal | | |
| Metabolic | | |
| Integument | | |
| Psychological Well-Being | | |

2. List the five functions of the skeletal system.

a. _____

_____

b. _____

_____

c. _____

_____

d. _____

_____

e. _____

_____

3. Explain how the following components of body mechanics affect body functioning.

a. Body alignment or posture: _____

_____

_____

_____

_____

b. Balance: _____

_____

_____

_____

_____

c. Coordinated body movement: _____

_____

_____

_____

_____

4. List five positive benefits of exercise.

a. _____

b. _____

c. _____

d. _____

e. _____

5. Mrs. Mulherin is a 60-year-old female client admitted to a health care facility for degenerative joint disease. For section a, make up a physical assessment by listing the components used to determine her mobility status. For sections b and c, write two sample nursing diagnoses. For section d, develop a sample exercise program for Mrs. Mulherin.

a. Physical assessment: _____

_____

_____

_____

_____

_____

_____

_____

b. Nursing diagnosis: _____

_____

_____

c. Nursing diagnosis: _____

_____

_____

c. Exercise program: _____

_____

_____

_____

_____

_____

6. Explain how the following devices can be used to promote correct alignment.

a. Rocking bed:_____

_____

_____

_____

b. Chair bed: _____

_____

_____

_____

c. Circular bed:_____

_____

_____

_____

_____

_____

d. Stryker frame:_____

_____

_____

_____

e. Footboards:_____

_____

_____

_____

f. Sandbags:_____

_____

_____

_____

g. Trochanter rolls: _____

_____

_____

_____

h. Trapeze bar: _____

_____

_____

_____

_____

7. Describe the following positioning techniques and list their therapeutic effect on body alignment.

a. Fowler's position: _____

_____

_____

_____

_____

b. Supine or dorsal recumbent position: _____

_____

_____

_____

_____

_____

c. Side-lying or lateral position:_____

_____

_____

_____

_____

d. Prone position: _____

_____

_____

_____

_____

8. List and describe four mechanical aids to assist a client with walking.

a. _____

_____

b. _____

_____

c. _____

_____

_____

d. _____

_____

_____

9. Mr. Morris is a 50-year-old male firefighter diagnosed with disuse osteoporosis following recovery from serious burns. Write three client goals for Mr. Morris.

a. _____

_____

b. _____

_____

c. _____

_____

## Case Study

Read the following case study and use your nursing process skills to answer the questions below.

Robert Witherspoon, a 42-year-old university professor, presented for his first "physical" shortly after his father's death. His father died of complications of coronary artery disease. Mr. Witherspoon is 5'9" tall, weighs 235 pounds, has a decided "paunch," and reports that until now, he has made no time for exercise because he preferred to utilize any free time he had reading or listening to classical music. He enjoys French cuisine, including rich desserts, and has a cholesterol level of 310 mg/dl [normal is 150 mg–250 mg/dl]. He expresses being frightened by his father's death and is appropriately concerned about his elevated cholesterol level. "I guess I've never given much thought to my health before. . . but my dad's death changed all that. I know coronary artery disease runs in families and I can tell you that I'm not ready to pack it all in yet. Tell me what I have to do to fight this thing." He admits that he used to tease a colleague—who lowered his cholesterol from 290 to 200 by diet and exercise alone—by accusing him of being a fitness freak. "Now I'm recognizing the wisdom of his health behaviors and wondering if diet and exercise won't do the trick for me. Can you help me design an exercise program that will work?"

1. Identify pertinent client data by placing a single underline beneath the *objective* data in the case study and a double underline beneath the *subjective* data.

2. Complete the Nursing Process Worksheet on the opposite page to develop a three-part diagnostic statement and related plan of care for this client.

3. Write down the client and personal nursing strengths you hope to draw upon as you assist this client to better health.

Client strengths:_____

_____

_____

_____

_____

Personal strengths: _____

_____

_____

_____

_____

4. Pretend that you are performing a nursing assessment of this client after the plan of care is implemented. Document your findings below.

_____

_____

_____

_____

_____

_____

_____

_____

## Nursing Process Worksheet

**Health Problem (Title)**

**Client Goal***

Related to

↓

**Etiology (Related Factors)**

**Nursing Interventions****

As Manifested by

↓

**Signs and Symptoms
(Defining Characteristics)**

**Evaluative Statement:**

*More than one client goal may be appropriate. For the purposes of this exercise, develop the one client goal that demonstrates a direct resolution of the client problem identified in the nursing diagnosis.
**Be sure you are able to list the scientific rationale for each nursing intervention you ordered.

# 31

## Rest and Sleep

Chapter 31 provides the learner with knowledge of the functions and physiology of sleep, dreams, and dream theories, and factors affecting sleep. Practical suggestions for performing a comprehensive sleep assessment are given. Sample interview questions for both a general and focused sleep history are presented, along with information on sleep diaries and pertinent physical assessment data. Client goals and specific nursing strategies for promoting rest and sleep are described.

### OBJECTIVES

After studying this chapter the learner will be able to:

Define key terms used in this chapter.

Describe the functions and physiology of sleep.

Identify variables that influence rest and sleep.

Describe nursing implications for age-related differencess in the sleep-wakefulness cycle.

Perform a comprehensive sleep assessment using appropriate interview questions, a sleep diary when indicated, and physical assessment skills.

Describe common sleep disorders, noting key assessment criteria.

Develop nursing diagnoses that correctly identify sleep problems that may be treated by independent nursing intervention.

Describe the nursing strategies to promote rest and sleep, and identify their rationale.

Plan, implement, and evaluate nursing care related to select nursing diagnoses involving sleep problems.

### EXERCISES

### Matching

Match the definition in Part B with its term listed in Part A.

Part A

a. rest

b. sleep

c. circadian rhythm

d. nonrapid eye movement sleep

e. rapid eye movement sleep

f. delta sleep

g. sleep cycle

h. fatigue

Part B

1. _____ A normal protective body mechanism and nature's way of warning that sleep is necessary.

2. _____ The stages of sleep a person passes through.

3. _____ Rhythmic biological clocks in humans that regulate select biologic and behavioral functions and complete a full cycle every 24 hours.

4. _____ A condition in which the body is in a decreased state of activity with the consequent feeling of being refreshed.

5. _____ Consists of four stages. Stages I and II consume about 5–50 percent of a person's sleep, respectively, and are light sleep; stages III and IV, each comprising about 10 percent of sleep times, are deep sleep states.

6. _____ Consumes 20–25 percent of a person's nightly sleep, during which a person dreams.

7. _____ A state of altered consciousness throughout which varying degrees of stimuli produce wakefulness.

8. _____ Deep sleep states or slow wave sleep.

Match the definition in Part B with the sleep disorder listed in Part A.

Part A

a. insomnia

b. hypersomnia

c. narcolepsy

d. sleep apnea

e. parasomnia

f. somnambulism

g. enuresis

h. sleep deprivation

i. bruxism

j. snoring

k. nocturnal myoclonus

Part B

9. _____ A condition characterized by excessive sleep, particularly sleep during the day-time.

10. _____ May result from decreased REM sleep, NREM sleep, or from total lack of sleep.

11. _____ Grinding of teeth, usually occuring during stage II sleep.

12. _____ Patterns of waking behavior that appear during sleep.

13. _____ Bedwetting during sleep.

14. _____ Sleepwalking.

15. _____ Periods of no breathing between snoring intervals.

16. _____ Marked muscle contractions, which result in the jerking of one or both legs during sleep.

17. _____ Caused by an obstruction to the air flow through the nose and mouth.

18. _____ A condition characterized by an uncontrollable desire to sleep.

19. _____ Characterized by difficulty in falling asleep, intermittent sleep, or early awakening from sleep.

## Multiple Choice

Circle the letter that corresponds to the best answer for each question.

1. Wakefulness occurs when which of the following systems is activated with stimuli from the cerebral cortex and from periphery sensory organs and cells.
   a. hypothalmic system
   b. reticular system
   c. cerebral regulatory system
   d. bulbar synchronizing system

2. Which of the following conditions exist when an individual's sleep-wake patterns follow the inner biologic clock?
   a. nonrapid eye movement
   b. delta sleep
   c. circadian synchronization
   d. somnambulism

3. Which of the following analytical tools is used to record eye movements?
   a. electromyograph
   b. electroencephalograph
   c. electrocardiogram
   d. electrooculograph

4. A client who is in a state of REM sleep would experience which of the following?
   a. Twenty to twenty-five percent of the client's nightly sleep would be spent in REM sleep.
   b. Decreased pulse, respiratory rate, blood pressure, and metabolic rate would occur.
   c. The client would experience little of no dreaming during this state.
   d. Deprivation of this REM sleep would result in a pattern of decreased REM sleep on successive nights.

5. Mrs Chang is admitted to your unit with severe sleep disorders. Her physician ordered Flurazepam (Dalmane) on a PRN basis. Which of the following should the nurse be aware of when administering this medication?
   a. Flurazepam (Dalmane) disturbs REM sleep.
   b. The sleep produced by hypnotic-sedatives is a natural sleep following regular sleep patterns.
   c. Flurazepam (Dalmane) disturbs NREM slow-wave sleep, which results in a morning "hang-over" effect.
   d. There are no withdrawal symptoms associated with the cessation of Flurazepam (Dalmane).

6. Difficulty in falling asleep or staying asleep which has existed for three weeks or less is known as which of the following?

   a. chronic insomnia

   b. intermediate insomnia

   c. sleep deprivation

   d. transient insomnia

7. Which of the following interventions would be recommended for a client with insomnia?

   a. Nap frequently during the day to make-up for the lost sleep at night.

   b. Eliminate caffeine and alcohol in the evening because both are associated with disturbance in the normal sleep cycle.

   c. Exercise vigorously prior to bedtime to promote drowsiness.

   d. Avoid high-protein food before bedtime.

8. Mrs. James, age 60, is a client in the Intensive Care Unit. After three days, you notice marked changes in her behavior. She has increased pain, is very irritable, has a poor appetite, and her judgment is poor. You determine she is reacting to a sleep pattern disturbance. What nursing measures would you initiate in order to assist Mrs. James achieve more normal sleep?

   a. Give her ordered Flurazepam (Dalmane).

   b. Keep Mrs. James awake during the latter portion of the night.

   c. Arrange your nursing interventions so that Mrs. James has longer periods of undisturbed rest.

   d. Ask for a psychiatric consultation for Mrs. James.

9. Mrs. Jones, age 48, comes to the health clinic complaining of insomnia. After your assessment, your nursing diagnosis is: sleep pattern disturbance, insomnia; difficulty returning to sleep after awakening related to anxiety about not sleeping. All of the following are appropriate nursing interventions for Mrs. Jones except which of the following?

   a. Tell her to take her sleeping medication when she awakens.

   b. Teach her to leave the bedroom and do something quietly when she begins to have difficulty returning to sleep.

   c. Teach her to try to sleep only when she is sleepy.

   d. Suggest that she eat a light, high protein snack before bedtime.

10. Mrs. Smith, a new admit to the medical-surgical unit, complains of difficulty sleeping. Mrs. Smith is scheduled for an exploratory laparotomy in the morning. Your diagnosis is: Sleep Pattern Disturbance: Insomnia related to fear of impending surgery. Which one of the following steps is the most appropriate in planning care for the above diagnosis?

    a. Help her maintain her normal bedtime routines and time for sleep.

    b. Provide opportunity for her to talk about her concerns.

    c. Utilize tactile relaxation techniques, such as massage.

    d. Bring her a warm glass of milk at bedtime.

## Completion

1. List two questions a nurse may ask when assessing a client for the following factors:

a. Usual sleeping and waking time: _____

_____

_____

_____

b. Number of hours of undisturbed sleep:_____

_____

_____

_____

c. Effect of sleep pattern on everyday functioning: ___

_____

_____

_____

d. Energy level (ability to perform activities of daily living): _____

_____

_____

_____

e. Sleep aids: _____

_____

_____

_____

f. Sleep disturbances/contributing factors: _____

_____

_____

_____

2. Write a sample nursing diagnosis for the following sleep problems:

a. Mr. Smith is admitted to the hospital for surgery. He normally has no problem falling asleep but the noise of the hospital and need for periodic treatments keeps him awake at night.

_____

_____

b. Mr. Loper, a 74-year-old client in a long-term health care facility, is bored during the day and admits taking a nap in the afternoon and early evening. He is not able to sleep at night.

_____

_____

c. Dr. Harris, a resident working varying shifts in the emergency room, complains that he is sleepy all the time but cannot sleep when he lies down after work.

_____

_____

d. Mrs. Maher, age 28, consumes four alcoholic drinks while watching television at night before bedtime. After eliminating the alcohol from her diet, she complains of waking after a short period of sleep and not being able to fall back to sleep.

_____

_____

e. Mrs. Eichorn, age 45, has two teenage sons who are often out late at night. She is unable to sleep until they are both home safely and even then continues to worry about their future.

_____

_____

3. Describe the six states of arousal in infants.

a. Regular sleep: _____

_____

_____

b. Irregular sleep: _____

_____

_____

c. Periodic sleep: _____

_____

_____

d. Drowsiness:_____

_____

_____

e. Alert inactivity: _____

_____

_____

f. Crying:_____

_____

_____

4. Describe normal sleep patterns for the following age groups:

a. Toddler: _____

_____

_____

_____

b. Preschoolers:_____

_____

_____

_____

c. School-aged children:_____

_____

_____

_____

d. Adolescents: _____

_____

_____

_____

e. Young adults: _____

_____

_____

_____

f. Middle adults: _____

_____

_____

_____

g. Older adults: _____

_____

_____

_____

_____

5. Briefly describe the characteristics of the following stages of NREM sleep. Be sure to list the percentage of sleep each stage comprises.

a. Stage I: _____

_____

_____

_____

b. Stage II: _____

_____

_____

_____

_____

c. Stage III: _____

_____

_____

_____

_____

d. Stage IV: _____

_____

_____

_____

_____

6. Describe the following characteristics of REM sleep:

a. Eyes: _____

_____

_____

b. Muscles: _____

_____

_____

c. Respirations: _____

_____

_____

d. Pulse: _____

_____

_____

e. Blood pressure: _____

_____

_____

f. Gastric secretions: _____

_____

_____

g. Metabolism: _____

_____

_____

h. Brain waves: _____

_____

_____

i. Sleep cycle: _____

_____

_____

7. Fill in the stages of sleep in a normal, single-sleep cycle, starting with wakefulness, on the chart provided on the next page.

7. *Cont'd*

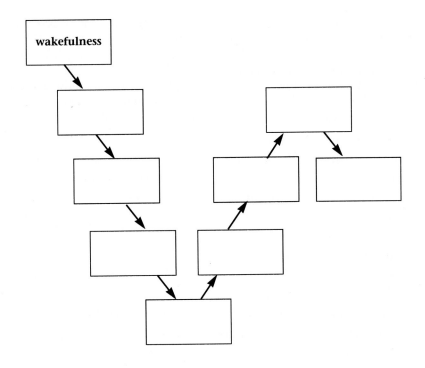

8. List five measures a nurse can take to correct a sleep problem in a client.

a. _____

b. _____

c. _____

d. _____

e. _____

## Case Study

Read the following case study and use your nursing process skills to answer the questions below.

Gina Cioffi, a 23-year-old graduate nurse, is three months in her new position as a critical care staff nurse in a large tertiary care medical center. "I was so excited about working three twelve-hour shifts a week when I started this job, thinking I'd have lots of time for other things I want to do, but I'm not so sure anymore. I've been doing extra shifts when we're short-staffed because the money is so good, and right now it seems I'm always tired and all I think about all day long is how soon I can get back to bed. Worst of all, when I do finally get into bed, I often can't fall asleep—especially if things have been busy at work and someone "went bad." Does everyone else feel like me?" Looking at Gina, you notice dark circles under her eyes and are suddenly struck by the change in her appearance from when she first started working. At that time, she "bounced into work" looking fresh each morning and her features were always animated. Now her skin color is pale, her hair and clothes look rumpled, and the "brightness" that was so characteristic of her earlier is strikingly absent. With some gentle questioning, you discover that she frequently goes out with new friends she has made at the hospital when her shift is over, and sometimes goes for 48 hours without sleep. "I know I've gotten myself into a rut. . . How do I get out of it? I used to think my sleep habits were bad at school, but this is a hundred times worse, because there never seems to be time to crash. . . . I have to just keep on going."

1. Identify pertinent client data by placing a single underline beneath the *objective* data in the case study and a double underline beneath the *subjective* data.

2. Complete the Nursing Process Worksheet on the opposite page to develop a three-part diagnostic statement and related plan of care for this client.

3. Write down the client and personal nursing strengths you hope to draw upon as you assist this client to better health.

Client strengths:_____

_____

_____

_____

_____

Personal strengths: _____

_____

_____

_____

_____

4. Pretend that you are performing a nursing assessment of this client after the plan of care is implemented. Document your findings below.

_____

_____

_____

_____

_____

_____

_____

_____

## Nursing Process Worksheet

**Health Problem (Title)**

**Client Goal***

Related to

↓

**Etiology (Related Factors)**

**Nursing Interventions****

As Manifested by

↓

**Signs and Symptoms
(Defining Characteristics)**

**Evaluative Statement:**

*More than one client goal may be appropriate. For the purposes of this exercise, develop the one client goal that demonstrates a direct resolution of the client problem identified in the nursing diagnosis.
**Be sure you are able to list the scientific rationale for each nursing intervention you ordered.

# 32

## Comfort

Study of Chapter 32 will provide the learner with knowledge of the pain experience and factors that influence it. A detailed guide to assessing alterations in comfort is presented, including specific questions and approaches to use when assessing various pain factors. Specific nursing strategies for promoting comfort and assisting clients to achieve pain management are detailed.

O B J E C T I V E S

After studying this chapter the learner will be able to:

Define key terms used in the chapter.

Describe specific elements in the pain experience.

Compare and contrast acute and chronic pain.

Identify factors that may affect an individual's pain experience.

Obtain a complete pain assessment utilizing appropriate interviewing and physical assessment skills.

Develop nursing diagnoses that correctly identify pain problems and demonstrate the relationship between pain and other areas of human functioning.

Demonstrate the correct use of noninvasive pain-relief measures: distraction, relaxation, cutaneous stimulation.

Administer analgesic agents safely to produce the desired level of analgesia without causing undesirable side effects.

Collaborate with the members of other health disciplines employing different treatment modalities to promote pain relief.

Plan, implement, and evaluate nursing care related to select nursing diagnoses for pain problems.

Utilize teaching and counseling skills to empower clients to direct their own pain management programs.

## E X E R C I S E S

### Matching

Match the definition in Part B with the term listed in Part A.

Part A

a. pain

b. psychogenic pain

c. nociceptors

d. phantom limb pain

e. gate control theory

f. pain threshold

g. neuromodulators

h. acute pain

i. chronic pain

j. pain tolerance

Part B

1. _____ The point beyond which a person is no longer willing to endure pain.

2. _____ Substances that regulate or modify the sensation of pain.

3. _____ The pain that is often referred to an amputated part, where receptor and nerves are clearly absent.

4. _____ One of the human body's defense mechanisms that indicates the person is experiencing a problem; a personal, private, sensation of hurt.

5. _____ Situation in which a physical cause for the pain cannot be found.

6. _____ A mechanism that determines which exciting and inhibiting signals pass through the spinal cord to the brain.

7. _____ Generally rapid in onset, varies in intensity from mild to severe, and lasts less than six months.

8. _____ The lowest intensity of a stimulus that causes the subject to recognize pain.

9. _____ Pain receptors.

10. _____ Pain that may be limited, intermittent, or persistent, but that lasts for six months or longer.

Match the examples in Part B with the type of pain listed in Part A. Answers may be used more than once.

Part A

a. cutaneous pain

b. deep somatic pain

c. visceral pain

d. referred pain

Part B

11. _____ Pain associated with cancer of the uterus.

12. _____ Pain associated with a myocardial infarction.

13. _____ Pain associated with a knee injury.

14. _____ Pain associated with burns.

15. _____ Pain associated with a brain tumor.

16. _____ Pain associated with a gash in the skin.

17. _____ Pain associated with a broken leg.

18. _____ Pain associated with ulcers.

Match the definitions of pain relief measures in Part B with the term listed in Part A.

Part A

a. imagery

b. relaxation techniques

c. contralateral stimulation

d. cutaneous stimulation

e. analgesic drug

f. opioid

g. patient controlled analgesia

h. epidural analgesia

i. continuous subcutaneous infusions

j. placebo

k. hypnosis

l. acupuncture

m. biofeedback

n. acupressure

Part B

19. _____ An inactive substance, often given to satisfy a person's demand for a drug.

20. _____ Pain relief during immediate, post-operative phase and for chronic pain, via a catheter inserted into the epidural space.

21. _____ Narcotic analgesics

22. _____ A technique that involves stimulating an area opposite the painful area.

23. _____ Technique that reduces skeletal muscle tension and lessens anxiety.

24. _____ A technique that utilizes a teaching machine with a feedback signal to help a client learn by trial and error to control the supposedly involuntary body mechanisms that may cause pain.

25. _____ A technique that produces a subconscious condition accomplished by suggestions.

26. _____ A technique developed to provide effective individualized, client-controlled analgesia and comfort.

27. _____ A technique that involves stimulating a painful area.

28. _____ A technique using mind/body interaction to decrease pain sensation by thinking of something that involves one or all of the senses and concentrating on that picture.

29. _____ A pharmaceutical agent that relieves pain.

30. _____ A route for pain medication that can effectively deliver small doses of narcotic/opioids controlled by an infusion pump.

31. _____ A technique that utilizes needles of various lengths to prick specific parts of the body to produce insensitivity to pain.

32. _____ The application of pressure or massage, or both, to usual acupuncture sites.

## Multiple Choice

Circle the letter that corresponds to the best answer for each question.

1. Which of the following substances that stimulate nociceptors releases histamine?
   a. bradykinin
   b. prostaglandins
   c. substance P
   d. lactic acid

2. Which of the following body parts is insensitive to pain?
   a. thorax
   b. cranium
   c. lungs
   d. uterus

3. Skin receptors in the area of a sunburn would be stimulated by which of the following stimuli?
   a. mechanical
   b. chemical
   c. electrical
   d. thermal

4. Which of the following is a mechanical stimulant?
   a. acid burn
   b. pressure from a cast
   c. sunburn
   d. cold water on a tooth with caries

5. Which of the following opioids are produced at neural synapses at various points in the central nervous system pathway?
   a. enkephalins
   b. dynorphins
   c. endorphins
   d. neurophins

6. Which of the following opioids are widespread throughout the brain and dorsal horn of the spinal cord?
   a. enkephalins
   b. dynorphins
   c. endorphins
   d. neurophins

7. Mr. Feldman, age 46, is a client experiencing acute pain following heart by-pass surgery. According to the study by Zborowski (1969), which of the following would be Mr. Feldman's response to this pain?
   a. He wants to be alone with his pain.
   b. He takes pride in his ability to handle his pain.
   c. He willingly accepts pain relief measures.
   d. He uses pain to elicit sympathy and support from others.

8. When treating a child who is in pain and cannot vocalize this pain, which of the following measures should the nurse employ?
   a. Ignore the child's pain if he is not complaining about it.
   b. Ask the child to draw a cartoon about the color or shape of his pain.
   c. Medicate the child with analgesics to reduce the anxiety of experiencing pain.
   d. Distract the child so he does not notice his pain.

9. Mr. Deer is in acute pain from a myocardial infarction. Which of the following pain control regimens would be recommended for him?
   a. analgesic administration
   b. distraction
   c. cutaneous stimulation
   d. relaxation technique

10. Three days post-surgery, Ms. Dodds continues to have moderate to severe incisional pain. According to the gate control theory, the nurse should do which of the following?
    a. Administer pain medications in smaller doses but more frequently.
    b. Decrease external stimuli in the room during painful episodes.
    c. Reposition Ms. Dodds and gently massage her back.
    d. Advise Ms. Dodds that she should try to sleep following administration of pain medication.

## Correct the False Statements

Circle the word *true* or *false* that follows the statement. If the word *false* has been circled, change the underlined word/words to make the statement true. Place your answer in the space provided.

1. A damaged cell releases <u>histamine</u>, which excites nerve endings.

   True    False    _____

2. <u>Bradykinin</u> is a hormone-like substance that sends additional pain stimuli to the central nervous system.

   True    False    _____

3. <u>C fibers</u> are free nerve ending pain receptors for fast-conducting, acute, well-localized pain.

   True    False    _____

4. There is integration of the sensory impulses of pain along its entire central nervous system route, but the highest level of integration occurs in the <u>cortex.</u>

   True    False    _____

5. <u>Neurectomy</u> is an interruption by surgical resection of the posterior root just outside the posterior horn cells of the spinal cord.

   True    False    _____

6. Causalgia is an example of a <u>peripheral pain syndrome.</u>

   True    False    _____

7. Thalamic syndrome is an example of <u>pain with underlying pathology syndrome.</u>

   True    False    _____

8. A pain that moves from one area to another, such as from the lower abdomen to the area over the stomach, is called a <u>diffuse pain.</u>

   True    False    _____

9. <u>Transient</u> pain is pain that starts and stops again.

   True    False    _____

10. Moving away from a painful stimulus is an example of a <u>behavioral response.</u>

    True    False    _____

11. Anxiety and depression is an example of a <u>behavioral response.</u>

    True    False    _____

## Completion

1. a. Read each of the situations below and use the accompanying chart to describe behavioral, physiological, and affective responses to pain which you might observe in these clients:

*Situation A:* Mrs. Novinger tells you that she frequently gets migraine headaches and feels one coming on.

*Situation B:* Ryan Goode, age three, reached out to get a stray cat who hissed and scratched his forearm.

*Situation C:* Mrs. Carol Chung is two days post-cesarean section and using her call light to request something for incisional pain.

*Situation D:* Joseph Miles, age 79, has a long history of degenerative joint disease and tells you this is a "bad morning" for his joints. He states: "I think the weather must be affecting my arthritis."

| Situation | Behavioral | Physiological | Affective |
|---|---|---|---|
| A | | | |
| B | | | |
| C | | | |
| D | | | |

b. Write a three-part diagnosis statement for each of the above clients, using the assessment data in the above chart.

Situation A:_____

_____

_____

Situation B:_____

_____

_____

Situation C: _____

_____

_____

Situation D: _____

_____

_____

2. Write an appropriate patient goal for each of the following nursing diagnoses.

a. Ineffective individual coping related to family inability to emotionally support client during pain experience. _____

_____

_____

b. Self-care deficit related to painful movement of joints. _____

_____

_____

_____

c. Pain: left leg related to fractured femur and multiple lacerations. _____

_____

_____

_____

d. Pain: acute postoperative related to fear of taking prescribed analgesics. _____

_____

_____

_____

e. Ineffective airway clearance related to acute postoperative pain. _____

_____

_____

_____

3. Using the table below, differentiate between the analgesic medications by listing the action, major side effect, and whether or not the medication is narcotic, in the appropriate box in the table below.

4. List eight characteristics of pain that are generally assessed.

a. _____

b. _____

c. _____

d. _____

e. _____

f. _____

g. _____

h. _____

| Medication | Action | Major Side Effect | Narcotic (Y/N) |
|---|---|---|---|
| a. Morphine | | | |
| b. Demerol | | | |
| c. Aspirin | | | |

## Case Study

Read the following case study and use your nursing process skills to answer the questions below.

Tabitha Wilson is a 24-month old infant with AIDS who is hospitalized, this admission, with infectious diarrhea. She is well known to the pediatric staff and there is real concern that she might not pull through this admission. She has suffered many of the complications of AIDS and is no stranger to pain. At the present time, the skin on her buttocks is raw and excoriated and tears stream down her face whenever she is moved. Her blood pressure also shoots up when she is touched. The severity of her illness has left her extremely weak and listless, and her foster mother reports that she no longer recognizes her child. When alone in her crib, she seldom moves and moans softly. Several nurses have expressed great frustration caring for Tabitha, because they find it hard to perform even simple nursing measures—like turning, diapering, and weighing her—when they see how much pain these procedures cause.

1. Identify pertinent client data by placing a single underline beneath the *objective* data in the case study and a double underline beneath the *subjective* data.

2. Complete the Nursing Process Worksheet on the opposite page to develop a three-part diagnostic statement and related plan of care for this client.

3. Write down the client and personal nursing strengths you hope to draw upon as you assist this client to better health.

Client strengths:_____

_____

_____

_____

_____

Personal strengths: _____

_____

_____

_____

_____

4. Pretend that you are performing a nursing assessment of this client after the plan of care is implemented. Document your findings below.

_____

_____

_____

_____

_____

_____

_____

_____

_____

## Nursing Process Worksheet

**Health Problem (Title)**

**Client Goal***

Related to

↓

**Etiology (Related Factors)**

**Nursing Interventions****

As Manifested by

↓

**Signs and Symptoms
(Defining Characteristics)**

**Evaluative Statement:**

*More than one client goal may be appropriate. For the purposes of this exercise, develop the one client goal that demonstrates a direct resolution of the client problem identified in the nursing diagnosis.
**Be sure you are able to list the scientific rationale for each nursing intervention you ordered.

# 33

# Nutrition

Chapter 33 provides the opportunity for the learner to gain a knowledge base of basic nutrition theory, focusing on the six classes of nutrients, energy balance, choosing an adequate diet, food patterns and habits, and factors affecting nutrition. Components of simple screening and in-depth nutritional assessments are outlined. Two sets of nursing diagnoses are provided, and client goals for healthy nutrition are discussed.

## OBJECTIVES

After studying this chapter the learner will be able to:

Define key terms used in the chapter.

List the six classes of nutrients and explain the significance of each, including variables affecting nutrient requirements.

Evaluate a diet using the food group approach.

Identify dietary, medical-socioeconomic, anthropometric, clinical, and biochemical risk factors for poor nutritional status.

Describe the nutritional implications of growth and development throughout the life cycle.

Perform a nutritional assessment using appropriate interview questions, a 24-hour food recall when indicated, and a nursing examination.

Describe common nutritional problems noting key assessment criteria.

Develop nursing diagnoses that correctly identify nutritional problems that may be treated by independent nursing intervention.

Describes nursing interventions to help clients achieve their nutritional goals.

Plan, implement, and evaluate nursing care related to selected nursing diagnoses involving nutritional problems.

Differentiate among the various types of enteral tubes.

## Exercises

### Matching

Match the definition in Part B with the term listed in Part A.

Part A

a. nutrition          h. amino acids

b. nutrients          i. vitamins

c. calories           j. minerals

d. basal metabolism   k. nitrogen balance

e. ideal body weight  l. lipids

f. body mass index    m. triglycerides

g. carbohydrates

Part B

1. _____ Organic compounds needed by the body in small amounts.

2. _____ The predominant form of fat in food; also the major storage form of fat in the body.

3. _____ An estimate of optimal weight for optimal health.

4. _____ The measurement of energy in the diet.

5. _____ The study of nutrients and how they are handled by the body, as well as the impact of human behavior and environment on the process of nourishment.

6. _____ The amount of energy required to carry on the involuntary activities of the body at rest.

7. _____ Sugars starches; organic compounds composed of carbon, hydrogen, and oxygen.

8. _____ Specific biochemical substances used by the body for growth, development, activity, reproduction, lactation, health maintenance, and recovery from illness or injury.

9. _____ A ratio of height to weight.

10. _____ Twenty-two basic building blocks.

11. _____ A comparison between catabolism and anabolism.

12. _____ Fats in the diet.

13. _____ Inorganic elements found in all body fluids and tissues in the form of salts, or combined with organic compounds.

Match the function in Part B with the micromineral listed in Part A. List one food source for each micromineral on the line provided at the end of the sentence.

Part A

a. iron

b. iodine

c. zinc

d. copper

e. manganese

f. fluoride

g. chromium

h. selenium

i. molybdenum

j. cobalt

Part B

14. _____ Tissue growth, development, and healing; sexual maturation and reproduction; enzyme formation; immune response.

_____

15. _____ Cofactor for insulin, proper glucose metabolism.

_____

16. _____ Oxygen transport via hemoglobin and myoglobin, constituent of enzyme systems.

_____

17. _____ Essential component of vitamin $B_{12}$.

_____

18. _____ Bone and blood formation, formation and activity of some enzymes, integrity of heart and large arteries.

_____

19. _____ Component of thyroid hormones.

_____

20. _____ Needed for bone formation, reproduction, and blood clotting; protein and energy metabolism.

_____

20. _____ Tooth formation and integrity, bone formation and integrity.

_____

22. _____ Oxidizes sulfur and products of sulfur and nucleic acid metabolism.

_____

23. _____ Antioxidant.

_____

Match the functions in Part B with the macrominerals listed in Part A. List one food source for each macromineral on the line provided at the end of the sentence.

Part A

a. calcium

b. phosphorus

c. magnesium

d. sulfur

e. sodium

f. potassium

g. chlorine

Part B

24. _____ Fluid balance, acid-base balance, nerve impulse transmission, striated skeletal and cardiac muscle activity, carbohydrate metabolism, protein synthesis catalyst for many metabolic reactions.

_____

25. _____ Bone and tooth formation, blood clotting, nerve transmission, muscle contraction, cell membrane permeability, activation of certain enzymes.

_____

26. _____ Component of HCl in the stomach, fluid balance, acid-base balance.

_____

27. _____ Bone and tooth formation, acid-base balance, energy metabolism, cell membrane structure, component of nucleic acids, regulates activity of hormones and coenzymes, fat absorption and transportation, glucose absorption.

_____

28. _____ Fluid balance, acid-base balance, muscular irritability, cell permeability, nerve impulse transmission.

_____

29. _____ Bone and tooth formation, smooth muscle relaxation, protein synthesis, carbohydrate metabolism, cell reproduction and growth, hormonal activity.

_____

30. _____ Store and release energy; structural component of nucleic acids, some vitamins, some amino acids, insulin, and heparin; promotes certain enzyme reactions; detoxification.

_____

Match the function in Part B with the vitamin listed in Part A. List one food source for each vitamin on the line provided at the end of the sentence.

Part A

a. vitamin C

b. vitamin $B_1$

c. vitamin $B_2$

d. vitamin $B_6$

e. folic acid

f. vitamin $B_{12}$

g. pantothenic acid

h. vitamin A

i. vitamin D

j. vitamin E

k. vitamin K

Part B

31. _____ Synthesis of certain proteins necessary for blood clotting.

_____

32. _____ Calcium and phosphorus metabolism, stimulates calcium absorption, mobilizes calcium and phosphorus from the bone, stimulates reabsorption of calcium and phosphorus by the kidney.

_____

33. _____ RNA and DNA synthesis, myelin formation; carbohydrate, protein, and fat metabolism; folic acid metabolism.

_____

34. _____ Visual acuity in dim light, formation and maintenance of skin and mucous membranes, normal growth and development of bones and teeth.

_____

5. \_\_\_\_ Collagen formation, protects other nutrients from oxidation, enhances iron absorption, converts folic acid to its active form, involved in the metabolism of certain amino acids.

6. \_\_\_\_ Amino acid metabolism, blood formation, maintenance of nervous tissue, conversion of tryptophan to niacin.

7. \_\_\_\_ Energy metabolism, especially the metabolism of carbohydrates, normal nervous system functioning.

8. \_\_\_\_ Carbohydrate, protein, and fat metabolism.

9. \_\_\_\_ Protects vitamin A and polyunsaturated fatty acids from oxidation, helps maintain cell membrane integrity, heme synthesis.

10. \_\_\_\_ Carbohydrate, protein, and fat metabolism, other metabolic functions.

11. \_\_\_\_ RNA and DNA synthesis, formation and maturation of RBC, amino acid metabolism.

## Multiple Choice

Circle the letter that corresponds to the best answer for each question.

1. Nutrients that supply energy and build tissue are referred to as which of the following?
   a. micronutrients
   b. super nutrients
   c. macronutrients
   d. carbohydrates

2. Which of the following nutrients provide energy to the body?
   a. carbohydrates
   b. vitamins
   c. minerals
   d. calcium

3. Mr. Edwards is a 75-year-old male hospitalized for a respiratory tract infection. Which of the following should a nutritionist consider when determining his basic metabolic requirements?
   a. As the amount of energy used on physical activity declines, the proportion of calories used for basal metabolism decreases.
   b. Infections, fever, emotional tension, extreme environmental temperatures, and elevated levels of certain hormones can increase BMR.
   c. Males have a lower basal metabolic rate than females.
   d. Aging, prolonged fasting, and sleep all increase BMR.

4. Mrs. Kuren is an obese 40-year-old female client— 5 feet 7 inches tall, 195 pounds—participating in a weight-reduction program. In assessing Mrs. Kuren's BMI, the nurse should do which of the following?
   a. Divide the client's weight in pounds by her height in inches.
   b. Multiply the client's weight in kilograms by her height in meters.
   c. Divide the client's weight in kilograms by her height in meters.

5. A diet for Mrs. Kuren should consider which of the following factors.
   a. Because Mrs. Kuren is more than twenty pounds overweight, her diet should result in a four-pound weight loss the first two weeks.
   b. To lose one pound in a week, her daily calorie intake should be decreased by 500 calories.
   c. Carbohydrates should be eliminated from Mrs. Kuren's diet until desired BMI is obtained.
   d. Most health experts recommend that carbohydrates provide 20–30 percent of the diet's total calories.

6. The main function of which of the following nutrients is to maintain body tissues that break down from normal "wear and tear"?
   a. carbohydrates
   b. minerals
   c. proteins
   d. fats

7. Which of the following foods would be considered high in saturated fatty acids?

   a. beef
   b. soybeans
   c. vegetable fats
   d. corn oil

8. Which of the following measures should be taken to decrease the cholesterol count of a client?

   a. eat less unsaturated fat
   b. decrease fiber in diet
   c. eat more saturated fat
   d. eat less total fat

9. Which of the following nutrients provides the most concentrated source of energy in the diet, providing 9 calories for every gram?

   a. proteins
   b. carbohydrates
   c. fats
   d. minerals

10. Which of the following vitamins are classified as water soluble?

    a. vitamins D and C
    b. vitamins C and B-complex
    c. vitamins A and K
    d. vitamins D and E

11. Which of the following is considered a micromineral?

    a. calcium
    b. phosphorous
    c. zinc
    d. magnesium

12. Which of the following elements accounts for 50–60 percent of the adult's total weight?

    a. water
    b. fat
    c. minerals
    d. bone matter

13. Glycosuria is a complication that may be seen in clients receiving gastric gavage for which of the following reasons?

    a. They develop diabetes mellitus while on gastric feedings.
    b. They receive a high carbohydrate load from the feeding.
    c. Gastric feedings have a high sugar content.
    d. Their kidneys cannot function normally.

## Correct the False Statements

Circle the word *true* or *false* that follows the statement. If the word *false* has been circled, change the underlined word/words to make the statement true. Place your answer in the space provided.

1. <u>Anthropometric measurements</u> measure body dimensions.

   True    False    _____

2. <u>Hematocrit</u> is the oxygen carrying protein of the red blood cells.

   True    False    _____

3. <u>Liquid diets</u> are adequate in calories and nutrients and may be used on a long-term basis.

   True    False    _____

4. <u>Enteral nutrition</u> involves passing a tube into the gastrointestinal tract in order to administer a formula containing adequate nutrients.

   True    False    _____

5. <u>Nasogastric feedings</u> have the advantage of allowing the stomach to be used as a natural reservoir regulating the amount of foods and liquids released into the small intestine.

   True    False    _____

6. <u>Parenteral nutrition</u> is required for clients who are comatose, have nonfunctioning G.I. tracts, or are recovering from serious burns.

   True    False    _____

7. Obesity is defined as body weight <u>30 percent</u> or more over ideal weight.

   True    False    _____

8. In the liver, monosaccharides are converted to <u>glucose.</u>

   True    False _____

9. Except for undigestable fiber, all carbohydrates provide <u>6</u> cal/g.

   True    False    _____

0. Underline Complete proteins contain sufficient amounts and proportions of all the essential amino acids to support growth.

    True    False    _____

1. The Food and Drug Administration is the federal agency charged with protecting our nation's food and drug supply.

    True    False    _____

## Completion

. Mr. Jones' ideal body weight is 170 lbs. He is moderately active. Calculate his calorie requirements by the three methods provided below.

a. Multiply ideal weight (IBW) by 10 to determine basal body requirements. Depending on activity level, multiply IBW by the appropriate number indicated below, and add the resulting number to the basal body requirements.

| Activity | Calories |
|----------|----------|
| sedentary | basal caloric needs x 3 |
| moderate | basal caloric needs x 5 |
| heavy | basal caloric needs x 10 |

_____

_____

_____

b. Depending on activity level, multiply IBW in pounds by the appropriate number of calories.

| Activity | Calories/Pounds of IBW |
|----------|------------------------|
| sedentary | 11–12 |
| light | 13–14 |
| moderate | 15–16 |
| heavy | 18–19 |

_____

_____

_____

c. Based on activity level, multiply IBW in pounds by the appropriate number of calories/pound, according to sex.

| Activity | Calories/Pounds of IBW | |
|----------|-------|---------|
| | Males | Females |
| sedentary | 16 | 14 |
| moderate | 21 | 18 |
| heavy | 28 | 22 |

_____

_____

_____

2. List five dietary guidelines for Americans and Canadians.

a. _____

b. _____

c. _____

d. _____

e. _____

3. Complete the number of servings required of each food group for the "basic four food group wheel" and the "food guide pyramid."

a. *Basic four food group wheel:*

Fruits and vegetables: _____ servings

Grains: _____ servings

Milk and milk products: _____ servings

Meat, poultry, and fish: _____ servings

b. *Food guide pyramid:*

Bread, cereal, grains, and pasta: _____ servings

Vegetables _____ servings

Fruits: _____ servings

Milk, yogurt, and cheese: _____ servings

Meat, poultry, fish, dry beans, eggs, and nuts:

_____ servings

Fats, oils, sweets: _____ servings

4. List five elements of a nutritional assessment.

a. _____

b. _____

c. _____

d. _____

e. _____

5. Describe four methods for checking placement of a feeding tube.

a. _____

_____

b. _____

_____

c. _____

_____

d. _____

_____

6. Describe four groups of people who may suffer mild or subclinical vitamin deficiencies in North America.

a. _____

_____

b. _____

_____

c. _____

_____

d. _____

_____

7. List four types of drugs that interfere with nutrient absorption.

a. _____

b. _____

c. _____

d. _____

8. Describe four dietary risk factors for poor nutritional status.

a. _____

_____

b. _____

_____

c. _____

_____

d. _____

_____

9. List five measures performed by a nurse that may help stimulate appetite.

a. _____

_____

_____

b. _____

_____

_____

c. _____

_____

_____

d. _____

_____

_____

e. _____

_____

10. Explain three ways that enteral nutrition is accomplished.

a. _____

_____

_____

b. _____

_____

_____

c. _____

_____

_____

11. Describe the use and insertion of a PEG tube.

_____

_____

_____

_____

_____

_____

2. List five complications of receiving nourishment by gastric gavage that the nurse has the responsibility to assess.

. _____

_____

_____

. _____

_____

_____

_____

. _____

_____

_____

_____

d. _____

_____

_____

_____

e. _____

_____

_____

_____

## Case Study

Read the following case study and use your nursing process skills to answer the questions below.

Mr. Church, a 74-year-old white male, is being admitted to the geriatric unit of the hospital for a diagnostic work-up. He was diagnosed as having Alzheimer's disease four years ago and just one year ago was admitted to a long-term care facility. His wife of 49 years is extremely devoted, and informed the nurse taking the admission history that she instigated his admission to the hospital because she was alarmed with the amount of weight he was losing. Assessment revealed a 6-foot tall, emaciated male, who weighed 149 pounds. His wife reported he lost 20 pounds in the last two months. The staff at the long-term care facility report that he was eating his meals, and his wife validated that this was the case. No one seemed sure, however, of the caloric content of his diet. His wife nodded her head vigorously when asked if her husband seemed more agitated and hyperactive recently. Mr. Church has dull, sparse hair, pale, dry skin, and dry mucous membranes.

1. Identify pertinent client data by placing a single underline beneath the *objective* data in the case study and a double underline beneath the *subjective* data.

2. Complete the Nursing Process Worksheet on the opposite page to develop a three-part diagnostic statement and related plan of care for this client.

3. Write down the client and personal nursing strengths you hope to draw upon as you assist this client to better health.

Client strengths:_____

_____

_____

_____

_____

Personal strengths: _____

_____

_____

_____

_____

4. Pretend that you are performing a nursing assessment of this client after the plan of care is implemented. Document your findings below.

_____

_____

_____

_____

_____

_____

_____

_____

# Nursing Process Worksheet

**Health Problem (Title)**

**Client Goal***

*Related to*

↓

**Etiology (Related Factors)**

**Nursing Interventions****

*As Manifested by*

↓

**Signs and Symptoms
(Defining Characteristics)**

**Evaluative Statement:**

*More than one client goal may be appropriate. For the purposes of this exercise, develop the one client goal that demonstrates a direct resolution of the client problem identified in the nursing diagnosis.
**Be sure you are able to list the scientific rationale for each nursing intervention you ordered.

# 34

# Urinary Elimination

Chapter 34 provides the learner with knowledge of the physiology of the urinary system and the multiple factors affecting urination. A practical guide to assessing urinary elimination is presented, as well as examples of nursing diagnoses. The learner is also introduced to focused assessment, diagnosis, planning, implementation, and evaluation guides for selecting nursing diagnoses of common urinary problems. These guides illustrate how the nurse's knowledge of the urinary system and urinary pathology is combined with specific nursing interventions to resolve urinary problems successfully.

## OBJECTIVES

After studying this chapter the learner will be able to:

Define key terms used in the chapter.

Describe the physiology of the urinary system.

Identify seven variables that influence urination.

Assess urinary elimination, using appropriate interview questions and physical assessment skills.

Execute the following assessment measures: measure urine output, collect urine specimens, determine the presence of select, abnormal urine constituents, determine urine specific gravity, and assist with diagnostic tests and procedures.

Develop nursing diagnoses that correctly identify urinary problems amenable to nursing therapy.

Demonstrate how to promote normal urination; facilitate use of the toilet, bedpan, urinal, and commode; perform catheterizations; and assist with urinary diversions.

Plan, implement, and evaluate nursing care related to select nursing diagnoses involving urinary problems.

# Exercises

## Matching

Match the definitions in Part B with the terms in Part A.

Part A

a. urine

b. nephron

c. bladder

d. micturition

e. kidney

f. detrusor muscle

g. involuntary sphincter

h. urethra

Part B

1. _____ The process of emptying the bladder.

2. _____ Conveys urine from the bladder to the exterior of the body.

3. _____ The waste product that the kidneys excrete.

4. _____ Organ that maintains the composition and volume of body fluids.

5. _____ Basic unit of kidney structure.

6. _____ Smooth muscle sac that serves as a reservoir for urine.

7. _____ The middle, circular layer of muscle tissue at the base of the bladder.

8. _____ The three layers of muscular tissue in the bladder.

Match the urine color in Part A with the medication that causes urine color change listed in Part B. (some colors may be used more than once.)

Part A

a. pale yellow

b. green or blue-green

c. orange, orange-red, pink

d. brown or black

Part B

9. _____ Pyridium (urinary tract analgesic)

10. _____ Diuretics

11. _____ Sulfonamides (anti-infectives)

12. _____ Injectable iron compounds

13. _____ B-complex vitamins

14. _____ Dilantin (anti-convulsant)

15. _____ Elavil (anti-depressant)

16. _____ Rifampin (anti-tuburcular)

17. _____ Levodopa (anti-Parkinsonian)

Match the difinition in Part B with the appropriate diagnostic procedure listed in Part A.

Part A

a. cystoscopy

b. intravenous pyelogram

c. retrograde pyelogram

Part B

18. _____ X-Ray films are taken of the kidney and ureters after a contrast material is injected into the renal pelvis through the ureter.

19. _____ An instrument provides a direct visualization of the bladder, the ureteral orifices, and the urethra.

20. _____ Injection of a contrast material intravenously followed by an X-ray examination of kidney and urethra.

Match the definition in Part B with the urinary tract problem listed in Part A.

Part A

a. dysuria

b. nocturnal enuresis

c. diurnal enuresis

d. primary enuresis

e. secondary enuresis

f. urinary incontinence

g. urinary retention

Part B

21. _____ The inability to retain urine in the bladder after the age of toilet training.

22. _____ A pattern of bedwetting that follows a period of dryness of weeks or months.

23. _____ Difficult urination associated with sensation of pain or burning.

24. _____ Bedwetting that occurs while a person is sleeping.

25. _____ Urine is produced normally, but is not excreted from the bladder.

26. _____ Involuntary urination occurring during the day.

27. _____ A pattern of bedwetting wherein the child never has a long period of dryness.

## Multiple Choice

Circle the letter that corresponds to the best answer for each question.

1. Which of the following statements is correct regarding the anatomy of the urinary bladder?
   a. There are two layers of muscular tissue in the bladder.
   b. The bladder is a striated muscular sac.
   c. The urethra carries urine from the bladder to the outside of the body.
   d. The inner layer of muscle tissue guards the opening between the bladder and the urethra.

2. The act of micturition, or urination, consists of which of the following?

   a. Contraction of the internal sphincter.
   b. Relaxation of the detrusor muscle.
   c. Relaxation of the abdominal wall.
   d. Lowering of the diaphragm.

3. The doctor has ordered the collection of a urine sample that is fresh, for a particular examination. Which urine sample would the nurse discard?

   a. The sample collected immediately after lunch.
   b. The first voiding of the day.
   c. The bedtime voiding.
   d. The voiding collected at 4:00 pm.

4. Mrs. Babbs has had four urinary tract infections in the past year. Which physiological change of aging is likely to be causing Mrs. Babbs' problem?

   a. decreased bladder contractility
   b. diminished kidney ability to concentrate urine
   c. decreased bladder muscle tone
   d. neuromuscular weakness

5. Mrs. Lukas is experiencing decreased urination. The intake of which food would likely cause decreased urination?

   a. potato chips
   b. a cup of coffee
   c. a glass of wine
   d. a cola drink

6. When making her assessment, the nurse notes that her client has costovertebral tenderness. Which of the following is indicated by this physical finding?

   a. a bladder infection
   b. bladder obstruction
   c. an inflamed kidney
   d. the presence of a kidney stone

7. Which of the following represents a normal urinary finding?

   a. dark, concentrated urine
   b. odor of ammonia
   c. presence of protein
   d. absence of glucose

8. Which of the following is the appropriate nursing response when a routine urinalysis is ordered?

   a. Collect the urine in a sterile container and send to the lab immediately.
   b. Collect the urine hourly for 24 hours and then send the specimen to the laboratory.
   c. Collect the specimen in an unsterile container and send to the laboratory immediately.
   d. Collect the urine early in the morning and send to the laboratory that evening.

9. Mr. Todd is transferred to the hospital from a nursing home with the diagnosis of dehydration and urinary bladder infection. His skin is also excoriated from urinary incontinence. Which of the following is the most appropriate nursing diagnosis for Mr. Todd?

   a. Impaired skin integrity related to functional incontinence.
   b. Impaired skin integrity related to urinary tract infection and dehydration.
   c. Urinary incontinence related to urinary tract infection.
   d. High risk for urinary tract infection related to dehydration.

10. Which of the following is the most prominent cause of nosocomial infection in hospitalized clients?

    a. skin excoriation
    b. urinary catheterization
    c. urinary incontinence
    d. parenteral fluid therapy

11. Which intervention is most appropriate for the client undergoing catheterization?

    a. Explain that the procedure is necessary and will be painful.
    b. Place the client in a soft, comfortable bed.
    c. Assure the client that unnecessary exposure will be avoided.
    d. Avoid explanation of the procedure because this produces anxiety.

12. Which nursing intervention would be the least effective when trying to maintain safety for the client with an indwelling catheter?

    a. Maintain closed drainage system.
    b. Apply a topical antibiotic ointment to urinary meatus.
    c. Restrict fluid intake.
    d. Report signs of infection promptly.

13. When the client complains of burning or pain on urination, it is referred to as which of the following?

    a. dysuria
    b. polyuria
    c. glycosuria
    d. pyuria

## Correct the False Statements

Circle the word *true* or *false* that follows the statement. If the word *false* has been circled, change the underlined word/words to make the statement true. Place your answer in the space provided.

1. A <u>bladder training program</u> teaches clients to void at short intervals and then gradually progress, over a period of time, to voiding at longer intervals.

   True   False   _____

2. <u>Urge incontinence</u> is the state in which an individual experiences a loss of urine of less than 50 ml, occurring with increased abdominal pressure.

   True   False   _____

3. The flushing of a tube, canal, or area with solution is called <u>irrigation.</u>

   True   False   _____

4. The bladder empties itself of urine regularly and maintains an <u>alkaline</u> environment, which has antibacterial advantages.

   True   False   _____

5. One reason for catheterization is to obtain a sterile urine speciman from a <u>man.</u>

   True   False   _____

6. An <u>indwelling catheter</u> has a balloon, which is inflated after the catheter is inserted into the bladder.

   True   False   _____

7. Assist both men and women into <u>Fowler's position</u> before catheterizing them.

   True   False   _____

8. In female catheterization, the catheter tip is inserted into the meatus <u>5–7.5 cm</u>, or until urine flows.

   True   False   _____

## Completion

1: Explain how the following factors affect micturition.

a. Developmental considerations: _____

_____

_____

_____

_____

b. Food and fluid: _____

_____

_____

_____

_____

c. Life style: _____

_____

_____

_____

_____

_____

d. Psychologic variables: _____

_____

_____

_____

_____

_____

e. Activity and muscle tone: _____

_____

_____

_____

_____

_____

f. Pathologic conditions: _____

_____

_____

_____

_____

_____

g. Medications:_____

_____

_____

_____

_____

2. List the four assessment measures the nurse uses to collect data related to urinary elimination.

a. _____

b. _____

c. _____

d. _____

3. Describe the types of catheters listed below and their uses.

a. Retention catheter or Foley catheter:_____

_____

_____

_____

b. Intermittent catheter: _____

_____

_____

_____

c. Suprapubic catheter:_____

_____

_____

_____

d. Condom catheter:_____

_____

_____

_____

_____

4. List five reasons a catheterization may be performed.

a. _____

_____

_____

_____

b. _____

_____

_____

_____

c. _____

_____

_____

_____

d. _____

_____

_____

_____

e. _____

_____

_____

_____

5. Describe an ileal conduit. _____

_____

_____

_____

_____

6. Name the body parts depicted in the following illustration.

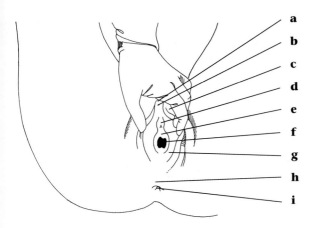

a
b
c
d
e
f
g
h
i

a. _____

b. _____

c. _____

d. _____

e. _____

f. _____

g. _____

h. _____

i. _____

7. Name the body parts depicted in the following illustration.

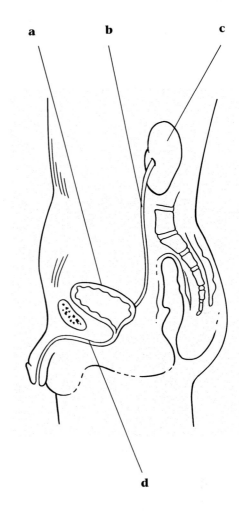

a          b          c

d

a. _____

b. _____

c. _____

d. _____

## Case Study

Read the following case study and use your nursing process skills to answer the questions below.

Mr. Eisenberg, age 84, was hurriedly admitted to a nursing home when his wife of 62 years died. He has two adult children, neither of whom feel prepared to care for him the way his wife did. "We don't know how mom did it year after year. After he retired from his law practice, he was terribly demanding and it just seemed nothing she did for him pleased him. His Parkinson's disease does make it a bit difficult for him to get around, but he's able to do a whole lot more than he is letting on. He's always been this way." You are talking with his son and daughter because the aides have reported to you that he is frequently incontinent of both urine and stool during the day as well as during the night. He is alert and appears capable of recognizing the need to void or defecate and signaling for any assistance he needs. His son and daughter report that this was never a problem at home—that he was able to go into the bathroom with assistance. He has been depressed about his admission to the home and seldom speaks, even when directly approached. He has refused to participate in any of the floor social events since his arrival.

1. Identify pertinent client data by placing a single underline beneath the *objective* data in the case study and a double underline beneath the *subjective* data.

2. Complete the Nursing Process Worksheet on the opposite page to develop a three-part diagnostic statement and related plan of care for this client.

3. Write down the client and personal nursing strengths you hope to draw upon as you assist this client to better health.

Client strengths:_____

_____

_____

_____

_____

Personal strengths: _____

_____

_____

_____

_____

4. Pretend that you are performing a nursing assessment of this client after the plan of care is implemented. Document your findings below.

_____

_____

_____

_____

_____

_____

_____

_____

# Nursing Process Worksheet

| Health Problem (Title) | Client Goal* |
|---|---|

Related to

↓

| Etiology (Related Factors) | Nursing Interventions** |
|---|---|

As Manifested by

↓

| Signs and Symptoms (Defining Characteristics) | Evaluative Statement: |
|---|---|

*More than one client goal may be appropriate. For the purposes of this exercise, develop the one client goal that demonstrates a direct resolution of the client problem identified in the nursing diagnosis.
**Be sure you are able to list the scientific rationale for each nursing intervention you ordered.

# 35

## Bowel Elimination

Chapter 35 provides the learner with knowledge of the physiology of bowel elimination and the multiple factors that influence this process. A practical guide to assess bowel elimination is presented, which includes a description of nursing responsibilities related to diagnostic studies of the gastrointestinal tract. Numerous examples of nursing diagnoses and goals are offered.

O B J E C T I V E S

After studying this chapter the learner will be able to:

Define key terms used in the chapter.

Describe the physiology of bowel elimination.

Identify ten variables that influence bowel elimination.

Assess bowel elimination using appropriate interview questions and physical assessment skills.

Assist with the following diagnostic measures: stool collection for laboratory analysis, and direct and indirect visualization studies of the gastrointestinal tract.

Develop nursing diagnoses that correctly identify bowel elimination problems amenable to nursing therapy.

Demonstrate how to (I) promote regular bowel habits (timing, positioning, privacy, nutrition, exercise); (2) use cathartics, laxatives, and antidiarrheals; (3) empty the colon of feces (enemas, rectal suppositories, rectal catheters, digital removal of stool); (4) design and implement bowel training programs; and (5) use comfort measures to ease defecation.

Plan, implement, and evaluate nursing care related to select nursing diagnoses involving bowel elimination.

## Exercises

### Matching

Match the definition in Part B with the term listed in Part A.

Part A

a. chyme              h. occult blood

b. feces              i. enema

c. stool              j. suppository

d. hemorrhoids        k. constipation

e. peristalsis        l. incontinence

f. flatus             m. diarrhea

g. bowel movement

Part B

1. _____ Abnormally distended veins in the vertical folds of the rectum.

2. _____ Hidden blood in the stool.

3. _____ Waste product of digestion.

4. _____ Intestinal gas.

5. _____ The emptying of the intestines.

6. _____ Contractions of the circular and longitudinal muscles of the intestines.

7. _____ The introduction of a solution into the large intestine, generallly for the purpose of removing feces.

8. _____ A conical or oval solid substance shaped for easy insertion into a body cavity and designed to melt at body temperature.

9. _____ The passage of dry, hard stools.

10. _____ Waste products that reach the distal end of the colon.

11. _____ The passage of excessively liquid and unformed stools.

12. _____ The inability of the anal sphincter to control the discharge of fecal and gaseous material.

13. _____ Excreted feces.

Match the type of enema in Part A with its desired effect listed in Part B.

Part A

a. carminative enemas

b. medicated enemas

c. antihelmintic enemas

d. nutritive enemas

Part B

14. _____ Enemas that are administered to destroy intestinal parasites.

15. _____ Enemas that help expel flatus from the rectum and provide relief from gaseous distention.

16. _____ Enemas used to administer fluids and nutrition rectally.

17. _____ Enemas used to administer medications that are absorbed through the rectal mucosa.

Match the type of laxative in Part A with its desired effect listed in Part B.

Part A

a. bulk-forming laxatives

b. emollient/stool softener

c. lubricant

d. stimulant

e. saline/osmotic

Part B

18. _____ Promote peristalsis by irritating the intestinal mucosa or stimulating nerve endings in the intestinal wall.

19. _____ Psyllium, grain, or synthetic product that causes stool to absorb water and swell, thus stimulating peristalsis.

20. _____ Draws water into the intestine and stimulates peristalsis.

21. _____ Agents with detergent activity that allow water and fat to penetrate and lubricate the stool.

22. _____ Absorbed from the intestinal tract, this agent softens the stool, making it easier to pass.

Match the organs of the gastrointestinal system listed
in Part A with the illustration in Part B.

Part A                                                    Part B

a. splenic flexure        j. hepatic duct          23._____      32._____

b. sigmoid colon          k. gallbladder           24._____      33._____

c. cecum                  l. duodenum              25._____      34._____

d. hepatic flexure        m. jejunum               26._____      35._____

e. common bile duct       n. rectum                27._____      36._____

f. stomach                o. ascending colon       28._____      37._____

g. esophagus              p. pancreatic duct       29._____      38._____

h. descending colon       q. ileocecal junction    30._____      39._____

i. ileum                  r. transverse colon      31._____      40._____

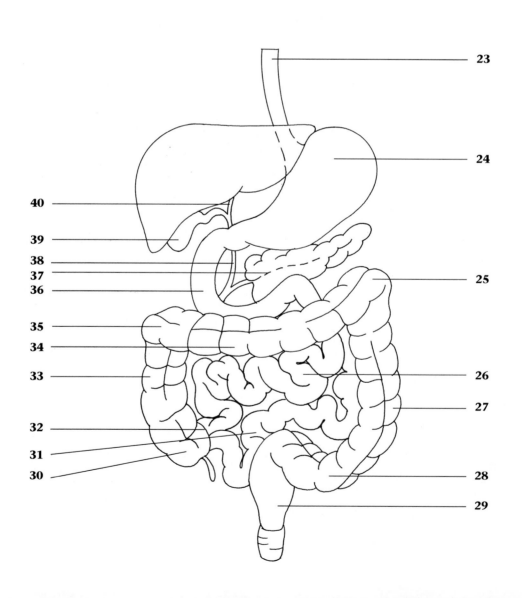

## Multiple Choice

1. Which of the following organs is the primary organ of bowel elimination, extending from the ileocecal valve to the anus?

   a. colon
   b. large intestine
   c. small intestine
   d. cecum

2. Which of the following is a function of the ileo-colic valve?

   a. Absorbing water.
   b. Expelling feces.
   c. Holding fecal material in the rectum temporarily.
   d. Preventing waste products from returning to the small intestine.

3. When informing a client about the functions of the intestines, the nurse should teach the client which of the following?

   a. Mass peristaltic sweeps occur one to four times each 24-hour period.
   b. Contractions of the circular and longitudinal muscles of the intestine occur every three to twelve hours and continually move waste products along the length of the intestine.
   c. The parasympathetic system inhibits movement and the sympathetic system stimulates movement in the intestines.
   d. Mass peristalsis seldom occurs after food has been ingested.

4. Mrs. Jackson is a client with a nursing diagnosis of constipation. Which of the following foods should she avoid?

   a. vegetables
   b. bran
   c. processed cheese
   d. cabbage

5. A nurse caring for a client on drug therapy should be aware of which of the following effects of medication on the appearance of stools?

   a. Any drug with the potential to cause GI bleeding (e.g., aspirin, anticoagulants) may result in the stool appearing pink to red to black.
   b. Iron salts result in a green stool from the oxidation of iron.
   c. Antacids may cause a bluish discoloration or speckling in the stool.
   d. Antibiotics may cause a black color because of impaired digestion.

6. Your client, John Brown, reports during your nursing history that his stools have been ribbonlike in shape. What would you suspect is a possible cause of this change in bowel habits?

   a. diverticulosis
   b. tumor in the ileum
   c. ulcerative colitis
   d. tumor in the colon

7. During abdominal surgery, direct manipulation of the bowel and inhaled anesthesia can cause a postop complication for the client. Which of the following would this complication be called?

   a. paralytic ileus
   b. pumping syndrome
   c. Crohn's disease
   d. megacolon

8. Tympany is the normal sound percussed over the abdomen. It is caused by which of the following?

   a. excess flatus
   b. hollow organs
   c. intestinal fluid
   d. fecal contents

9. A proctosigmoidoscopy is an examination involving use of which type of equipment?

   a. fiberoptic endoscope
   b. Miller-Abbott tube
   c. Salem-sump tube
   d. rigid metal scope

## Correct the False Statements

Circle the word *true* or *false* that follows the statement. If the word *false* has been circled, change the underlined word/words to make the statement true. Place your answer in the space provided.

1. <u>Proctosigmoidoscopy</u> is the visual examination of the lining of the esophagus, the stomach, and the upper duodenum with a flexible, fiberoptic endoscope.

   True    False    _____

2. In the <u>upper gastrointestinal examination (UGI) and lower bowel series,</u> barium sulfate is instilled into the large intestine by means of a rectal tube inserted through the anus.

   True    False    _____

3. When gas is not expelled and accumulates in the intestinal tract, the condition is referred to as typanites.

True    False    _____

4. Cathartics are drugs that induce emptying of intestinal tract.

True    False    _____

5. Opiates are medications that help to relieve constipation.

True    False    _____

6. Cleansing enemas are given to remove feces from the colon.

True    False    _____

7. Return flow enemas are used to expel flatus.

True    False    _____

8. A fecal incontinence pouch can be secured around the anal opening and attached to gravity drainage, allowing liquid stool to accumulate in a collection bag.

True    False    _____

9. Fecal compaction is the prolonged retention, or an accumulation, of fecal material, which forms a hardened mass in the rectum.

True    False    _____

10. The purpose of a bowel training program is to manipulate factors within the individual's control to produce the elimination of a soft, formed stool at regular intervals without laxative support.

True    False    _____

## Completion

1. List the type of colostomy or ileostomy depicted in illustrations A–E.

A. _____

B. _____

C. _____

D. _____

E. _____

2. Describe how the following factors affect bowel elimination.

a. Developmental considerations: _____

_____

_____

_____

_____

b. Daily patterns: _____

_____

_____

_____

_____

c. Food and fluid: _____

_____

_____

_____

d. Activity and muscle tone: _____

_____

_____

_____

_____

e. Life style: _____

_____

_____

_____

_____

f. Psychologic variables: _____

_____

_____

_____

_____

g. Pathologic conditions:_____

_____

_____

_____

_____

h. Medications:_____

_____

_____

_____

_____

3. List the four techniques used to assess the abdomen.

a. _____

b. _____

c. _____

d. _____

4. Describe four instructions a nurse may give the client when collecting a stool sample.

a. _____

_____

_____

b. _____

_____

_____

c. _____

_____

_____

d. _____

_____

_____

5. Write two client goals for clients without specific bowel elimination problems.

a. _____

_____

_____

b. _____

_____

6. List five factors that affect the promotion of regular bowel habits.

a. _____

b. _____

c. _____

d. _____

e. _____

7. List five common warning signs of colon cancer.

a. _____

b. _____

c. _____

d. _____

e. _____

## Sequencing

Place each step in the correct sequence by numbering the following steps for inserting a rectal suppository.

1. _____ Introduce the suppository well beyond the internal sphincter, so that the suppository is in the retum, where its effect is desired.

2. _____ Be sure the client understands that he is to retain, usually 30–45 minutes after insertion. Encourage the client to walk about if he is ambulatory; this often helps promote peristalsis.

3. _____ Use a glove to protect the hand while inserting the suppository.

4. _____ Lubricate the suppository and finger tips to reduce irritation on intestinal mucosa while inserting the suppository.

5. _____ Avoid embedding the suppository in the fecal mass. Correct placement, when there is stool in the rectum, should be between the stool and rectal mucosa.

6. _____ Separate the buttocks, and then have the client relax by breathing through the mouth while the suppository is inserted.

7. _____ Have the client lie on either side, and pie-fold top linens over him.

## Case Study

Read the following case study and use your nursing process skills to answer the questions below.

Ms. Elgaresta, age 54, a single, Hispanic woman, is being followed by a cardiologist who monitors her heart arrhythmia. Last month, she was started on a new heart medication. This visit, she complains to the nurse practitioner who works with the cardiologist; "Right after I started taking that medication, I got terribly constipated and nothing seems to help. I'm desperate and about ready to try dynamite unless you can think of something else!" She reports a change in her bowel movements from one soft formed stool daily to one to two hard stools weekly—stools that cause much straining. The nurse practitioner realizes that regulating Ms. Elgaresta's heart is difficult and that her best cardiac response to date has been with the medication now causing the constipa-

tion. Reluctant to suggest substituting another medication too quickly, she asks more questions and discovers the following. "I've never been much of a drinker. Two cups of coffee in the morning and maybe a glass of wine at night. Water? Almost never. And I don't drink juices or soft drinks." Analysis of her diet reveals a diet low in fiber; "I never was one much for vegetables, and they can just keep all this bran stuff that's out on the market! Coffee and a cigarette. That's for me!" Ms. Elgaresta is a workaholic computer programmer who has little leisure time and who spends what she has watching TV. She reports tiring after walking one flight of stairs, and states that she avoids all forms of vigorous exercise.

1. Identify pertinent client data by placing a single underline beneath the *objective* data in the case study and a double underline beneath the *subjective* data.

2. Complete the Nursing Process Worksheet on the opposite page to develop a three-part diagnostic statement and related plan of care for this client.

3. Write down the client and personal nursing strengths you hope to draw upon as you assist this client to better health.

Client strengths:_____

_____

_____

_____

_____

Personal strengths: _____

_____

_____

_____

_____

4. Pretend that you are performing a nursing assessment of this client after the plan of care is implemented. Document your findings below.

_____

_____

_____

_____

_____

_____

_____

_____

# Nursing Process Worksheet

**Health Problem (Title)**

Related to

↓

**Etiology (Related Factors)**

As Manifested by

↓

**Signs and Symptoms
(Defining Characteristics)**

**Client Goal***

**Nursing Interventions****

**Evaluative Statement:**

*More than one client goal may be appropriate. For the purposes of this exercise, develop the one client goal that demonstrates a direct resolution of the client problem identified in the nursing diagnosis.
**Be sure you are able to list the scientific rationale for each nursing intervention you ordered.

# 36

# Oxygenation

Chapter 36 introduces the learner to the physiology, general purpose, and general factors affecting respiratory functioning. Practical suggestions for performing a comprehensive respiratory assessment are given and client goals and specific nursing strategies for implementation are described. Sample interview questions for both a general and focused respiratory history are presented, along with information on collecting data from the nursing examination.

O B J E C T I V E S

After studying this chapter the learner will be able to:

Define key terms used in the chapter.

Describe the principles of respiratory physiology.

Describe age-related differences that influence care of the client with respiratory problems.

Identify six factors that influence respiratory function.

Perform a comprehensive respiratory assessment using appropriate interview questions and physical assessment skills.

Develop nursing diagnoses that correctly identify problems that may be treated by independent nursing interviews.

Describe eleven nursing strategies to promote adequate respiratory functioning, identifying their rationale.

Plan, implement, and evaluate nursing care related to select nursing diagnoses involving respiratory problems.

## Matching

Match the definition in Part B with the term listed in Part A.

Part A

a. ventilation

b. atelectasis

c. perfusion

d. hypoxia

e. hypoventilation

f. hyperventilation

g. crackles

h. gurgles

i. wheezes

j. pleural friction rub

Part B

1. __b__ Incomplete lung expansion or lung collapse.

2. __e__ A decreased rate or depth of air movement into the lungs.

3. _____ High-pitched squeaky sounds heard on expiration and sometimes on inspiration.

4. __d__ An inadequate amount of oxygen is available to cells.

5. __j__ A dry grating sound caused by inflammation of pleural surfaces.

6. __f__ The increased rate and depth of ventilation above the body's normal metabolic requirements.

7. _____ Continuous, musical sounds audible in expiration, inspiration, or both.

8. __g__ Noncontinuous sounds that occur when air moves through airways that contain fluid.

9. __c__ The passing of fluid through tissue.

10. __a__ The movement of air in and out of the lungs.

Match the organs of the respiratory tract listed in Part
A with the illustration in Part B.

Part A

a. right main bronchus

b. epiglottis

c. terminal bronchioles

d. esophagus

e. pleura

f. left main bronchus

g. nasal cavity

h. thyroid cartilege

i. trachea

j. oral cavity

Part B

11. _____

12. _____

13. _____

14. _____

15. _____

16. _____

17. _____

18. _____

19. _____

20. _____

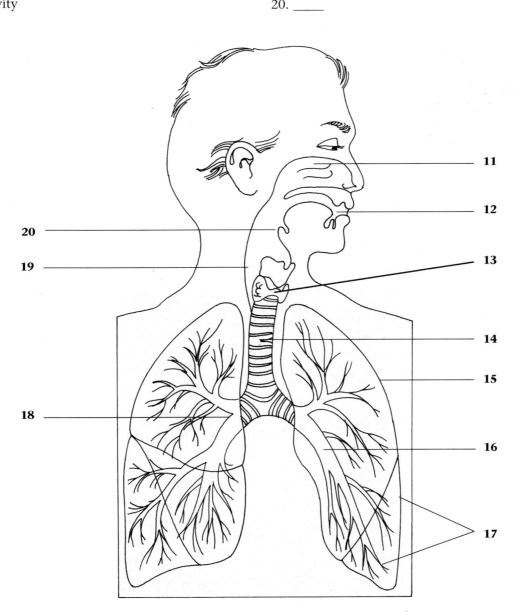

Match the definition of lung volumes and capacities listed in Part B with their terms listed in Part A. At the end of each definition, list the normal rate in the space provided.

Part A

a. tidal volume

b. inspiratory reserve volume

c. expiratory reserve volume

d. residual volume

e. vital capacity

f. forced vital capacity

g. functional residual capacity

h. total lung capacity

Part B

21. _____ This capacity is equal to the expiratory reserve volume plus the residual volume.

Normal is _____

22. _____ The amount of air inspired and expired in a normal respiration.

Normal is _____

23. _____ The tidal volume plus the residual volume.

Normal is _____

24. _____ The amount of air that can be inspired beyond tidal volume. Normal is The maximal amount of air that can be inhaled followed by a fast maximal forced exhalation with greatest effort.

Normal is _____

25. _____ The amount of air remaining in the lungs after a maximal expiration.

Normal is _____

26. _____ The amount of air that can be exhaled beyond tidal volume.

Normal is _____

27. _____ The maximal amount of air that can be exhaled following a maximal inhalation.

Normal is _____

Match the tests in Part A with their definitions listed in Part B.

Part A

a. pulse oximetry

b. cytologic study

c. endoscopy

d. skin tests

e. radiography

f. thoracentesis

Part B

28. _____ An aspiration of fluid or air from the pleural space to provide a fluid sample for diagnostic purposes of a tissue sample for biopsy.

29. _____ The direct visualization of a body cavity used to view lesions, obtain a biopsy, improve drainage, remove foreign substances, and drain abscesses.

30. _____ A non-invasive technique that measures the oxygen saturation ($SaO_2$) or arterial blood useful for monitoring persons on oxygen, those at risk for hypoxia, and postoperative clients.

31. _____ A study of sputum and cells it contains done primarily to study cells that may be malignant, determine organisms causing infection, and identify blood or pus in the sputum.

32. _____ Antigens are injected into the superficial layer of skin with a needle and syringe or a sterile fourpronged lance to evaluate immune response.

33. _____ An X-ray examination of the lungs and thoracic cavity to help diagnose pulmonary diseases and to determine the progress of development of the disease.

## Multiple Choice

Circle the letter that corresponds to the best answer for each question.

1. Which of the following nursing interventions would be appropriate for a client receiving corticosteroids?

   a. Position client upright to prevent aspiration if vomiting occurs; monitor heart rate, respirations, breath sounds and BP every 15 minutes.

   b. Reduce sodium intake; weigh daily in morning; monitor BP and blood sugar; make client and family aware of potential for labile emotions.

   c. Observe clients for prolonged bleeding if thay are using warfarin anticoagulants; do not mix with alcohol, tranquilizers or sedatives; warn client to use only with physician advice in presence of bronchial asthma.

   d. Remind client this is used to prevent asthma attacks, not to treat acute episodes; warn client this drug contains lactose and will cause diarrhea in lactose-deficient clients

2. Which of the following side effects are associated with the drug epinephrine?

   a. nausea, vomiting, rapid heart rate, diuresis, irritability, vertigo, convulsions

   b. drowsiness, anorexia, constipation, dry mouth, blurred vision, urinary retention

   c. cough, fluid retention, hypertension, mood swings

   d. tremors, anxiety, insomnia, headache, palpitations, elevated BP, vomiting

3. Which of the following drugs is *not* a bronchodilator?

   a. antihistamines

   b. isoproterenol

   c. metaproterenol

   d. theophylline

4. Which of the following is administered through an inhaler?

   a. epinephrine

   b. theophylline

   c. cromolyn sodium

   d. antihistamines

5. Which of the following characteristics of respiration are accurate for an infant?

   a. respiratory rate of 30–60

   b. thoracic breathing is regular

   c. elliptical shape of thorax

   d. respiratory rate of 15–25

6. Which of the following positions facilitates postural drainage of the lower lobes, superior segments?

   a. Lying supine with pillows under buttocks.

   b. Lying face down with pillows supporting abdomen.

   c. Lying on right side with pillows supporting right hip.

   d. Lying on left side with pillows supporting left hip.

7. Which of the following describes the purpose of the alveoli in respiration?

   a. Acts as a lubricant and as an adhesive agent to hold the lungs in an expanded position.

   b. Conduction of air, mucociliary clearance, and production of plumonary surfactant.

   c. Reduces surface tension of the fluid lining the alveoli.

   d. The site of gas exchange.

8. Which of the following statements about the general principles of respiration are accurate?

   a. All living cells need oxygen, which can be stored in the body.

   b. Muscles of the abdomen, back, and neck provide the physical force necessary for respiration.

   c. Ventilation depends on the extent of perfusion in the area.

   d. Oxygen and carbon dioxide must move through the alveoli and be carried to and from body cells by the respiratory gases.

9. When the nurse places her palms to the patient's chest wall and has him say "ninety-nine," she is palpating for which of the following?

   a. vocal fremitus

   b. vocal cacophony

   c. crepitation

   d. pleural tympany

10. Mr. Parks has chronic obstructive pulmonary disease. His nurse has taught him pursed-lip breathing, which helps him in which of the following ways?

    a. Increases carbon dioxide, which stimulates breathing.
    b. Teaches him to prolong inspiration and shorten expiration.
    c. Helps liquefy his secretions.
    d. Decreases the amount of air trapping and resistance.

11. What is the safest flow rate of oxygen for the patient with a chronic lung disease who retains carbon dioxide?

    a. 7 liters/minute
    b. 10 liters/minute
    c. 2 liters/minute
    d. 5 liters/minute

12. Which of the following is the objective data (SOAP) documented in Johnny White, a 2-year-old with asthma, admitted to the emergency room?

    a. Rhonchi and expiratory wheezes auscultated over entire chest.
    b. "Can't breathe mommy, can't breathe."
    c. Reduce coughing episodes.
    d. Client will have less labored respirations in two hours.

13. Nancy Nelson was suctioning her client through a tracheostomy tube and was very careful not to occlude the Y-port when inserting the suction catheter, because it would do which of the following?

    a. Prevent suctioning from occurring.
    b. Cause trauma to the tracheal mucosa.
    c. Break the sterile technique.
    d. Suction out all the carbon dioxide.

14. Which of the following tests is done to measure the integrity of pulmonary blood vessels and evaluate blood-flow abnormalities?

    a. pulmonary angiogram
    b. tomogram
    c. Q scan
    d. V scan

15. The client's health history is an essential element of respiratory functioning assessment. Which interview question is most likely to elicit relevant respiratory data from the client?

    a. "Do you do a significant amount of heavy labor?"
    b. "Tell me about your favorite leisure time activities."
    c. "Do you have frequent colds, coughs, or painful breathing?"
    d. "You aren't a smoker, are you?"

16. Which of the following blood–gas values are considered within the normal range?

    a. pH 7.25–7.35
       $P_{CO_2}$ 25–35 mmHg
       $P_{O_2}$ 50–100 mmHg
    b. pH 7.35–7.45
       $P_{CO_2}$ 45–50 mmHg
       $P_{O_2}$ 90–100 mmHg
    c. pH 7.30–7.40
       $P_{CO_2}$ 30–45 mmHg
       $P_{O_2}$ 70–100 mmHg
    d. pH 7.35–7.45
       $P_{CO_2}$ 35–45 mmHg
       $P_{O_2}$ 80–100 mmHg

17. Which of the following statements concerning tracheotomized clients is accurate?

    a. The wound around the tube and the inner cannula, if one is present, should be cleaned at least once every 24 hours.
    b. The tracheotomized client has no impaired speaking function.
    c. A newly inserted tracheostomy tube requires no immediate attention.
    d. Suctioning of the tracheostomy tube must be done under sterile technique.

# Correct the False Statements

Circle the word *true* or *false* that follows the statement. If the word *false* has been circled, change the underlined word/words to make the statement true. Place your answer in the space provided.

1. <u>Percussion</u> is the examination of the lungs in which the nurse moves from apex to base with a stethoscope, comparing one side with the other side for normal breath sounds.

   True    False    _____

2. A <u>pulse oximetry unit</u> is used for measuring oxygen saturation (SaO2) of arterial blood.

   True    False    _____

3. The presence of excessive fluids or secretions in an organ or body tissue is called <u>congestion</u>.

   True    False    _____

4. <u>Expectorants</u> are drugs that depress a body function, such as the cough reflex.

   True    False    _____

5. <u>Cupping</u> is the manual percussion of lung areas to loosen pulmonary secretions so that they can be expectorated with greater ease.

   True    False    _____

6. <u>Postural drainage</u> involves the nurse's true rhythmic contraction and relaxation of the arm and shoulder muscles while holding the hands flat on the client's chest wall.

   True    False    _____

7. <u>Poor nutrition</u> is the most important risk factor in pulmonary disease.

   True    False    _____

8. A <u>nasal cannula</u> is a disposable, plastic device with two protruding prongs for insertion into the nostrils, connected to an oxygen source with a humidifier and flowmeter.

   True    False    _____

9. A <u>transtracheal oxygen delivery system</u> involves the insertion of a catheter into the throat through one nostril, which must be changed to the other nostril every eight hours.

   True    False    _____

10. A <u>nasopharyngeal airway</u> is a semicircular tube of plastic or rubber inserted into the back of the pharynx, through the mouth or nose, in the spontaneously breathing client.

    True    False    _____

11. A <u>tracheostomy tube</u> is a polyvinylchloride airway that is inserted through the nose or the mouth into the trachea, using a laryngoscope as a guide.

    True    False    _____

## Completion

1. List and describe the ABCs of basic life support.

A: _____

_____

_____

B: _____

_____

_____

C: _____

_____

_____

2. List three client goals for the client experiencing an actual or potential loss of adequate ventilation, related to an altered breathing pattern.

a. _____

_____

b. _____

_____

c. _____

_____

3. Write a sample client statement and defining characteristics for the following respiratory problems.

a. Ineffective airway clearance:_____

_____

b. Impaired gas exchange: _____

_____

c. Ineffective breathing pattern:_____

_____

4. Write two interview questions for the following elements of a respiratory assessment.

a. Usual patterns of respiration:_____

_____

_____

b. Cough: _____

_____

_____

c. Chest pain: _____

_____

_____

d. Dyspnea: _____

_____

_____

e. Fatigue: _____

_____

_____

5. List three factors that normal respiratory functioning depends on.

a. _____

b. _____

c. _____

6. Describe the two phases of ventilation.

a. _____

_____

b. _____

_____

. Explain how the following factors affect respira-
ory functioning.

. Levels of health: _____

_____

_____

_____

. Development:_____

_____

_____

_____

. Life style:_____

_____

_____

_____

_____

. Environment:_____

_____

_____

_____

e. Psychologic health:_____

_____

_____

_____

8. List five precautions for administering oxygen to a
client.

a. _____

b. _____

c. _____

d. _____

e. _____

## Case Study

Read the following case study and use your nursing process skills to answer the questions below.

Toni is a 14-year-old who is on the adolescent mental health unit following a suicide attempt. Her chart reveals that on several occasions when her mother was visiting, she began hyperventilating (increased respiratory rate [42] and increased depth). Gasping for breath on these occasions, she nevertheless pushed away all who approached her to assist. Her mother confided that she and her husband are in the midst of a divorce and that it hasn't been easy for Toni at home. "I know she's been having a rough time at school and I guess I've been too caught up in my own troubles to be there for her." When you attempt to discuss this with Toni and mention her mother's concern, she begins hyperventilating again.

1. Identify pertinent client data by placing a single underline beneath the *objective* data in the case study and a double underline beneath the *subjective* data.

2. Complete the Nursing Process Worksheet on the opposite page to develop a three-part diagnostic statement and related plan of care for this client.

3. Write down the client and personal nursing strengths you hope to draw upon as you assist this client to better health.

Client strengths:_____

_____

_____

_____

_____

Personal strengths: _____

_____

_____

_____

_____

4. Pretend that you are performing a nursing assessment of this client after the plan of care is implemented. Document your findings below.

_____

_____

_____

_____

_____

_____

_____

_____

# Nursing Process Worksheet

| Health Problem (Title) | Client Goal* |
|---|---|

Related to

↓

| Etiology (Related Factors) | Nursing Interventions** |
|---|---|

As Manifested by

↓

| Signs and Symptoms (Defining Characteristics) | Evaluative Statement: |
|---|---|

*More than one client goal may be appropriate. For the purposes of this exercise, develop the one client goal that demonstrates a direct resolution of the client problem identified in the nursing diagnosis.

**Be sure you are able to list the scientific rationale for each nursing intervention you ordered.

# 37

## Fluid, Electrolyte, and Acid-Base Balance

Chapter 37 provides the learner with basic knowledge of the principles of fluid, electrolyte, and acid-base balance; and the etiologies, defining characteristics, and nursing interventions for common disturbances. Sample interview questions for performing a fluid balance nursing history are presented, along with information on specific physical assessment measures and laboratory studies. Numerous examples of nursing diagnoses are offered and client goals and specific nursing strategies for promoting fluid balance are described.

O B J E C T I V E S

After studying this chapter the learner will be able to:
Define key terms used in the chapter.
Describe the functions of body fluids, the two main compartments where fluids are located in the body, and factors that affect variations in fluid compartments.
Describe the functions, sources and losses, and regulation of main electrolytes of the body.
Explain the principles of osmosis, diffusion, active transport, and filtration.
Describe how thirst and the organs of homeostasis function to maintain fluid homeostasis.
Describe the role of buffer systems, and respiratory and renal mechanisms in achieving acid-base balance.
Identify the etiologies, defining characteristics, and treatment modalities for common fluid, electrolyte, and acid-base disturbances.
Perform a fluid, electrolyte, and acid-base balance assessment.
Describe the role of dietary modification, modification of fluid intake, medication administration, intravenous therapy, blood replacement, and total parenteral nutrition in resolving fluid, electrolyte, and acid-base imbalances.
Plan, implement, and evaluate nursing care related to select nursing diagnoses involving fluid, electrolyte, and acid-base imbalances.

## Exercises

### Matching

Match the definition in Part B with the term listed in Part A.

Part A

a. intracellular fluid

b. extracellular fluid

c. intravascular fluid

d. interstitial fluid

e. ion

f. electrolytes

g. cations

h. anions

i. solvents

j. solutes

Part B

1. _____ Liquids that hold a substance in solution.

2. __f__ Substances capable of releasing electrically charged ions when dissolved in a solution

3. __d__ The fluid within the cell, which comprises approximately 70 percent of the total body water.

4. __c__ The liquid constituent of blood or fluid found within the vascular system.

5. __g__ Ions that develop a positive charge.

6. __d__ The fluid in which tissue cells are bathed; includes lymph.

7. __j__ Substances that are dissolved in a solution

8. __e__ An atom or molecule carrying an electric charge in solution.

9. __b__ All the fluid outside of cell walls, which comprises approximately 30 percent of total body water.

10. __h__ Ions that develop a negative charge.

Match the functions of electrolytes in Part B with the electrolytes listed in Part A.

Part A

a. sodium

b. potassium

c. calcium

d. magnesium

e. chloride

f. bicarbonate

g. phosphate

Part B

11. _F_ The major chemical base buffer within the body, found in both extracellular and intracellular fluid; it is essential for acid-base balance.

12. _a_ The chief electrolyte of extracellular fluid; many chemical reactions in the body are influenced by this cation, particularly in nervous-tissue cells and muscle-tissue cells.

13. _____ A cation found within body cells, it is the second most important cation of intracellular fluid, and is present in the heart, bone, nerve and muscle tissues.

14. _____ The major cation of intracellular fluid, it works with sodium reciprocally and is the chief regulator of cellular enzyme activity and cellular water content.

15. _____ The major anion in body cells, it is a buffer anion in both intracellular and extracellular fluid. Its functions include maintainence of acid-base balance, important chemical reactions in the body, and cell division and transmission of hereditary traits.

16. _____ The chief extracellular anion found in blood, interstitial fluid, and lymph, and in very small amounts in intracellular fluid. Some of its functions are: It acts with sodium to maintain the osmotic pressure of the blood and is essential for the production of hydrochloric acid in gastric juices.

17. _____ The most abundant electrolyte in the body, up to 99 percent of the total amount is found in bones and teeth in ionized form. It works intimately with phosphorus and its functions include: responsibility for nerve-impulse transmissions, blood clotting, and muscle contraction, and establishing thickness and strength of cell membranes.

Match the organ function in Part B with the primary organ of homeostasis listed in Part A.

Part A

a. kidneys

b. cardiovascular system

c. lungs

d. adrenal glands

e. pituitary gland

f. thyroid gland

g. parathyroid glands

h. gastrointestinal tract

i. nervous system

Part B

18. _____ Secretes parathormone, which regulates the level of calcium in extracellular fluid.

19. _____ Responsible for pumping and carrying nutrients and water throughout the body.

20. _____ Normally filters 179 liters of plasma daily in the adult while excreting only 1.5 liters of urine.

21. _____ Acts as a switchboard and inhibits and stimulates mechanisms that influence fluid balance.

22._____ Absorbs water and nutrients that enter the body through the intestines.

23. _____ Regulate oxygen and carbon dioxide levels of the blood.

24. _____ Stores antidiuretic hormone, which is manufactured in the hypothalmus.

25. _____ Secrete aldosterone, which is known as the great sodium conserver of the body.

26. _____ Releases thyroxin, which increases blood flow in the body.

Match the equations in Part B with the type of imbalance listed in Part A.

Part A

a. respiratory acidosis

b. metabolic acidosis

c. respiratory alkalosis

d. metabolic alkalosis

Part B

27. low pH, normal $P_{CO_2}$, low $HCO_3^-$

28. low pH, high $P_{CO_2}$, normal $HCO_3^-$

29. high pH, normal $P_{CO_2}$, high $HCO_3^-$

30. high pH, low $P_{CO_2}$, normal $HCO_3^-$

## Multiple Choice

Circle the letter that corresponds to the best answer for each question.

1. Which of the following is one of the three buffer systems found in the body?
   a. hydrogen buffer system
   b. protein buffer system
   c. calcium buffer system
   d. bicarbonate acid buffer system

2. Which of the following short or long-term venous access devices is usually introduced into the subclavian or internal jugular veins and passed to the superior vena cava just above the right atrium?
   a. peripherally inserted central catheters
   b. implanted port
   c. central venous catheter
   d. electronic infusion devices

3. Which of the following devices automatically regulates the flow rate at preset limits and notifies the nurse by an alarm when air is in the tubing, the flow is obstructed, or solution level of the bottle or bag is getting low?
   a. electronic infusion devices
   b. implanted port
   c. central venous catheter
   d. peripherally inserted central catheters

4. In which of these people would you expect his/her body water to make up the greatest percentage of body weight?
   a. a 20-year-old marathon runner
   b. a 30-year-old female secretary
   c. a frail, elderly female
   d. a 30-year-old sedentary man

5. In teaching a client about foods that affect his fluid balance, the nurse will keep in mind that the electrolyte, which primarily controls water distribution throughout the body, is which of the following?
   a. $Na^+$
   b. $K^+$
   c. $Ca^{++}$
   d. $Mg^{++}$

6. A healthy client eats a regular, balanced diet, and drinks 3,000 cc of liquids during a 24-hour period. In evaluating his urine output for the same 24-hour period, the nurse realizes that it should total approximately how many cc's?
   a. 3,750 cc
   b. 3,000 cc
   c. 1,000 cc
   d. 500 cc

7. The movement of fluids out of the arterioles into the interstitial spaces is accomplished by which of the following processes?
   a. diffusion
   b. osmosis
   c. active transport
   d. filtration

8. When there is a decrease in blood volume (as in dehydration or blood loss), the body reacts by retaining sodium, and thus water. This occurs mainly as a result of adrenal gland secretions of which of the following?
   a. antidiuretic hormone (ADH)
   b. cortisol
   c. aldosterone
   d. parathyroid hormone

9. Which of the following is produced in the kidney and is a part of a mechanism to control the acid-base balance in the body?
   a. carbonic acid
   b. ammonia
   c. carbon dioxide
   d. ketones

10. The nurse would refer to the results of an arterial blood analysis to look for indications of which of the following?
    a. acid-base imbalance
    b. electrolyte imbalance
    c. fluid-volume excess
    d. fluid-volume deficit

11. Which of the following values would indicate that efforts to hydrate a patient were successful? A urine specific gravity of:
    a. 1.001–1.010
    b. 1.025–1.030
    c. 1.035+
    d. 1.003–1.035

12. The nurse has diagnosed a patient as having "fluid volume excess" related to compromised regulatory mechanism (kidneys). Which of the following symptoms probably alerted the nurse to this diagnosis?
    a. muscular twitching
    b. distended neck veins
    c. fingerprinting over sternum
    d. nausea and vomiting

13. Which of the following nursing diagnoses would you expect to be caused by the effects of fluid and electrolyte imbalance on human functioning?
    a. Constipation related to immobility.
    b. Pain related to surgical incision.
    c. Altered thought processes related to cerebral edema, mental confusion, and disorientation
    d. Health risk for infection related to inadequate personal hygiene.

14. For the client with "hyperkalemia related to decreased renal excretion secondary to potassium-conserving diuretic therapy," an appropriate goal would be which of the following?
    a. Bowel motility will be restored within 24 hours after beginning supplemental K$^+$.
    b. ECG will show no cardiac arrhythmias within 48 hours after removing salt substitutes, coffee, tea, and other K$^+$ foods from diet.
    c. ECG will show no cardiac arrhythmias within 24 hours after beginning supplemental K$^+$.
    d. Bowel motility will be restored within 24 hours after eliminating salt substitutes, coffee, tea, and other high K$^+$ foods from diet.

## Correct the False Statements

Circle the word *true* or *false* that follows the statement. If the word *false* has been circled, change the underlined word/words to make the statement true. Place your answer in the space provided.

1. <u>Hypervolemia</u> is the deficiency in the amount of both water and electrolytes in the extracellular fluid, but the water and electrolyte proportions remain near normal.

   True    False    _____

2. <u>Hydration</u> is the union of a substance with water and is often used to indicate that there is normal water volume in the body.

   True    False    _____

3. <u>Overhydration</u> refers to a distributional shift of body fluids into body spaces such as the pleural, peritoneal, pericardial or joint cavities, the bowel, or into the interstitial space.

   True    False    _____

4. A nursing intervention for a client with <u>hypocalcemia</u> would be: discourage excessive consumption of milk products and other high-calcium foods.

   True    False    _____

5. A nursing intervention for a client with <u>hyperkalemia</u> would be: caution client to avoid foods high in potassium content, such as coffee, cocoa, tea, dried fruits, dried beans, whole grain breads and milk desserts.

   True    False    _____

6. For clients with <u>hyponatremia,</u> encourage foods and fluids with a high sodium content.

   True    False    _____

7. Early signs of <u>hypomagnesemia</u> include a serum magnesium level of 3–5 mEq/liter or 1.5–2.5 mmol/liter, flushing and a sense of skin warmth, hypotension, and nausea and vomiting.

   True    False    _____

8. Clients at risk for <u>hypophosphatemia</u> include extremely malnourished clients being started on TPN or large caloric intake by tube feeding, alcoholic clients undergoing withdrawal therapy, and clients with diabetic ketoacidosis during the early treatment period with insulin and intravenous fluids.

   True    False    _____

9. Clients at risk for <u>chronic respiratory acidosis</u> include: clients with emphysema, cystic fibrosis, advanced multiple sclerosis, bronchiectasis, and bronchial asthma.

   True    False    _____

10. Treatment for <u>metabolic acidosis</u> is directed toward correcting the metabolic defect. If the cause of the problem is excessive intake of chloride, the treatment focuses on eliminating the source. When necessary, bicarbonate is administered.

    True    False    _____

11. The kidneys form phosphate salts by exchanging a <u>K$^+$</u> ion for an H$^+$ ion when acid sodium phosphate is converted to alkaline sodium phosphate.

    True    False    _____

12. In the lungs, carbon dioxide and water are acted upon by carbonic anhydrase to produce <u>carbonic acid.</u>

    True    False    _____

## Completion

1. List and describe the four most common routes for transporting materials to and from intracellular compartments.

a. _____

_____

_____

b. _____

_____

_____

_____

c. _____

_____

_____

_____

d. _____

_____

_____

_____

2. List three sources of water for the body.

a. _____

b. _____

c. _____

3. List the three major homeostatic regulators of hydrogen ions that help the body achieve the narrow range of normal pH.

a. _____

b. _____

c. _____

4. Identify four clients at risk for fluid, electrolyte, and/or acid-base imbalances.

a. _____

_____

_____

_____

b. _____

_____

_____

_____

c. _____

_____

_____

_____

d. _____

_____

_____

5. Name four significant values for hemoglobin and hematocrit provided by a complete blood count.

a. _____

_____

b. _____

_____

c. _____

_____

d. _____

_____

6. List five responsibilities of the nurse when mineral-electrolyte preparations are prescribed to correct electrolyte imbalances in a client.

a. _____

_____

b. _____

_____

c. _____

_____

d. _____

_____

e. _____

_____

7. List four factors that should be considered to determine the suitability of veins for intravenous infusion.

a. _____

b. _____

c. _____

d. _____

8. Define the following terms associated with replacing blood and blood products.

a. Blood transfusion:_____

_____

_____

b. Typing:_____

_____

_____

c. Crossmatching: _____

_____

_____

d. Antigen:_____

_____

_____

e. Antibody: _____

_____

_____

f. Agglutinin: _____

_____

_____

g. Rh factor:_____

_____

_____

h. RhoGam: _____

_____

_____

9. Write a preoperative and postoperative client goal for maintaining electrolyte balance in a client receiving cardiac by-pass surgery.

a. Preoperative:_____

_____

_____

_____

_____

b. Postoperative:_____

_____

_____

_____

_____

10. List three duties of the nurse caring for a client receiving a blood transfusion.

a. _____

_____

b. _____

_____

c. _____

_____

11. List three hypertonic solutions capable of reestablishing positive nitrogen balance and weight gain that are infused using a central vein in total parenteral nutrition.

a. _____

_____

b. _____

_____

c. _____

_____

12. Define the condition experienced by the following clients receiving intravenous infusions and provide a nursing intervention to relieve the symptoms.

a. Client has local, acute tenderness, redness, warmth, and slight edema of the vein above the insertion site:

_____

_____

_____

_____

b. Client has pounding headache, fainting, rapid pulse rate, apprehension, chills, back pains, and dyspnea: _____

_____

_____

_____

c. Client has engorged neck veins, increased blood pressure, and difficulty in breathing (dyspnea): _____

_____

_____

_____

_____

d. Client has hives, itching, and anaphylaxis: _____

_____

_____

_____

_____

e. Client has fever, hypertension, dry, flushed skin, and abdominal pain:_____

_____

_____

_____

In the following cases, determine the acid-base imbalance. Refer to the chart below entitled Rules of ABG interpretation for your answers.

13. Mr. W. is a 90-year-old man who had a successful cardiopulmonary resuscitation a few hours ago. He received bicarbonate during that resuscitation.

ABGs: pH = 7.55; $P_{CO_2}$ = 43; $HCO_3^-$ = 36

14. Mr. F. is a 56-year-old with a known history of COPD.

a. ABGs: pH = 7.36; $P_{CO_2}$ = 60; $HCO_3^-$ = 35

15. A 55-year-old woman is admitted with chronic renal failure. She is weak and tired.

ABGs: pH = 7.24; $P_{CO_2}$ = 30; $HCO_3^-$ = 12

16. Mrs. S. is a 55-year-old with heart failure and dyspnea. She complains of pleuritic pain.

ABGs: pH = 7.56; $P_{CO_2}$ = 22; $HCO_3^-$ = 24

17. Ms. S. is a 21-year-old who has been found by her friends on the floor of her room. She is "out of it."

ABGs: pH = 7.18; $P_{CO_2}$ = 79; $HCO_3^-$ = 26

---

**Rules of ABG Interpretation**

| pH | Paco₂ | HCO₃ |
|---|---|---|
| <7.35 acidosis | >45 mmHg = respiratory acidosis | <22 mEq/liter = metabolic acidosis |
| >7.45 = alkalosis | <35 mmHg = respiratory alkalosis | >26 mEq/liter = metabolic alkalosis |

---

- It is <u>OK</u> to use what you know about your patient.
- The body usually does the smart thing to compensate: metabolic disorders—compensated by the lung; respiratory disorders—compensated by the kidney.
- Any pH below 7.35—state of acidosis; Any pH greater than 7.45—state of alkalosis; $CO_2$ is an acid—$HCO_3^-$ is a base. Any change in $CO_2$ reflects a respiratory change. Any change in $HCO_3^-$ reflects a metabolic change.

- Usually, the initiating abnormality is the predominate abnormality.
- If the pH has returned to <u>normal</u>, compensation has taken place.
- If the primary event is a fall in pH—whether respiratory or metabolic in origin—the arterial pH stays on the <u>acid</u> side after compensation. If the primary event is an increase in pH—whether respiratory or metabolic in origin—the arterial pH stays on the <u>base</u> side after compensation.

18. Indicate in the following chart: the nature of the acid-base disturbance; whether compensation is present or not; and if present, whether compensation is renal or respiratory, and partial or complete.

| pH | Pco₂ | HCO₃⁻ | Nature of Disturbance | Comp. Present? Yes | No | If Yes Renal | Respiratory | If Yes Partial | Complete |
|------|------|-------|-----------------------|-------|-----|-------|-------------|---------|----------|
| 7.28 | 63 | 25 | | | | | | | |
| 7.20 | 40 | 14 | | | | | | | |
| 7.52 | 40 | 35 | | | | | | | |
| 7.48 | 30 | 31 | | | | | | | |
| 7.16 | 82 | 30 | | | | | | | |
| 7.36 | 68 | 35 | | | | | | | |
| 7.56 | 23 | 26 | | | | | | | |
| 7.40 | 40 | 26 | | | | | | | |
| 7.56 | 23 | 26 | | | | | | | |
| 7.26 | 70 | 25 | | | | | | | |
| 7.52 | 44 | 38 | | | | | | | |
| 7.32 | 30 | 18 | | | | | | | |
| 7.49 | 34 | 26 | | | | | | | |
| 6.98 | 84 | 18 | | | | | | | |

## Sequencing

Place each step in the correct sequence by numbering the following steps in regulating IV flow rate.

1. _____ Verify drop factor (number of drops in lml) of the equipment in use.

2. _____ Adjust IV clamp as needed and recount the drops per minute.

3. _____ Monitor IV flow rate at frequent intervals. Document client's response to infusion at prescribed rate.

4. _____ Check physician's order for IV solution.

5. _____ Calculate the flow rate.

6. _____ Check patency of IV line and needle.

7. _____ Count drops per minute in drip chamber (# of gtts/15-second interval × 4 = gtts per minute). Hold watch beside drip chamber.

8. _____ Mark IV container according to agency policy and manufacturer's recommendations. Use a time tape or label to measure amount to be infused at timed intervals.

## Case Study

Read the following case study and use your nursing process skills to answer the questions below.

Rebecca is a college freshman who, on the night she had her wisdom teeth removed, had an oral temperature of 39.5°C (103.1°F). She had a sore throat several days prior to the extraction, but neglected to mention this to the oral surgeon. Because of the soreness in her throat she reported that she had greatly decreased both her food and fluid intake. Friends that night gave her some Tylenol, which brought her temperature down, and encouraged her to drink more fluids. When they checked on her in the morning her temperature was elevated again and she said she had felt too weak during the night to drink. She was brought to the student health service where the admitting nurse noticed her dry mucous membranes, decreased skin turgor, and rapid pulse. At 5'2" and 98 pounds, Rebecca was always petite but she had lost four pounds in the last week.

1. Identify pertinent client data by placing a single underline beneath the *objective* data in the case study and a double underline beneath the *subjective* data.

2. Complete the Nursing Process Worksheet on the opposite page to develop a three-part diagnostic statement and related plan of care for this client.

3. Write down the client and personal nursing strengths you hope to draw upon as you assist this client to better health.

Client strengths:_____

_____

_____

_____

_____

Personal strengths: _____

_____

_____

_____

_____

4. Pretend that you are performing a nursing assessment of this client after the plan of care is implemented. Document your findings below.

_____

_____

_____

_____

_____

_____

_____

_____

## Nursing Process Worksheet

**Health Problem (Title)**

**Client Goal***

Related to

↓

**Etiology (Related Factors)**

**Nursing Interventions****

As Manifested by

↓

**Signs and Symptoms
(Defining Characteristics)**

**Evaluative Statement:**

*More than one client goal may be appropriate. For the purposes of this exercise, develop the one client goal that demonstrates a direct resolution of the client problem identified in the nursing diagnosis.
**Be sure you are able to list the scientific rationale for each nursing intervention you ordered.

# 38

## Self-Concept

Chapter 38 introduces the learner to self-concept: its dimensions, how it is formed, and the key factors affecting self-concept. Practical interview guides are offered for assessing self-concept; strategies for enhancing the self-esteem of the nurse are also explored. Numerous examples of nursing diagnoses are presented along with specific nursing strategies for assisting clients to meet self-concept goals.

O B J E C T I V E S

After studying this chapter the learner will be able to:

Define key terms used in the chapter.

Identify three dimensions of self-concept: self-knowledge, self-expectation, self-evaluation (self-esteem).

Describe major steps in the development of self-concept.

Differentiate positive and negative self-concept and high and low self-esteem.

Identify six variables that influence self-concept.

Use appropriate interview questions and observations to assess a client's self-concept.

Develop nursing diagnoses to correctly identify disturbances in self-concept (body image, self-esteem, role performance, self-identity).

Describe nursing strategies that are effective in resolving self-concept problems.

Plan, implement, and evaluate nursing care related to select nursing diagnoses for disturbances in self-concept.

## Matching

Match the definition in Part B with the term listed in Part A.

Part A

a. self-esteem

b. self-actualization

c. self-concept

d. body image

e. subjective self

f. ideal self

g. social self

Part B

1. _____ The need to feel good about one's self and believe others also hold one in high regard.

2. _____ How I see myself, who I think I am.

3. _____ How I experience my body.

4. _____ The need to reach one's potential through development of one's unique capability.

5. _____ The way I feel others see me.

6. _____ The self I would like to be or feel I should be.

7. _____ The mental image or picture of self.

Match the examples of self concept in Part B with the appropriate dimension listed in Part A.

Part A

a. self-knowledge

b. self-expectations

c. self-evaluation

Part B

8. _____ Children identify sports figures as their heroes.

9. _____ An adult describes himself as intelligent, kind, and ambitious.

10. _____ An adolescent wants to be a model when she graduates from high school.

11. _____ A man states that he spends his leisure time alone, enjoying his hobbies.

12. _____ A woman executive has pride in her salary and social status.

13. _____ An alcoholic is unhappy with his lack of willpower and has low self-esteem.

Match the examples of high risk factors for self-concept disturbances in Part B with the factors listed in Part A.

Part A

a. personal identity disturbances

b. body image disturbances

c. self-esteem disturbances

d. altered role performance

Part B

14. _____ A 55-year-old executive is laid off from his job due to cutbacks.

15. _____ A 45-year-old woman undergoes a radical mastectomy.

16. _____ A 30-year-old woman finds herself in a relationship with an abusive husband.

17. _____ An exchange student from France attends high school in America to learn a new language and customs.

18. _____ A new mother discovers she is terrified of taking care of her newborn son on her own.

19. _____ An 11-year-old girl starts menstruating and developing earlier than her peers.

20. _____ A 65-year-old retired lawyer regrets that he was unable to become a judge as he had always dreamed of doing.

21. _____ An athlete loses his pitching arm to cancer.

## Multiple Choice

1. According to Coopersmith, which of the following is *not* one of the four bases for self-esteem?

   a. virtue
   b. power
   c. significance
   d. wealth

2. Which of the following questions would you expect to find on a self-concept assessment related to body image?

   a. Do you like who you are?
   b. Who has influenced you the most growing up?
   c. Tell me how you feel about any physical changes you noticed recently.
   d. Who would you most like to be?

3. Which of the following questions would best relate to self-identity on a focused self-concept assessment?

   a. Who would you like to be?
   b. What are your personal strengths?
   c. What do you like most about your body?
   d. Do you like being a teacher?

4. Which of the following elements are you *least* likely to find in a focused self-concept assessment?

   a. self-identity
   b. medical diagnosis
   c. self-esteem
   d. role performance

5. Which of the following is *not* an example of a negative self-concept disturbance?

   a. faulty categorizing
   b. distortions
   c. role modeling
   d. old standards

6. Which of the following nursing diagnoses lacks a self-concept disturbance etiology?

   a. Noncompliance related to low self-esteem.
   b. Post-trauma response related to disturbance in personal identify.
   c. Self-care deficit related to paralysis following TIA.
   d. Altered health maintenance related to altered role performances.

## Completion

1. List four concepts a nurse explores in a detailed assessment of self-esteem.

   a. _____
   b. _____
   c. _____
   d. _____

2. List four strategies a nurse can use to help clients identify and use personal strengths.

   a. _____

   _____

   b. _____

   _____

   c. _____

   d. _____

   _____

3. Describe two major types of boundary disturbances according to McClosky (1976).

   a. _____

   _____

   b. _____

   _____

4. List four factors that affect self-concept.

   a. _____
   b. _____
   c. _____
   d. _____

5. Describe nursing strategies to develop self-esteem that you might use to meet the needs of the following elderly clients with disturbances in self-concept:

a. An 88-year-old woman, newly admitted to a nursing home, who states she has lost all sense of self; self-identity disturbance.

_____

_____

_____

b. A 75-year-old man with crippling arthritis who tells you that he no longer recognizes himself when he looks in the mirror; body image disturbance.

_____

_____

_____

c. A 62-year-old-man who is recovering from a stroke that has paralyzed his right side states: "I don't know if I can live like this"; self-esteem disturbance.

_____

_____

_____

d. A 67-year-old woman who complains that she no longer has the patience to baby-sit for her grandchildren whom she loves; role performance disturbance.

_____

_____

_____

## Sequencing

Rank the order, from birth to death, in which achievement of a positive self-concept occurs.

1. _____    Incorporates into him/herself the parent's attitudes toward self.

2. _____    Internalizes the standards of society into self.

3. _____    Identifies with, and tries out roles and behaviors, of "heroes."

4. _____    Differentiates physical self from environment and others.

5. _____    Internalizes the attitudes of teachers and peers towards self.

6. _____    Has no self-concept.

## Case Study

Read the following case study and use your nursing process skills to answer the questions below.

An English teacher asks you, the school nurse, to see one of her students whose grades have recently dropped and who no longer seems to be interested in school—or anything else. "She was one of my best students and I can't figure out what's going on. She seems reluctant to talk about this change." When Julie, a 16-year-old junior, walks into your office you are immediately struck by her stooped posture, unstyled hair, and sloppy appearance. Julie is attractive, but at 5 feet 3 inches and 150 pounds, she is overweight. Although Julie is initially reluctant to talk, she breaks down at one point and confides that for the first time in her life she feels "absolutely awful" about herself. "I've always concentrated on getting good grades and achieved this easily. But right now this doesn't seem so important. I don't have any friends. All I hear the girls talking about is boys and I was never even asked out by a boy—which I guess isn't surprising. Look at me. . . ." After a few questions, it becomes clear that Julie has new expectations for herself based on what she observes in her peers, and she finds herself falling far short of her new, ideal self. Julie admits that in the past, once she set a goal for herself she was always able to achieve it, because she is strongly self-motivated. Although she has withdrawn from her parents and teachers, she admits that she does have trusted adults who have been a big support to her in the past. "If only I could become the kind of teenager other kids like and have lots of friends!"

1. Identify pertinent client data by placing a single underline beneath the *objective* data in the case study and a double underline beneath the *subjective* data.

2. Complete the Nursing Process Worksheet on the opposite page to develop a three-part diagnostic statement and related plan of care for this client.

3. Write down the client and personal nursing strengths you hope to draw upon as you assist this client to better health.

Client strengths:_____

_____

_____

_____

_____

Personal strengths: _____

_____

_____

_____

_____

4. Pretend that you are performing a nursing assessment of this client after the plan of care is implemented. Document your findings below.

_____

_____

_____

_____

_____

_____

_____

_____

## Nursing Process Worksheet

| Health Problem (Title) | Client Goal* |
|---|---|

Related to

↓

| Etiology (Related Factors) | Nursing Interventions** |
|---|---|

As Manifested by

↓

| Signs and Symptoms (Defining Characteristics) | Evaluative Statement: |
|---|---|

*More than one client goal may be appropriate. For the purposes of this exercise, develop the one client goal that demonstrates a direct resolution of the client problem identified in the nursing diagnosis.
**Be sure you are able to list the scientific rationale for each nursing intervention you ordered.

# 39

# Sensory Stimulation

Chapter 39 introduces the learner to the process of sensation, the role of arousal mechanisms, sensory alterations, and factors affecting sensory stimulation. Examples are given of nursing diagnoses identifying specific sensory-perceptual alterations, as well as diagnoses describing the effects of altered sensory functioning on other areas of human functioning. Client goals for preventing and managing sensory alterations are presented, as well as specialized nursing interventions for vision or hearing-impaired, confused, or unconscious clients.

## OBJECTIVES

After studying this chapter the learner will be able to:

Define key terms in this chapter.

Describe the four conditions that must be met in each sensory experience.

Explain the role of the reticular activating system in sensory experience.

Identify etiologies and perceptual, cognitive, and emotional responses to sensory deprivation and sensory overload.

Perform a comprehensive assessment of sensory functioning utilizing appropriate interview questions and physical assessment skills.

Develop nursing diagnoses that correctly identify sensory-perceptual alterations that may be treated by independent nursing intervention.

Describe specific nursing strategies to prevent sensory alterations, to stimulate the senses, and to assist clients with sensory difficulties.

Develop a plan of nursing care to assist clients in meeting individualized sensory-perceptual goals.

Implement individualized nursing strategies that successfully resolve the client's individualized sensory-perception alterations.

Evaluate the plan of nursing care using specified criteria.

## EXERCISES

## Matching

Match the examples in Part B with the appropriate stimulation listed in Part A.

Part A

a. visual stimulation

b. auditory stimulation

c. gustatory/olfactory stimulation

d. tactile stimulation

Part B

1. _____ A nurse wears a brightly colored top when caring for clients confined to bed.

2. _____ A nurse collaborates with the hospital nutritionist to prepare meals with varied seasonings and textures.

3. _____ A client confined to bed is given daily massages.

4. _____ Soft music is played in the room of a client who has eye patches following his surgery.

5. _____ A nurse checks clients for properly fitting dentures in a long-term facility.

6_____ A nurse hugs a depressed client who makes the effort to bathe and dress herself.

7. _____ A nurse explains a procedure to a comotose patient.

8. _____ A nurse arranges a client's cards in a heart shape on her walls.

## Correct the False Statements

Circle the word *true* or *false* that follows the statement. If the word *false* has been circled, change the underlined word/words to make the statement true. Place your answer in the space provided.

1. The <u>reticular activating system</u>, located in the core of the brain stem, mediates arousal of the brain.

   True    False    _____

2. <u>Sensory reception</u> is the conscious processs of selecting, organizing, and interpreting data from the senses into meaningful information.

   True    False    _____

3. <u>Adaptation</u> is the phenomenon whereby a body quickly adapts to constant stimuli.

   True    False    _____

4. A <u>perceptual response</u> to sensory deprivation would be inaccurate perception of sight, sound, tastes, smells, and body position.

   True    False    _____

5. A <u>cognitive response</u> to sensory deprivation would include inappropriate emotional responses.

   True    False    _____

6. <u>Sensory overload</u> is the condition that results when a person experiences so much sensory stimuli that the brain is unable to meaningfully respond to, or ignore, the stimuli.

   True    False    _____

7. When sensory disturbances can be treated independently by nursing interventions, nursing diagnoses are developed, and labeled <u>sensory perceptual</u> alterations.

   True    False    _____

8. <u>Conductive</u> hearing loss is caused by inner ear or central nervous system problems.

   True    False    _____

9. <u>Presbycusis</u> is a condition of aging in which decreased elasticity of the lens hinders accommodation to close vision.

   True    False    _____

## Completion

1. Illustrate how the following factors influence the amount and quality of stimuli needed to maintain cortical arousal.

   a. Developmental considerations: _____

   _____

   _____

   _____

   _____

   b. Culture: _____

   _____

   _____

   _____

   _____

   c. Personality/life style: _____

   _____

   _____

   _____

   _____

   d. Stress: _____

   _____

   _____

   _____

   _____

   e. Illness/medications: _____

   _____

   _____

   _____

   _____

2. List four nursing measures to prevent sensory alteration.

   a. _____

   b. _____

   c. _____

   d. _____

3. List four guidelines for communicating with an unconscious client.

a. _____

_____

b. _____

_____

c. _____

_____

d. _____

_____

4. Describe two common types of age-related sensory deprivation problems.

a. _____

_____

b. _____

_____

5. List seven areas in which Gioiella and Bevil recommend data collection to define the extent of chronic sensory deprivation in an elderly client.

a. _____
b. _____
c. _____
d. _____
e. _____
f. _____
g. _____

## Case Study

Read the following case study and use your nursing process skills to answer the questions below.

Mr. Gibson, an 81-year-old married African-American, with much prodding from his wife, reluctantly reports that he seems not to be hearing as well as he used to be. "I don't know what the trouble is. I'm in perfect health—always have been. More and more people just seem to be mumbling instead of talking." You notice that he is seated on the edge of his chair and strains toward you when you speak to him. His wife reports that he has stopped going out and pretty much stays in his room whenever people come to the house to visit—because he is embarrassed by his inability to hear. "This is really a shame because George was always the life of the party." You ask Mr. Gibson if he has ever had his hearing evaluated and he tells you, "no," that until now he's been trying to convince himself that nothing's wrong with his hearing.

1. Identify pertinent client data by placing a single underline beneath the *objective* data in the case study and a double underline beneath the *subjective* data.

2. Complete the Nursing Process Worksheet on the opposite page to develop a three-part diagnostic statement and related plan of care for this client.

3. Write down the client and personal nursing strengths you hope to draw upon as you assist this client to better health.

Client strengths:_____

_____

_____

_____

Personal strengths: _____

_____

_____

_____

_____

4. Pretend that you are performing a nursing assessment of this client after the plan of care is implemented. Document your findings below.

_____

_____

_____

_____

_____

_____

_____

## Nursing Process Worksheet

**Health Problem (Title)**

Related to

↓

**Etiology (Related Factors)**

As Manifested by

↓

**Signs and Symptoms
(Defining Characteristics)**

**Client Goal\***

**Nursing Interventions\*\***

**Evaluative Statement:**

\*More than one client goal may be appropriate. For the purposes of this exercise, develop the one client goal that demonstrates a direct resolution of the client problem identified in the nursing diagnosis.
\*\*Be sure you are able to list the scientific rationale for each nursing intervention you ordered.

# 40

## Sexuality

Chapter 40 explores sexuality: the degree to which a person exhibits and experiences maleness or femaleness physically, emotionally, and mentally. Reproductive anatomy and physiology, the sexual response cycles, and factors that affect sexuality are discussed in this chapter. The learner is also introduced to the development of a sexual history as part of a comprehensive client history, and the use of specific interview questions to address a client with sexual dysfunctions.

O B J E C T I V E S

After studying this chapter the learner will be able to:

Define key terms used in the chapter.

Describe male and female reproductive anatomy and physiology.

Describe the sexual response cycles, differentiating male and female responses.

Identify factors that affect an individual's sexuality.

Perform a sexual assessment utilizing suggested interview questions and appropriate physical assessment skills.

Describe types of sexual dysfunctions and assessment priorities for each one.

Develop nursing diagnoses identifying a problem with sexuality that may be remedied by independent nursing actions.

Describe five areas in which the nurse can provide the client with education to promote knowledge of sexuality.

Plan, implement, and evaluate nursing care related to select nursing diagnoses involving problems of sexuality.

# E X E R C I S E S

## Matching

Match the examples of sexuality in Part B with the appropriate age level listed in Part A.

Part A

a. 0–18 months

b. 1–3 years

c. 4–6 years

d. 6–10 years

e. 10–13 years

f. 13–19 years

g. 20–35 years

h. 35–55 years

i. 55+ years

Part B

1. _____ Begins to develop opposite sex relationships.

2. _____ Gradually can differentiate self from others.

3. _____ Orgasms may become shorter and less intense in men and women.

4. _____ Establishes control over bowels and bladder.

5. _____ Puberty begins for most boys and girls with development of secondary sex characteristics.

6. _____ Bodily changes as a result of menopause.

7. _____ Methods of play and dress in accordance with gender.

8. _____ Premarital sex is common.

9. _____ Attachment to parent of opposite sex.

Match the symptoms of disease in Part B with the STD listed in Part A.

Part A

a. AIDS

b. cervical cancer

c. chlamydia

d. cytomegalovirus

e. non-specific vaginitis

f. gonorrhea

g. herpes

h. venereal warts

i. syphilis

j. trichomonas vaginalis

Part B

10. _____ A virus in the same family as herpes and Epstein Barr; may be asymptomatic or may be confused with other diseases like pneumonia, mononucleosis, or hepatitis.

11. _____ Foul smelling vaginal discharge, thin, foamy green color, itching of vulva and vagina, burning on urination, dyspareunia.

12. _____ Lesions develop mostly in oral and genital area.

13. _____ Fatique, diarrhea, weight loss, enlarged lymph nodes, fever, anorexia, and night sweats.

14. _____ Three stages to disease if left untreated: primary—single, painless genital lesion 10 days–3 months after exposure; secondary—skin rash, fever, enlarged lymph nodes; latent—may evolve and damage neurological and cardiovascular organs.

15. _____ Asymptomatic; possible vaginal bleeding or spotting.

16. _____ Pale, soft papillary lesions found around internal and external genitalia and perianal and rectal areas, profuse watery vaginal discharge, dyspareunia, intense pruritus, and vulvar irritation.

17. _____ Foul smelling, thin, grayish-white vaginal discharge; males—asymptomatic.

18. _____ Vaginal discharge, burning on urination, urinary frequency, dysuria, and urethral soreness.

19. _____ Men—purulent penile discharge, dysuria, frequency of urination; women—dysuria, abnormal menses, vaginal discharge, pelvic inflammatory disease.

Match the descriptions in Part B with the female body part listed in Part A.

Part A

a. mons pubis

b. pubic hair

c. labia majora

d. labia minora

e. clitoris

f. clitoral hood

g. hymen

h. ovaries

i. uterus

j. vagina

k. fallopian tubes

l. cervix

Part B

20. _____ A thick membrane contained in the vaginal opening with no apparent function.

21. _____ Slender structures that extend from either side of the uterus and end in a fringed fashion near each ovary, and which transport mature ova from the ovary to the uterus.

22. _____ A pear-shaped organ located between the urinary bladder and rectum which houses and nurtures a pregnancy.

23. _____ Structure at lower portion of uterus that connects the uterus and vagina.

24. _____ A pad of fatty tissue that lies over the part of the bony pelvis called the symphysis pubis.

25. _____ Consists of two rounded folds of fatty tissue that separates downward from mons pubis and meets again below vaginal introitus.

26. _____ A small, button-like structure similar to the male penis in reaction to stimuli, that contains erectile tissue, blood vessels,. and nerves; found above urinary meatus.

27. _____ A tubular, hollow organ that lies between the urinary urethra and rectum.

28. _____ Two almond-shaped organs on either side of the female body that secrete estrogen and progesterone.

29. _____ Coarse hair covering the mons pubis.

30. _____ Smaller lips located within the labia majora.

31. _____ Contains the clitoris at the joining of the labia minora.

Match the description in Part B with the appropriate male body function/organ listed in Part A.

Part A

a. testes

b. sperm

c. scrotum

d. vas deferens

e. semen

f. seminal plasma

g. foreskin

h. erection

i. ejaculation

j. nocturnal emission

Part B

32. _____ Ejaculatory episode that occurs during sleep without physical stimulation.

33. _____ Smooth structure (usually two), approximately the size of walnuts, that are freely movable within the scrotum and that produce sperm.

34. _____ A liquid produced by seminal vesicles, prostrate glands and Cowpers glands that aid in transport of sperm and provide nutrients for sperm.

35. _____ Male reproductive cell produced by the testes.

36. _____ The process by which the blood vessels in the shaft of the penis congest and penis becomes hard.

37. _____ Loose, bag-like structure that houses the testes.

38. _____ Expulsion of semen by the rhythmic contraction of the penis.

39. _____ Acts as a reservoir for sperm between ejaculations.

40. _____ Loose skin covering the glans that can be retracted.

41. _____ Seminal plasma and sperm combined.

**Multiple Choice**

Circle the letter that corresponds to the best answer for each question.

1. Male orgasm always consists of which of the following?
   a. ejaculation of semen
   b. 15–20 contractions
   c. 4–10 contractions
   d. Involuntary spasmodic contractions of the genitals.

2. Which of the following is least likely to be the cause of vaginismus in a client?
   a. Use of cosmetic or chemical irritants, such as deodorant tampons, contraceptive creams, or jellies.
   b. History of rape, sexual abuse or trauma.
   c. Fear of pregnancy, anxiety, or guilt.
   d. Presence of other sexual dysfunction.

3. Which of the following examples best supports the diagnosis, "sexual dysfunction: dyspareunia"?
   a. Client with colostomy feels she is unable to have sexual relationship with her husband as she feels he will be repulsed by her stoma.
   b. A 50-year-old woman with a history of stroke is afraid to have sex with her partner and elevate her blood pressure.
   c. A 50-year-old woman in the process of menopause has pain and burning during intercourse.
   d. A 39-year-old alcoholic woman is no longer interested in sex with her partner.

4. Which of the following refers to a woman's inability to reach orgasm?
   a. dyspareunia
   b. orgasmic dysfunction
   c. vaginismus
   d. inhibited sexual desire

5. Which of the following phases in the sexual response cycle is initiated by erotic stimlation and arousal?
   a. excitement phase
   b. plateau phase
   c. orgasm phase
   d. resolution phase

6. In which of the following phases does the climax and sexual explosion built on the preceding phases occur?

   a. excitement phase
   b. plateau phase
   c. orgasm phase
   d. resolution phase

7. A thorough sexual history should be obtained from all but which of the following clients?

   a. A client recovering from an STD.
   b. A client receiving care for pregnancy.
   c. A client recovering from a spinal cord injury.
   d. A client receiving care for an ulcer.

8. Which of the following is the inability of a man to attain or maintain an erection to such an extent that he cannot have satisfactory intercourse?

   a. impotence
   b. premature ejaculation
   c. retarded ejaculation
   d. penile incompetence

9. Which of the following would be given as a reason for a client to perform routine breast self-examination?

   a. To feel for lumps.
   b. To become familiar with her normal breast tissue.
   c. To be alert for cancer.
   d. To examine breasts in a tic-tac-toe fashion.

10. Premenstrual syndrome (PMS) is a term used to denote which of the following conditions?

    a. The appearance of swelling and mood changes during ovulation.
    b. The thickening of the cervix prior to menstruation.
    c. Irritability, emotional tension, mood swings, and water retention several days prior to menstruation.
    d. The sharp, cramping pain experienced during ovulation.

## Completion

1. List four measures used to stop sexual harrassment

   a. _____

   b. _____

   c. _____

   d. _____

2. List the four steps in the model for counseling clients with sexual problems (PLISSIT).

   a. _____

   b. _____

   c. _____

   d. _____

3. List five factors affecting sexuality; explain how each factor affects sexuality, using a concrete example.

   a. _____

   _____

   _____

   b. _____

   _____

   _____

   _____

   c. _____

   _____

   _____

   d. _____

   _____

   _____

   e. _____

   _____

   _____

4. List four responsibilities of the nurse during the examination of a woman's reproductive system.

a. _____

b. _____

c. _____

d. _____

5. List the advantages and disadvantages associated with the following contraceptive methods:

a. Natural family planning

Advantages: _____

_____

_____

_____

Disadvantages: _____

_____

_____

_____

b. Barrier methods

Advantages: _____

_____

_____

Disadvantages: _____

_____

_____

_____

c. Intrauterine devices

Advantages: _____

_____

_____

_____

Disadvantages: _____

_____

_____

d. Hormonal methods

Advantages: _____

_____

_____

_____

Disadvantages: _____

_____

e. Sterilization

Advantages: _____

_____

_____

_____

Disadvantages: _____

_____

_____

_____

## Sequencing

Place in order of occurrence the events that take place in the menstrual cycle.

1. _____ The luteal phase occurs in the ovaries—leftover follicle fills up with corpus luteum to produce hormones to encourage egg to grow. This phase coincides with the secretory phase in the uterus.

2. _____ Ovulation occurs—a mature ovum ruptures from follicles and surface of ovary and is swept into fallopian tube. If sperm are present, fertilization occurs.

3. _____ In absence of fertilized egg, the corpus luteum dies and endometrial lining disintegrates; menses begins.

4. _____ In the follicular phase, a number of follicles will mature, but only one will produce a mature ovum. At the same time, the proliferation phase is occurring in the uterus, wherein the endometrium is becoming thick and velvety in preparation for receiving a fertilized egg.

## Case Study

Read the following case study and use your nursing process skills to answer the questions below.

Anthony Piscatelli, a 6-foot tall, well-muscled, healthy, 19-year-old college freshman in the school of nursing, confides to his nursing advisor that "everything is great" about college life—with one exception. "All of a sudden I find myself questioning the values I learned at home about sex and marriage. My mom was really insistent that each of her sons should respect women and that intercourse was something you saved until you were ready to get married. If she told us once she told us a hundred times that we'd save ourselves, the girls in our lives, and her and dad a lot of heartache if we could just learn to control ourselves sexually. Problem is that no one here seems to subscribe to this philosophy. I feel like I'm abnormal in some way to even think like this. There's a lot of sexual activity in the dorms and no one even thinks you're serious if you talk about virginity positively. What do you think? Did my mom sell me a bill of goods? Is it true that if you take the proper precautions no one gets hurt and everyone has a good time?" Tony reports that he is a virgin and that he does really miss his close family back home. "I do get lonely at times, and would love to just cuddle with someone or even give and get a big hug—but no one seems to understand this."

1. Identify pertinent client data by placing a single underline beneath the *objective* data in the case study and a double underline beneath the *subjective* data.

2. Complete the Nursing Process Worksheet on the opposite page to develop a three-part diagnostic statement and related plan of care for this client.

3. Write down the client and personal nursing strengths you hope to draw upon as you assist this client to better health.

Client strengths:_____

_____

_____

_____

_____

Personal strengths: _____

_____

_____

_____

_____

4. Pretend that you are performing a nursing assessment of this client after the plan of care is implemented. Document your findings below.

_____

_____

_____

_____

_____

_____

_____

_____

_____

## Nursing Process Worksheet

**Health Problem (Title)**

**Client Goal***

Related to

↓

**Etiology (Related Factors)**

**Nursing Interventions****

As Manifested by

↓

**Signs and Symptoms
(Defining Characteristics)**

**Evaluative Statement:**

*More than one client goal may be appropriate. For the purposes of this exercise, develop the one client goal that demonstrates a direct resolution of the client problem identified in the nursing diagnosis.
**Be sure you are able to list the scientific rationale for each nursing intervention you ordered.

# 41

# Spirituality

Chapter 41 provides the learner with a knowledge base related to spirituality needs. Practical suggestions for performing a spiritual assessment and specific interview questions are presented. Sample nursing diagnoses are provided for common problems of spiritual distress, and evaluation guides are offered for clients experiencing spiritual distress related to challenged beliefs and value systems.

O B J E C T I V E S

After studying this chapter the learner will be able to:

Define key terms used in the chapter.

Identify three spiritual needs believed to be common to all persons.

Describe the influences of spirituality on everyday living, and on health and illness.

Differentiate life-affirming influences of religious beliefs from life-denying influences.

Distinguish the spiritual beliefs and practices of the major religions practiced in the United States and Canada.

Identify five factors that influence spirituality.

Perform a nursing assessment of spiritual health, utilizing appropriate interview questions and observation skills.

Develop nursing diagnoses that correctly identify spiritual problems.

Describe nursing strategies to promote spiritual health and state their rationale.

Plan, implement, and evaluate nursing care related to select nursing diagnoses involving spiritual problems.

## E X E R C I S E S

### Matching

Match the definitions in Part B with the term listed in Part A.

Part A

a. spirituality     d. spiritual distress

b. atheist     e. religion

c. agnostic     f. faith

Part B

1. _____ Confident belief in something for which there is no proof or material evidence.

2. _____ Anything that pertains to a person's relationship with a nonmaterial force or higher power.

3. _____ A person who denies the existence of God.

4. _____ A person who holds that nothing can be known about the existence of God.

5. _____ Results when an individual is unable to meet one or more of the basic spiritual needs for meaning or purpose, for love and relatedness, or for forgiveness.

6. _____ An organized system of beliefs about a higher power.

Match the religious belief which may affect prevalent health care practices listed in Part B with the religion listed in Part A. Use each answer only once.

Part A

a. Jehovah's Witnesses

b. Conservative Judaism

c. Roman Catholic

d. Islam

e. American Muslim Mission

f. Native American Religion

g. Christian Scientist

h. Buddhism

Part B

7. _____ A nurse should be aware of the importance of sacraments and the potential importance of private devotion to these clients.

8. _____ Blood transfusions are prohibited.

9. _____ Women are not allowed to make independent decisions and husbands need to be present when informed consent is sought.

10. _____ Treatments and procedures should not be scheduled on Sabbath, provided this will not hurt the client.

11. _____ Members are encouraged to obtain health care provided by the black community.

12. _____ The doctrine of avoidance of extreme is applied to the use of drugs, blood, and vaccines.

13. _____ Sucking, blowing, and drawing out with a feather fan are designed to remove the agent of the disease.

14. _____ They will utilize orthopedic services to set bones, but decline drugs and, in general, other medical or surgical procedures.

Match the example of a religious belief in Part B with the religion listed in Part A. Use each answer only once.

Part A

a. Seventh Day Adventists

b. Christian Scientist

c. Church of Jesus Christ of Latter Day Saints

d. Jehovah's Witnesses

e. Unification Church

f. Unitarian Universal Association

g. Buddhism

h. Confucianism

i. Daoism

j. Hinduism

Part B

15. _____ Denies the existence of health crises. Sickness, sin and death are errors of the human mind and can be destroyed by altering thoughts, not by drugs or medicines.

16. _____ Doctrine of transmigration—Moral factors linked with all-embracing doctrine of Karma were believed to be significant in promoting health or causing disease.

17. _____ Belief in individual choice and God's sovereignty; the body is believed to be a temple of the Holy Spirit.

18. _____ Health is a manifestation of harmony of the universe obtained through proper balancing of internal and external forces.

19. _____ Devout adherents believe in divine healing through laying on of hands, although many do not prohibit medical therapy.

20. _____ Encourages creativity, reason, and living an ethical life; no member is required to adhere to a given creed or set of religious beliefs; inherent worth and dignity of every human being is affirmed.

21. _____ Appreciation of life and desire to keep body from untimely or unnecessary death.

22. _____ They oppose the "false teachings" of other sects; opposition often extends to modern science, including medicine.

23. _____ God is the living, external person who represents universal love and care; God created the world and humans to reflect his nature; their goal is to unite Christians everywhere as one family under God.

24. _____ The "Great Physician" taught the four noble truths in order to indicate the range of "suffering," its "origin," its "cessation," and the "way" which leads to its cessation.

## Multiple Choice

Circle the letter that corresponds to the best answer for each question.

1. Which of the following is a spiritual need underlying all religious traditions according to Fish and Shelly (1978)?

   a. Need for meaning and purpose.
   b. Need for formal ceremony.
   c. Need for power in relationship with God.
   d. Need for justice.

2. Which of the following is a major religion with a Western philosophy?

   a. Christian Scientists
   b. Jehovah's Witnesses
   c. Native American Religions
   d. Islam

3. Which of the following religions is the foundation on which Christianity and Islam were built?

   a. Roman Catholicism
   b. Jehovah's Witnesses
   c. American Muslim Mission
   d. Judaism

4. Which of the following is <u>not</u> a form of Judaism?

   a. reform
   b. conservative
   c. traditional
   d. orthodox

5. Which of the following was a factor contributing to the split between Eastern and Western churches?

   a. Belief that wine and bread were symbols of Jesus Christ's body and blood.
   b. Selection of hymns.
   c. Use of pictures and statues in church.
   d. Use of different-colored vestements to symbolize emotions.

6. Which of the following is a religous duty of the Islamic faith?

   a. Almsgiving.
   b. A prayer to Muhammed, morning and evening.
   c. A yearly retreat to reinforce the tenents of Islam.
   d. Receiving sacraments.

7. The chief difference between the Shoshoni and Zuni religion is which of the following?

   a. Shoshoni look to natural spirits as a source of revelation, whereas the Zuni believe in supernatural spirits.
   b. Shoshoni seek plants and the underground as a source of power and the Zuni seek animals and the sky as a source of power.
   c. Shoshoni believe in life after death in the underground and Zuni believe in life after death among the clouds.
   d. Shoshoni's source of power and revelation can be found in animals and the sky and the Zuni source of power and revelation is located in plants and the underground.

## Completion

1. Describe a client conversation that would reflect the following unmet spiritual needs:

   a. Need for meaning and purpose: _____

   _____

   _____

   _____

   b. Need for love and relatedness: _____

   _____

   _____

   c. Need for forgiveness: _____

   _____

   _____

2. Give a clinical example of the following areas of spiritual distress:

a. Spiritual pain: _____

_____

_____

_____

b. Spiritual alienation: _____

_____

_____

_____

_____

c. Spiritual anxiety: _____

_____

_____

_____

d. Spiritual guilt: _____

_____

_____

_____

e. Spiritual anger: _____

_____

_____

_____

_____

f. Spiritual loss: _____

_____

_____

_____

_____

g. Spiritual despair: _____

_____

_____

_____

_____

3. List four measures a nurse can take to assist a client to meet his spiritual needs.

a. _____

_____

b. _____

_____

c. _____

_____

d. _____

_____

4. List four measures a nurse can use to assist a religlious counselor attending a client.

a. _____

_____

b. _____

_____

c. _____

_____

d. _____

_____

## Case Study

Read the following case study and use your nursing process skills to answer the questions below.

Jeffrey Stein is a 31-year-old attorney who is presently in a step-down unit following his transfer from cardiac care unit, where he was treated for a massive heart attack. "Bad hearts run in my family but I never thought it would happen to me. I jog several times a week and work out at the gym, eat a low fat diet, and I don't smoke." Jeffrey is 5 feet 7 inches tall, weighs about 150 pounds, and is well-built. His second night in the step-down unit, he is unable to sleep and tells the nurse, "I've really got a lot on my mind tonight. I can't stop thinking about how close I was to death. If I wasn't with someone who knew how to do CPR when I keeled over, I probably wouldn't be here today." Gentle questioning reveals that Mr. Stein is worried about what would have played out had he died. "I don't think I've ever thought seriously about my mortality and I sure don't think much about God. My parents were semi-observant Jews but I don't go to synagogue myself. I celebrate the holidays but that's about all. If there is a God, I wonder what he thinks about me." He asks if there is a rabbi or anyone he can talk with in the morning who could answer some questions for him and perhaps help him get himself back on track. "For the last couple of years, all I've been concerned about is paying off my school debts and making money. I guess there's a whole lot more to life, and maybe this was my invitation to sort out my priorities."

1. Identify pertinent client data by placing a single underline beneath the *objective* data in the case study and a double underline beneath the *subjective* data.

2. Complete the Nursing Process Worksheet on the opposite page to develop a three-part diagnostic statement and related plan of care for this client.

3. Write down the client and personal nursing strengths you hope to draw upon as you assist this client to better health.

Client strengths:_____

_____

_____

_____

_____

Personal strengths: _____

_____

_____

_____

_____

4. Pretend that you are performing a nursing assessment of this client after the plan of care is implemented. Document your findings below.

_____

_____

_____

_____

_____

_____

_____

_____

## Nursing Process Worksheet

| Health Problem (Title) | Client Goal* |
|---|---|

Related to

↓

| Etiology (Related Factors) | Nursing Interventions** |
|---|---|

As Manifested by

↓

| Signs and Symptoms (Defining Characteristics) | Evaluative Statement: |
|---|---|

*More than one client goal may be appropriate. For the purposes of this exercise, develop the one client goal that demonstrates a direct resolution of the client problem identified in the nursing diagnosis.

**Be sure you are able to list the scientific rationale for each nursing intervention you ordered.

# 42

# Medications

Chapter 42 provides the learner with a knowledge base related to the preparation and administration of medications. Drug names, preparations, classifications, adverse effects, and physiologic factors affecting drug action are presented in this chapter. Assessments entailing a comprehensive medication history as well as ongoing assessments of the client's response, nursing diagnoses, and client-centered outcomes are discussed.

O B J E C T I V E S

After studying this chapter the learner will be able to:

Define key terms used in the chapter.

Discuss drug legislation in the United States and Canada.

Describe drug names, types of preparation, and types of drug orders.

Identify drug classifications and actions.

Discuss adverse effects of drugs, including allergy, tolerance, cumulative effect, idiosyncratic effect, and interactions.

Obtain client information necessary to establish a medication history.

Calculate drug dosages, using the various systems of equivalents.

Describe prinicples used to safely prepare and administer medications orally, parenterally, topically, and by inhalation.

Develop teaching plans to meet client needs specific to medication administration.

## Exercises

## Matching

Match the definition in Part B with the term listed in Part A.

Part A

a. drug

b. pharmacology

c. prescription

d. chemical name

e. generic name

f. official name

g. trade name

h. pharmacodynamics

i. pharmacokinetics

j. absorption

k. distribution

l. metabolism

Part B

1. _____  An order conveying the medication plans to others.

2. _____  Copyrighted name selected by the drug company selling the drug.

3. _____  The study of the movement of drug molecules in the body in relation to the drug's absorption, distribution, metabolism, and excretion.

4. _____  The movement of a drug throughout the body after it has been absorbed into the bloodstream.

5. _____  Any substance that modifies body functions when taken into the living organism.

6. _____  The name of a drug assigned by the manufacturer who first develops the drug; often derived from the chemical name.

7. _____  The process by which a drug is transferred from its site of entry into the body to the bloodstream.

8. _____  The breakdown of a drug into an inactive form.

9. _____  The study that deals with chemicals affecting the body's functioning.

10. _____  A very precise description of the drug's chemical composition, identifying the drug's atomic and molecular structure.

11. _____  The name by which the drug is identified in the official publication.

12. _____  The process by which drugs alter cell physiology.

Match the drug effect in Part B with the term listed in Part A.

Part A

a. iatrogenic disease

b. drug allergy

c. anaphylactic reaction

d. drug tolerance

e. cumulative effect

f. idiosyncratic effect

g. antagonistic effect

h. synergistic effect

i. drug interaction

Part B

13. _____  The combined effect of two or more drugs acting simultaneously, producing an effect greater than that of each drug alone.

14. _____  Disease caused unintentionally by drug therapy.

15. _____  Exists when the body becomes accustomed to a particular drug over a period of time.

16. _____  An abnormal or peculiar response to a drug that may manifest itself by overresponse, underresponse, or response different from the expected outcome.

17. _____  Occurs in an individual who has been previously exposed to the drug and has developed antibodies.

18. _____  The combined effect of two or more drugs acting simultaneously, producing an effect less than that of each drug alone.

19. _____  A life-threatening, immediate drug allergy that results in respiratory distress, sudden severe bronchospasm, and cardiovascular collapse.

20. _____  The combined effect of two or more drugs acting simultaneously.

21. _____  Occurs when the body cannot metabolize one dose of a drug before another dose is administered.

Match the description of drug preparations in Part B with the drug form listed in Part A.

## Part A

a. capsule

b. elixir

c. extended release

d. liniment

e. lotion

f. lozenge

g. ointment

h. patch

i. pill

j. powder

k. solution

l. suppository

m. suspension

n. syrup

o. tablet

## Part B

22. _____ Finely divided, undissolved particles in a liquid medium; should be shaken before use.

23. _____ Powder or gel form of an active drug enclosed in a gelatinous container.

24. _____ Small, solid dosage of medication, compressed or molded; may be any color, size, or shape.

25. _____ Preparation of a medication that allows for slow and continuous release over a predetermined period of time.

26. _____ Medication combined in a water and sugar solution.

27. _____ Medication in a clear liquid containing water, alcohol, sweeteners, and flavor.

28. _____ A drug dissolved in another substance.

29. _____ Drug particles in a solution for topical use.

30. _____ Mixture of a powdered drug with a cohesive material; may be round or oval in shape.

31. _____ An easily melted medicated preparation in a firm base such as gelatin that is inserted into the body.

32. _____ Medication mixed with alcohol, oil, or soap, which is rubbed on the skin.

33. _____ Unit dose of medication applied directly to skin for diffusion through skin and absorption into the blood stream.

34. _____ Small, oval, round, or oblong preparation containing a drug in a flavored or sweetened base, which dissolves in the mouth and releases medication.

35. _____ Semi-solid preparation containing a drug to be applied externally, also called an unction.

36. _____ Drugs finely ground, singly or in a mixture.

Match the measurement in Part B with its abbreviated form listed in Part A.

Part A

a. ℥

b. gt

c. gtt

d. g

e. mg or mgm

f. ml or mL

g. m or min

h. ℥

i. tbsp

j. tsp

k. gr

Part B

37. _____ Grain

38. _____ Dram

39. _____ Teaspoon

40. _____ Drop

41. _____ Ounce

42. _____ Minim

43. _____ Drops

44. _____ Gram

45. _____ Milliliter

46. _____ Milligram

47. _____ Tablespoon

Match the parts of a needle and syringe listed in Part B with their location on the diagram in Part A.

Part A

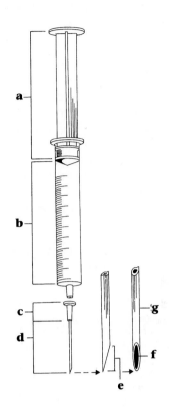

Part B

48. _____ Lumen

49. _____ Shaft

50. _____ Plunger

51. _____ Needle

52. _____ Bevel

53. _____ Barrel

54. _____ Needle hilt

## Multiple Choice

Circle the letter that corresponds to the best answer for each question.

1. When administering a drug to a client, the nurse should know which of the following facts about drug absorption?

   a. Oral medications are more rapidly absorbed than injected medications.

   b. Solid preparations are absorbed more rapidly than liquid medications.

   c. The more extensive the absorbing surface, the greater the absorption of the drug and the more rapid the effect.

   d. Enteric coated preparations are easily digested in the stomach.

2. Which of the following organs is a primary site for the metabolism of drugs?

   a. heart

   b. liver

   c. pancreas

   d. intestine

3. Mrs. Harris is a 78-year-old woman admitted to your unit after experiencing symptoms of stroke. When administering the medication prescribed for Mrs. Harris, the nurse should be aware that this client has an increased possibility of drug toxicity due to which of the following age-related factors?

   a. A decreased adipose tissue and increased total body fluid in proportion to the total body mass.

   b. Increased number of protein-binding sites.

   c. Increased kidney function resulting in excessive filtration and excretion.

   d. Decline in liver function and enzyme production needed for drug metabolism.

4. Which of the following is a type of medication order the physician may write indicating that a medication be given immediately?

   a. stat order

   b. prn order

   c. double order

   d. standard order

5. Which of the following is considered part of a medication order?

   a. client's age

   b. client's name, address, and phone number

   c. signature of the client

   d. date and time order is written

6. Your client's physician writes an order for antibiotics stat that you feel is too high a dosage for that client. What should your reaction to this order be?

   a. Administer the drug as prescribed since the physician is legally responsible for any mistakes in the order.

   b. Check with the prescribing physician before administering the drug.

   c. Administer the drug first since it is a stat drug, and then check with the physician.

   d. Check with the client about dosages administered to him/her in the past and compare this response to the ordered dosage.

7. Which of the following is a medication supply system?

   a. group supply system

   b. single dose system

   c. stock supply system

   d. apothecary system

8. Which of the following is a measurement for administering medications?

   a. household system

   b. standard weight system

   c. pharmacologic system

   d. stock supply system

9. In order to convert 0.8 grams to milligrams, the nurse should do which of the following?

   a. Move the decimal point two places to the right.

   b. Move the decimal point two places to the left.

   c. Move the decimal point three places to the right.

   d. Move the decimal point three places to the left.

10. Which of the following measurements would be included in the apothecary system?

    a. mg

    b. tsp

    c. glass

    d. m

11. Mr. Downs is given a dose of gentamycin and has an immediate reaction of hypotension, bronchospasms, and rapid, thready pulse. Which of the following would be the drugs of choice for this situation?

    a. antibiotic, antihistamines, and isuprel

    b. epinephrine, antihistamines, bronchodilators

    c. bronchodilators, antihistamines, and vasodilators

    d. antihistamines, vasodilators, and bronchoconstrictors

12. Mrs. Banks has an order for chloromycetin 500mg. q 6 hours. The drug comes in 250 mg per capsule. Which of the following would be the correct dosage?

   a. 1 tab
   b. 2 tab
   c. 3 tab
   d. 4 tab

13. Mr. Moran has oral medication ordered. He has a nasogastric tube in place. Which of the following would increase the safety of medication administration?

   a. Check the tube placement prior to administration.
   b. Have Mr. Moran swallow the pills around the tube.
   c. Flush the tube with 30 to 40 cc prior to medication administration.
   d. Bring the liquids to room temperature before administration.

14. Mr. Doyle asks you to give an intramuscular injection in his deltoid muscle. Which of the following would be the best response?

   a. "The deltoid has more blood vessels and nerves."
   b. "The deltoid site is more painful"
   c. "The deltoid is very quick to bruise."
   d. "The deltoid is very small."

15. George Riley is a 46-year-old man in the hospital for COPD. He has an order for penicillin to be given intramuscularly. Which of the following would be the correct angle to use for the dorsogluteal site?

   a. 45 degree angle
   b. 60 degree angle
   c. 90 degree angle
   d. 75 degree angle

## Correct the False Statements

Circle the word *true* or *false* that follows the statement. If the word *false* has been circled, change the underlined word/words to make the statement true. Place your answer in the space provided.

1. The formula for calculating pediatric dosages according to Clark's rule is:

$$\frac{BSA\ (child)}{BSA\ (adult)} \times adult\ dose = child\ dose$$

   True    False    _____

2. Drugs given <u>orally</u> are intended for absorption in the stomach and small intestine.

   True    False    _____

3. The term <u>enteral</u> means outside the intestines.

   True    False    _____

4. The technique of adding a diluent to a powdered drug is called <u>reabsorption.</u>

   True    False    _____

5. The <u>intradermal route</u> has the longest absorption time of all parenteral routes.

   True    False    _____

6. <u>Subcutaneous tissue</u> lies between the epidermis and the muscle.

   True    False    _____

7. An <u>intradermal site</u> is often used for drugs that are irritating, since there are few nerve endings in this deep tissue.

   True    False    _____

8. The <u>dorsogluteal site,</u> located in the buttock, is a common site for administering intramuscular injections.

   True    False    _____

9. The <u>ventrogluteal site</u> involves the gluteus medius and gluteus minimus muscles in the hip area.

   True    False    _____

10. The <u>vastus lateralis site</u> is on the anterior part of the thigh.

    True      False _____

11. The <u>deltoid muscle site</u> is located in the lateral aspect of the upper arm.

    True      False _____

12. Not more than <u>5ml</u> should be injected into a single injection site.

    True      False _____

13. The <u>oral</u> route of medication administration is the most dangerous route.

    True      False _____

14. The intravenous <u>tandem</u> delivery system requires the intermittent or additive solution to be placed higher than the primary solution container.

    True      False _____

15. A <u>heparin lock</u> is used for a client who requires intermittent intravenous medication but not a continuous intravenous infusion.

    True      False _____

16. When a drug is applied directly to a body site, it is called a <u>topical application.</u>

    True      False _____

17. When a drug is incorporated into an agent, such as an ointment, and is rubbed into the skin for absorption, the procedure is referred to as an <u>inunction.</u>

    True      False _____

18. The outer layer of the eyeball is called the <u>canthus.</u>

    True      False _____

19. Drugs classified as bronchodilators, and decongestants are frequently administered by <u>inhalation.</u>

    True      False _____

## Completion

1. In administering medications, you find a certain amount of the medication has been ordered by the physician and you have a different amount on hand. Make the necessary conversions and state what you will give to each patient.

   a. Order: Gentamicin 60 mg. On hand is gentamicin 80mg/2 cc.

   Give: _____

   b. Order: aspirin gr V. On hand is aspirin 300 mg/tab.

   Give: _____

   c. Order: Mestinon 30 mg. On hand is Mestinon 60 mg/tab.

   Give: _____

   d. Order: amitriptyline 75 mg. On hand is amitriptyline 25 mg/tab.

   Give: _____

   e. Order: phenylbutazone 250 mg. On hand is phenylbutazone 500 mg/tab.

   Give: _____

   f. Order: ProBanthine 15 mg. On hand is ProBanthine 5 mg/tab.

   Give: _____

   g. Order: Penicillin V 250 mg. On hand is Penicillin V 500 mg/tab.

   Give: _____

   h. Order: Lanoxin 0.125 mg. On hand is Lanoxin 0.250 mg/tab.

   Give: _____

   i. Order: metaproterenol sulfate 20 mg. On hand is metaproterenol sulfate 10 mg/tab.

   Give: _____

   j. Order: ACTH 40 mg. On hand is ACTH 10 mg/cc.

   Give: _____

2. You are preparing Jim Toole for discharge. He will be taking the following medications at home. Use the chart below to identify the information you will need to teach him about these medications. Use a pharmacology text to look up Xanax, Zantac, and Cipro.

| | Xanax | Zantac | Cipro |
|---|---|---|---|
| Dosage | | | |
| Route of administration | | | |
| Frequency/schedule | | | |
| Desired effects | | | |
| Possible adverse effects | | | |
| S&S of toxic drug effects | | | |
| Special instructions | | | |
| Recommended course of action with problems | | | |

3. Transcribe the following medication orders on the client medication record and sign for the medications you would administer in a 24-hour period. Be prepared to discuss administration guidelines.

Tenormin, 50 mg, PO od
Hydrodiuril, 50 mg, PO od
NPH Insulin U-l00, 45 units SQ daily in AM

Regular Insulin U-100, l0 units SQ STAT
Cipro, 500 mg, PO q 12 h
Timoptic 0.25% ☦ gtt OD bid
Dalmane, 30 mg, po hs, PRN
Nitro-paste 1/2 ", q 8 h to chest wall
Tylenol with codeine #2, ☦ PO q 4 h, PRN
Colace, l00 mg, PO od

---

**Medical Administration Record**

| ORD DATE | PRN MEDS. | |
|---|---|---|
| | | Date |
| | | Time |
| | | Init / Site |
| | | Date |
| | | Time |
| | | Init / Site |

| | SINGLE ORDERS—PREOPERATIVES | | |
|---|---|---|---|
| ORD DATE | MEDICATION—DOSAGE—ROUTE OF ADMIN | DATE/TIME | SITE/INITITALS |
| | | | |
| | | | |

INJECTION SITES MUST BE CHARTED

| | ROUTINE MEDICATIONS | | DATE/TIME | | | | | | |
|---|---|---|---|---|---|---|---|---|---|
| ORD DATE | MEDICATION—DOSAGE—ROUTE OF ADMIN | HR | | | | | | | |
| | | | | | | | | | |
| | | | | | | | | | |
| | | | | | | | | | |
| | | | | | | | | | |
| | | | | | | | | | |
| | | | | | | | | | |
| | | | | | | | | | |
| | | | | | | | | | |
| | | | | | | | | | |
| | | | | | | | | | |
| | | | | | | | | | |
| | | | | | | | | | |
| | | | | | | | | | |
| | | | | | | | | | |
| | | | | | | | | | |
| | | | | | | | | | |
| | | | | | | | | | |

4. List the "three checks and five rights" when administering medications.

a. Three "checks": Check the label on the medication—

_____

_____

_____

b. Five "rights": The nurse gives the—

_____

_____

_____

_____

_____

5. List five factors the nurse should consider before choosing the equipment needed for an injection.

a. _____

b. _____

c. _____

d. _____

e. _____

6. Describe three methods used for dispensing injectible drugs.

a. _____

_____

b. _____

_____

c. _____

_____

7. Complete the chart below by listing the terms used to describe the following routes of administration of drugs.

| Route | Term Used to Describe Route |
| --- | --- |
| Given by mouth | |
| Given via respiratory tract | |
| Given by injection (types of injections) | |
| Given on skin or mucous membrane (types of administration) | |

8. Give the abbreviations for the following words used in prescribing medications.

a. of each _____

b. before meals _____

c. twice a day _____

d. with_____

e. capsule _____

f. hour of sleep_____

g. intramuscular _____

h. intravenous_____

i. every other day _____

j. by mouth_____

k. as needed_____

l. every day _____

m. every hour _____

n. 4 times a day_____

o. immediately _____

9. Describe the location on the human body used for administering the following injections:

a. Subcutaneous site injections:_____

_____

_____

_____

b. Dorsogluteal site injections:_____

_____

_____

_____

c. Ventrogluteal site injections:_____

_____

_____

_____

d. Vastus lateralis site injections:_____

_____

_____

_____

e. Rectus femoris site injections:_____

_____

_____

_____

f. Deltoid muscle site injections:_____

_____

_____

_____

10. Describe the following injection procedures:

a. Z-track technique:_____

_____

_____

_____

_____

b. Heparin lock:_____

_____

_____

_____

_____

## Sequence

For items 1–11, place each step in the correct sequence by numbering the following steps in removing medication from a vial.

1. _____ Swab the rubber top with the alcohol swab.

2. _____ Pierce the rubber stopper in the center with the needle tip and inject the measured air into the space above the solution. The vial may be positioned upright on a flat surface or inverted.

3. _____ Wash your hands.

4. _____ Draw up the prescribed amount of medication while holding the syringe at eye level and vertically.

5. _____ Once the correct dose is withdrawn, remove the needle from the vial and cap it. If a multiple dose vial is being used, store the vial containing the remaining medication, according to agency policy.

6. _____ Gather equipment. Check medication order against the physician's order, according to agency policy.

7. _____ Remove the metal or plastic cap on the vial that protects the rubber stopper.

8. _____ Invert the vial and withdraw the needle tip slightly so that it is below the fluid level.

9. _____ Wash your hands.

10. _____ Remove the cap from the needle by pulling it straight off.

11. _____ If any air bubbles accumulate in the syringe, tap the barrel of the syringe sharply and move the needle past the fluid into the air space to reinject the air bubble into the vial. Return the needle tip to the solution and continue wilthdrawal of the medication.

# 43

# Care of Wounds

Chapter 43 discusses all aspects of the care of wounds. The reaction of the body to trauma (wounds) is discussed in terms of types of wounds, wound healing, wound complications, and psychologic effects of wounds. The role of the nurse in wound care is presented, including applying bandages and binders, changing the dressing, and applying heat and cold.

## OBJECTIVES

After studying this chapter the learner will be able to:

Define key terms used in the chapter.

Describe the physical and psychologic effects of trauma to the body, with resultant wounds.

Discuss the processes involved in wound healing.

Describe wound complications, integrating factors affecting wound healing.

Summarize emergency wound assessment and care.

Describe the effects of the application of heat and cold.

Use the nursing process to knowledgeably derive an individualized plan of care for the client with a wound, including the application of dressings and hear or cold.

## EXERCISES

### Matching

Match the term in Part A with the correct definition in Part B.

Part A

a. intentional wound

b. unintentional wound

c. open wound

d. closed wound

e. contusion

f. laceration

g. clean wound

h. contaminated wound

i. infected wound

j. incision

Part B

1. __i__ A wound with demonstrated pathogens. *infected*

2. __b__ A wound that occurs from unexpected trauma. *unintentional wound*

3. __e__ A closed wound resulting from a blow with a hard object. *contusion*

4. __a__ The result of planned invasive therapy or treatment. *intentional*

5. __j__ An intentional wound made with a sharp instrument. *infected wound*

6. __c__ The skin surface is broken; occurs from intentional or accidental trauma. *open wound*

7. __g__ A surgical incision or closed wound. *clean wound*

8. __d__ The skin surface is not broken; the result of a blow, force, or strain. *closed wound*

9. __f__ An unintentional wound that has torn tissues and ragged edges. *laceration*

10. __h__ May occur during surgery with major contamination from the gastrointestinal system; high risk of infection. *contaminated*

Match the term in Part A with the correct definition in Part B.

Part A

a. granulation tissue

b. scar

c. serous

d. sanguineous

e. purulent

Part B

11. __e__ Is thick, often has a foul odor, and has varying colors, depending on the causative organism.

12. __a__ Highly vascular, reddish in color, and bleeds easily.

13. __b__ Avascular collagen tissue that will not sweat, grow hair, or tan in sunlight.

14. __d__ Consists of large numbers of red blood cells; looks like blood.

15. __c__ Is clear and watery.

## Multiple Choice

Circle the letter that corresponds to the best answer for each question.

1. Which of the following clients would be most at risk for developing a wound infection?
   a. A toddler having a hernia repair.
   b. An adolescent who is malnourished.
   c. A 40-year-old of normal weight.
   d. A 55-year-old having back surgery.

2. Which of the following nursing actions is probably most effective in preventing wound infection?
   a. Careful hand washing.
   b. Wearing rubber gloves.
   c. Doing sterile dressing changes.
   d. Teaching proper skin care.

3. On the first postoperative day following abdominal surgery, your client has several responses as a result of the inflammatory phase of wound healing. Which of the following assessments is a normal part of this phase?
   a. purulent drainage from the wound
   b. bradycardia
   c. oral temperature elevated one degree
   d. disorientation

4. Most surgical incisions and small sutured lacerations heal by what process?
   a. first intention
   b. secondary intention
   c. tertiary intention
   d. quintile intention

5. Which of the following assessments is a normal body response to cold?
   a. pallor
   b. cyanosis
   c. pain
   d. shivering

6. Which of the normal physiologic changes that occur in the older adult would be a factor affecting wound healing?
   a. loss of near vision
   b. decreased gastric motility and constipation
   c. slower cognitive response time
   d. loss of skin turgor, with increased fragility

7. You are removing staples from an incision. What pattern of removal would you use?
   a. Remove all of the top half first.
   b. Remove all of the bottom half first.
   c. Remove every other staple first.
   d. Remove all of the staples at once.

8. You are initiating a physician order to apply heat to a lower extremity. When you assess the leg, you find it to be pale and cold, with weak pulses and absent sensation. What will you do now?
   a. Question the order.
   b. Continue with the heat application.
   c. Substitute a cold application.
   d. Ignore the order.

9. Mrs. Jolle is taking a sitz bath. She tells you she is feeling dizzy and looks pale. You check her blood pressure and find it to be 86/42; her pulse is 106. What will you do now?
   a. Continue with the sitz bath.
   b. Recognize these as normal signs.
   c. Discontinue the sitz bath.
   d. Continue to monitor her vital signs.

10. What is the maximum length of time for one application of an ice bag?
    a. 10 minutes
    b. 30 minutes
    c. one hour
    d. four hours

## Correct the False Statements

Circle the word *true* or *false* that follows the statement. If the word *false* has been circled, change the underlined word/words to make the statement true. Place your answer in the space provided.

1. A localized collection of pus is called an <u>abscess.</u>

   True     False     _____

2. A <u>scar</u> forms during the proliferation phase of wound healing.

   True     False     _____

3. Wounds that heal by <u>tertiary</u> intention will have minimal scarring.

   True     False     _____

4. The partial or total disruption of wound layers is <u>dehiscence.</u>

   True     False     _____

5. <u>Skin sutures</u> are used to provide extra support for wounds in obese clients.

   True     False     _____

6. <u>Bandages</u> are strips of cloth, gauze, or elasticized material used to wrap a body part.

   True     False     _____

7. A sling is an example of a <u>bandage.</u>

   True     False     _____

8. The <u>figure-of-eight turn</u> is effective for the application of a bandage to a joint.

   True     False     _____

9. New trends in dressings for open wounds are the <u>"wet-to-damp"</u> packing.

   True     False     _____

10. Heat causes <u>vasoconstriction</u> of peripheral blood vessels.

    True     False     _____

## Completion

1. List the general principles of tissue healing included in the chapter:

   a. _____

   _____

   _____

   b. _____

   _____

   c. _____

   _____

   _____

   d. _____

   _____

   _____

   e. _____

   _____

   _____

   f. _____

   _____

   _____

2. Fill in the blanks in the paragraph about the maturation phase of wound healing with the correct word or words.

This final stage of healing begins about day

(a) _____ and can continue for as long as

(b) _____ years after injury. (c) _____

that has been haphazardly deposited in the wound is

remodeled, making the healed wound

(d) _____. New collagen continues to be

deposited, which compresses (e) _____ in the

healing wound, so that the (f) _____ eventu-

ally is a thin, flat, line.

3. Provide the rationale for the way these factors affect wound healing:

a. Obesity: _____

_____

_____

_____

b. Peripheral vascular disease: _____

_____

_____

c. Chronic smokers: _____

_____

_____

4. List seven symptoms of wound infection.

a. _____

b. _____

c. _____

d. _____

e. _____

f. _____

g. _____

5. List four possible causes of hemorrhage in the client with a wound.

a. _____

b. _____

c. _____

d. _____

6. What should the nurse do if evisceration occurs?

_____

_____

_____

7. The first priority in the emergency assessment and care of a wound is "ABC." What do these letters stand for?

a. A: _____

b. B: _____

c. C: _____

8. In formulating nursing diagnoses for the client with a wound, what data would be necessary?

a. _____

b. _____

c. _____

d. _____

e. _____

9. List the questions that should be asked before initiating heat or cold applications.

a. _____

_____

b. _____

_____

c. _____

_____

d. _____

_____

e. _____

_____

f. _____

_____

10. List the broad indications for heat applications:

a. _____

b. _____

c. _____

d. _____

e. _____

11. List the broad indications for cold applications:

a. _____

b. _____

c. _____

12. Provide the rationale for each of the following actions in heat and cold applications.

a. Do not use pins to secure a heating pad. _____

_____

_____

_____

b. Prevent wet conditions around a heating pad. _____

_____

_____

_____

c. Clean and dry the area before applying a heat lamp._____

_____

_____

d. Cover warm, moist compresses with plastic wrap or a heating agent._____

_____

_____

e. Place a cover on the ice bag._____

_____

_____

f. Drape the client properly during an alcohol sponge bath. _____

_____

_____

g. Cover, but do not dry, each area that is sponged. __

_____

_____

_____

13. List the six advantages of wound dressings listed in the chapter.

a. _____

_____

_____

b. _____

_____

_____

c. _____

_____

_____

d. _____

_____

_____

e. _____

_____

_____

f. _____

_____

_____

# 44

## Perioperative Nursing

Chapter 44 discusses the surgical experience, including the preoperative, intraoperative, and postoperative periods. Classification of surgical procedures, anesthesia, and informed consent are described. Preoperative nursing care is discussed, including assessing life-style and preparing the client psychologically and physically for surgery. Intraoperative nursing care is described. Postoperative nursing care includes immediate care, prevention of complications during ongoing care, and promoting a return to health.

### OBJECTIVES

After studying this chapter the learner will be able to:

Define key terms used in the chapter.

Describe the surgical experience; including perioperative phases, categories of surgery, types of anesthesia, and informed consent.

Conduct a preoperative nursing history and nursing examination to identify client strengths as well as factors increasing surgical and postoperative complication risk.

Demonstrate preoperative exercises: deep-breathing, coughing, and leg exercises.

Prepare a client physically and psychologically for surgery.

Describe the nurse's role in the intraoperative phase.

Identify assessments specific to the prevention of complications in the immediate postoperative phase.

Plan and implement interventions for ongoing postoperative care to prevent complications, promote a return to health, and facilitate coping with alterations.

Use the nursing process to knowledgeably develop an individualized plan of care for the surgical client during each phase of the perioperative period.

### EXERCISES

#### Matching

In sets A–C, match the terms for surgery classifications with the definitions provided.

Set A

a. urgent

b. elective

c. emergency

1. _____ Performed to preserve life

2. _____ Coronary artery by-pass

3. _____ Intestinal obstruction

4. _____ Performed to improve self-concept

5. _____ Performed to restore function

6. _____ Mammoplasty

Set B

a. major

b. minor

7. _____ May be either elective or emergency

8. _____ abdominal hysterectomy

9. _____ Cataract extraction

10. _____ To remove a body part

11. _____ To correct deformities

*(cont'd)*

Set C

a. diagnostic

b. ablative

c. palliative

d. reconstructive

e. transplant

f. constructive

12. _____ Performed to replace organs

13. _____ Debridement of necrotic tissue

14. _____ Restores function in congenital anomalies

15. _____ Bronchoscopy

16. _____ To improve self-concept

17. _____ Colon resection

18. _____ Is not curative surgery

19. _____ Skin graft for burns

20. _____ To make or confirm a diagnosis

21. _____ Cleft palate repair

Match the term in Part A with the correct definition in Part B relating to possible complication in the post-operative surgical phase.

Part A

a. hypovolemic shock

b. thrombophlebitis

c. embolus

d. pneumonia

e. atelectasis

f. paralytic ileus

g. hemorrhage

Part B

22. _____ Absence of peristalsis.

23. _____ Inflammation of the alveoli.

24. _____ Inflammation of a vein associated with blood clot formation.

25. _____ A decrease in blood volume.

26. _____ Excessive blood loss.

27. _____ A blood clot, or other substance, that is dislodged and travels through the blood stream.

28. _____ The incomplete expansion or collapse of alveoli.

## Multiple Choice

Circle the letter that corresponds to the best answer for each question.

1. When a client is given drugs by inhalation, intravenous, rectal, or oral routes to produce central nervous system depression, it is termed:
   a. local anesthesia
   b. regional anesthesia
   c. general anesthesia
   d. surface anesthesia

2. Homan's sign is assessed by having the client dorsiflex the foot and asking if pain occurs in the:
   a. calf
   b. arch of the foot
   c. thigh
   d. toes

3. Your postoperative client suddenly begins having chest pain, dyspnea, cough, cyanosis, and tachypnea, and appears very anxious. What would you do?
   a. Carry out cough and deep-breathing exercises.
   b. Ask the client how he/she feels every 10 minutes.
   c. Monitor vital signs.
   d. Notify the physician.

4. Nursing interventions of encouraging coughing, deep breathing, and use of incentive spirometry are performed with the goal of preventing:
   a. cardiovascular complications.
   b. respiratory complications.
   c. wound infection.
   d. elimination problems.

5. Which of the following is the most common emergency during the post-anesthesia recovery period?
   a. hemorrhage
   b. infection
   c. respiratory obstruction
   d. renal shutdown

## Correct the False Statements

Circle the word *true* or *false* that follows the statement. If the word *false* has been circled, change the underlined word/words to make the statement true. Place your answer in the space provided.

1. Regional anesthesia occurs when an agent is injected or applied near a nerve, inhibiting the transmission of <u>motor stimuli</u>.

   True    False    _____

2. An informed consent for surgery is a <u>legal document.</u>

   True    False    _____

3. Those at greatest risk from surgery are <u>children</u> and <u>young to middle-age adults.</u>

   True    False    _____

4. Clients who have a history of of alcohol abuse will require <u>smaller</u> doses of anesthetic.

   True    False    _____

5. Any surgical procedure causes <u>anxiety and fear.</u>

   True    False    _____

6. A client who has been in the lithotomy position during surgery is at increased risk for <u>thrombophlebitis.</u>

   True    False    _____

7. On returning from the PAR, your client is lethargic. You would place the client in a <u>supine</u> position.

   True    False    _____

8. A common assessment of fluid status in the postoperative client is <u>intake and output.</u>

   True    False    _____

9. Assessments for <u>pain</u> should include location, intensity, and duration

   True    False    _____

10. Reaction to loss of a body part by surgery can result in <u>grieving.</u>

    True    False    _____

## Completion

1. List the types of clients for which a signed consent form is not legal.

a. _____

b. _____

c. _____

d. _____

e. _____

6. Fill in the blank with the category of drug that increases surgical risk.

a. _____ Long-term users may have cardiovascular collapse if the drug is abruptly withdrawn.

b. _____ May precipitate hemorrhage.

c. _____ May increase the hypotensive effect of anesthetic agents.

d. _____ If mycin group, may cause respiratory paralysis if combined with certain muscle relaxants.

e. _____ May cause electrolyte imbalances, with resulting respiratory depression from anesthesia.

3. Describe the three phases of general anesthesia.

a. Induction: _____

_____

_____

b. Maintenance: _____

_____

_____

c. Emergence: _____

_____

_____

Describe the physiologic changes with aging that increase surgical risk.

4. Cardiovascular:

a. _____

b. _____

c. _____

5. Respiratory:

a. _____

b. _____

c. _____

6. Neurologic:

a. _____

b. _____

7. Renal:

a. _____

b. _____

8. Integument

a. _____

b. _____

9. List the common fears of the preoperative client.

a. _____

b. _____

c. _____

10. List specific goals for planning the care of the surgical client.

a. _____

_____

b. _____

_____

c. _____

_____

d. _____

_____

11. List the purposes of deep breathing exercises.

a. _____

b. _____

c. _____

d. _____

12. List the purposes of turning in bed.

a. _____

b. _____

c. _____

13. Provide the correct rationale for the following pre-operative nursing responsibilities:

a. Take and record vital signs: _____

_____

_____

b. Remove make-up and fingernail polish: _____

_____

_____

c. Remove dentures: _____

_____

_____

d. Remove jewelry: _____

_____

_____

14. Describe the rationale for the following preoperative medications:

a. Sedatives/tranquilizers: _____

_____

_____

b. Anticholinergics: _____

_____

_____

c. Narcotic analgesics: _____

_____

_____

d. Antihistaminics: _____

_____

_____

15. What are the aims of nursing interventions during the postoperative phase?

a. _____

_____

_____

b. _____

_____

_____

c. _____

_____

_____

d. _____

_____

_____

e. _____

_____

_____

# Answers

# Chapter 1

## Matching

1. f  2. k  3. j  4. e  5. c  6. a  7. i  8. g
9. b  10. h  11. d  12. f  13. g  14. d  15. c  16. h
17. a  18. e  19. b  20. j  21. i

## Completion

1. The nine contributions Florence Nightengale made to nursing are:
   a. Recognized nutrition as a part of nursing care.
   b. Defined nursing as separate and distinct from medicine.
   c. Recognized importance of continuing education for nurses.
   d. Instituted occupational and recreational therapy for the sick.
   e. Expanded role of the nurse to include identifying and meeting the personal needs of the patient.
   f. Established standards for hospital management.
   g. Established a respected occupation for women.
   h. Established nursing education.
   i. Recognized the two components of nursing: health and illness.

2. Nursing is the demonstration of nonpossessive *caring* for and about others.

3. Nursing is *sharing* self with patients, other health-team members, and other nurses.

4. Nursing is *touching* to provide comfort and give care.

5. Nursing is sharing with clients in the human *feelings* of sorrow, joy, frustration, and satisfaction.

6. Nursing is *listening* attentively to the verbal and nonverbal communication signals of others.

7. Nursing is *accepting* of self in order to accept others.

8. Nursing is *respecting* of individual differences through unconditional acceptance, ensuring confidences and privacy, and individualizing care.

9. American Nurses' Association

10. International Council of Nurses

11. National League for Nursing

12. National Student Nurses' Association

13. Canadian Nurses' Association

14. The four broad aims of nursing are:
    a. promoting wellness
    b. preventing illness
    c. restoring health
    d. facilitating coping

15. caregiver

16. teacher

17. counselor

18. advocate

19. leader

20. researcher

21. communicator

22. nurse midwife
    a. certificate or advanced degree
    b. provides pre-/postnatal care; delivers babies in uncomplicated pregnancies

23. Nurse Practitioner
    a. advanced degree, certification
    b. Works in a variety of settings providing health assessment and primary care.

24. Nurse Anesthetist
    a. advanced degree
    b. Administers and monitors anesthesia.

# C h a p t e r 2

## Matching

| 1. f | 2. i | 3. c | 4. l | 5. e | 6. j | 7. b |
|------|------|------|------|------|------|------|
| 8. g | 9. m | 10. d | 11. n | 12. o | 13. a | 14. k |

## Multiple Choice

1. b    2. c    3. d    4. a    5. b

## Completion

1. Health is a state of complete physical, mental, and social well-being, not merely the absence of disease or infirmity.
2. *Disease* is a medical term, meaning that there is a pathologic change in the structure or function of the body or mind; a condition with specific symptoms and boundaries. *Illness* is an abnormal process in which the person's level of functioning is changed as compared to a previous level; an individualized perception and definition of self in relation to health.
3. The six human dimensions are:
   a. physical
   b. emotional
   c. intellectual
   d. environmental
   e. sociocultural
   f. spiritual
4. ◄------- Health  Good  Normal  Illness  Death -------►
5. Compare your response with the examples given in the textbook.
6. Common causes of disease are:
   a. genetic defects
   b. biologic toxins or agents
   c. physical agents
   d. developmental defects
   e. hormone/enzyme imbalance
   f. tissue response to injury or irritation
   g. reaction to stress
7-16. *Primary:* 11, 12, 13. *Secondary:* 7, 9, 10, 14, 15. *Tertiary:* 8, 16.

# C h a p t e r   3

## Matching

| | | | | | | | |
|---|---|---|---|---|---|---|---|
| 1. d | 2. a | 3. e | 4. b | 5. c | 6. d | 7. c | 8. a |
| 9. b | 10. e | | | | | | |

## Multiple Choice

| | | | | | | | |
|---|---|---|---|---|---|---|---|
| 1. b | 2. c | 3. d | 4. a | 5. c | 6. d | 7. a | 8. c |
| 9. a | 10. d | | | | | | |

## Completion

1. Government health care agencies are financed by national, state, local, or provincial taxes.
2. a. Supplies funds to health care for migrant workers and the poor or uninsured. Also supplies health care professionals for federal prisons, and is involved in programs for drug/alcohol abuse and mental health.
   b. Focuses on the epidemiology, prevention, control, and treatment of communicable disease, including sexually transmitted diseases.
   c. Engaged in various research activities.
3. a. skilled care
   b. social services
   c. counseling
   d. personal services
4. Pharmacist
   a. formulate and dispense medications
   b. college degree
   c. license
5. Physical Therapist
   a. restore function or prevent disability
   b. college degree
   c. PT, state license
6. Physicians' Assistant
   a. depend on the physician supervising the activities
   b. specific courses or program
   c. PA
7. Occupational Therapist
   a. assist the disabled client to adapt to limitations
   b. college degree
   c. OT, state license
8. Dietitian
   a. responsible for managing and planning for client dietary needs
   b. college degree
   c. RD, registration
9. Respiratory Therapist
   a. improve pulmonary function and oxygenation
   b. specific courses, program
   c. RT
10. Diagnostic related groups are a prospective payment plan implemented by the federal government to try to control rising health care costs. This plan pays the hospital a fixed rate that is predetermined by the medical diagnosis or specific procedure rather than by actual hospitalization costs.
11. The Canada Health Act is a law that clarifies and defines the conditions of Canadian health insurance: universality, accessibility, comprehensiveness, and portability among provinces.
12. a. determine staffing needs
    b. direct nursing documentation
    c. computerized nursing care plans
    d. automated staff scheduling
    e. medication documentation records
    f. availability of diagnostic test results
    g. direct order processing
    h. analysis of budget and positions

# C h a p t e r   4

## Matching

1. b    2. e    3. a    4. c    5. d    6. g    7. d    8. b
9. c    10. a    11. e    12. f

## Completion

1. a. parts
   b. self
   c. others
   d. biochemical reactions
2. a. orderly
   b. predictable
3. The five basic characteristics of nursing theory are:
   a. interrelated concepts
   b. logical in nature
   c. simple and general
   d. increase nursing's body of knowledge
   e. guide and improve practice
4. a. person
   b. environment
   c. health
   d. nursing
5. Primary goal is to foster balance within an individual, specific to the behavioral system, when illness occurs.
6. A process of human interactions between nurse and client whereby each perceives the other and the situation; and through communication, together set goals, explore means, and agree on means to achieve goals.
7. A humanistic art and science that focuses on personalized care behaviors and processes that are directed toward promoting and maintaining health behaviors or recovery from illness, and which have physical, psychocultural, and social significance or meaning.
8. The giving of direct assistance to a person who is unable to meet his own self-care needs, developed through nursing education and experiences.
9. A theoretical system in which knowledge prescribes a process of analysis and action related to the care of the ill or potentially ill person.
10. An art and science of a human-to-human care process with a spiritual dimension. Nursing consists of knowledge, thought, values, philosophy, commitment, and action.

# Chapter 5

## Matching

1. b    2. e    3. d    4. f    5. c    6. a
7. (d) *Social:* values human beings in terms of love; is kind, sympathetic and unselfish.
8. (b) *Religious:* values unity.
9. (c) *Theoretical:* values truth and tends to be empirical, critical and rational.
10. (f) *Political:* values power.
11. (a) *Economical:* values what is practical and useful.
12. (e) *Aesthetic:* values beauty, form, and harmony.
13. f    14. h    15. a    16. d    17. g    18. b    19. e    20. c

## Multiple Choice

1. b    2. c    3. b    4. d

## Correct the False Statements

1. true
2. false—utilitarian
3. true
4. true
5. false—human dignity
6. true

## Completion

1. Sample answers:
   a. (1) allocation of scarce nursing resources; (2) conflict between clients and nurse's interests, for example, caring for a patient with AIDS.
   b. (1) disagreement about proposed medical regimen for a client; (2) physician incompetence.
   c. (1) claims of loyalty to a friend; (2) nurse incompetence.
2. The six-step procedure for ethical decision making is:
   Step 1. Identify the problem.
   Step 2. Gather data.
   Step 3. Identify options.
   Step 4. Think the ethical problem through.
   Step 5. Make a decision.
   Step 6. Act and assess.
3. Four chief functions of institutional ethics committees are:
   a. education
   b. policy formation
   c. case review
   d. consultations
4. The five common modes of value transmission are:
   a. Modeling: a child learns what is of high or low value by observing parents, peers and significant others.
   b. Rewarding and punishing: a child is rewarded when demonstrating values held by parents and punished when demonstrating unacceptable values.
   c. Laissez-faire: a child is left to explore values and to develop a personal value system.
   d. Moralizing: a child is taught a complete value system by parents or an institution that allows little opportunity for the child to weigh different values.
   e. Responsible choice: a child is encouraged to explore different values and weigh their consequences with support and guidance.
5. a. Altruism: concern for the rights of others.
   b. Aesthetics: qualities of objects, events, and persons that provide satisfaction.
   c. Equality: having same rights, privileges, or status.
   d. Freedom: capacity to exercise choice.
   e. Human dignity: inherent worth and uniqueness of an individual.
   f. Justice: upholding moral and legal principles.
   g. Truth: faithfulness to fact or reality.

## Sequencing

1. Step 3: chooses after careful consideration of each alternative.
2. Step 1: chooses freely.
3. Step 5: prizes with public affirmation.
4. Step 2: chooses from alternatives.
5. Step 6: acting with incorporation of choice into one's behavior.
6. Step 4: prizing with pride and happiness.
7. Step 7: acting with consistency and regularity on the value.

# C h a p t e r   6

## Matching

1. (c) Slander: An untruthful, oral statement about a person that subjects him to ridicule or contempt.
2. (e) Fraud: The willful or purposeful misrepresentation that could cause, or has caused, loss or harm to a person or property.
3. (b) Battery: An assault carried out that includes willful, angry, violent, or negligent touching of another's person, or clothes, or anything attached to or held by that person.
4. (a) Assault: A threat or attempt to make bodily contact with another person without that person's consent.
5. (d) False imprisonment: Unjustified retention or prevention of movement of another person without proper consent.
6. (g) Invasion of privacy: The right of privacy, or to be left alone, guaranteed by the U.S. Fourth Ammendment.
7. (f) Libel: written defamation.
8. d   9. a   10. e   11. h   12. i   13. f   14. c   15. b
16. g
17. (f) Nurses are legally responsible to carry out orders of physicians in charge unless the order would lead a reasonable person to anticipate injury if carried out.
18. (g) Programs designed to identify, analyze and treat risks.
19. (b) The exchange of a promise between two parties which is legally enforceable.
20. (e) Writing down the complete facts of a situation.
21. (d) Making sure that educational background and clinical experience are adequate to fulfill the nursing responsibilities described in the job description.
22. (c) Protects the nurse in event of a malpractice claim.
23. (a) Discuss the nursing care plan with the client and his family and identify their learning needs and learning readiness.

## Multiple Choice

1. c   2. b   3. a   4. c

## Correct the False Statements

1. true
2. false—voluntary
3. true
4. false—it is needed for each specific diagnostic or surgical procedure
5. false—durable power of attorney for health care
6. true
7. false—U.S. Self Determination Act of 1990
8. true

## Completion

1. a. duty
   b. breach of duty
   c. causation
   d. damages
2. a. Indicate how their governments are created and given authority and state the principles and provisions for establishing specific laws.
   b. Enacted by a legislative body; in the United States, must be in keeping with the state and federal government.
   c. Executive officers designate various agencies that, among other functions, are responsible for law enforcement.
   d. A judiciary system responsible for reconciling controversies; it interprets legislation at the local, state, and national level as applied to specific instances and makes decisions concerning law enforcement.
3. a. Living Wills: Provide specific instruction about the kinds of health care that should be provided or foregone in a particular situation.
   b. Durable Power of Attorney: Appoints an agent that the person trusts to make decisions in event of the appointing person's subsequent incapacity.
4. The eight elements of competent nursing practice are:
   a. Respecting legal boundaries of nursing.
   b. Following institutional procedures and policies.
   c. Owning personal strengths and being aware of weaknesses.
   d. Evaluating proposed assignments.
   e. Keeping current.
   f. Respecting clients' rights and developing rapport with clients.
   g. Careful documentation.
   h. Working with nursing managements to develop and implement programs to improve quality care and decrease risks of client injury.
5. a. Do not discuss the case with anyone at your hospital.
   b. Do not discuss the case with the plaintiff's lawyer.
   c. √ Do not disscuss the case with reporters.
   d. Do not alter the client's records.
   e. √ Go to the witness stand prepared.
   f. Do not volunteer any information.
   g. √ Be courteous on the witness stand.
   h. √ Do not hide any information from your lawyer.

# C h a p t e r   7

## Matching

1. B     2. L     3. S     4. S     5. S     6. L     7. L     8. B
9. B     10. S     11. E     12. g     13. a     14. f     15. b     16. e
17. d     18. c

## Completion

1. self-actualization
2. self-esteem
3. love and belonging
4. safety and security
5. physiologic
6. The 10 community risk factors are:
   a. number and availability of health care services
   b. housing code; fire and police departments
   c. nutritional services
   d. zoning regulations
   e. waste disposal services and locations
   f. pollution guidelines
   g. food sanitation guidelines
   h. health education services
   i. recreational opportunities
   j. prevalence of violent crimes, drug use
7. traditional
8. blended
9. step
10. nuclear
11. extended
12. provide safe, comfortable environment
13. financial aid for family members, monetary needs of society
14. birth of children
15. emotional comfort; help members establish an identity and maintain that identity in times of stress
16. teaching; transmittal of beliefs, values, attitudes, and coping mechanisms; provide feedback and guidance in problem-solving.

# C h a p t e r   8

## Matching

1. g    2. b    3. d    4. a    5. c    6. h    7. f    8. e

## Multiple Choice

1. c    2. d    3. b    4. a    5. b    6. d    7. c    8. a
9. b    10. b

## Correct the False Statements

1. true
2. false—females
3. false—African or Mediterranean
4. True
5. True

## Completion

1. language and dialect
2. religious practices
3. literature
4. folklore
5. music
6. political interests
7. food preferences
8. employment patterns
9. *Yin:* feminine, negative, dark, cold; *Yang:* Masculine, positive, light, warm.
10. Hyperkinetic seizure activity.
11. Technique by which fine needles are inserted into the body at energy pathway points.
12. Special bond between a child's parents and his/her grandparents.
13. Folk healers who base treatments on humoral pathology.
14. a. human cultures
    b. universalities (similarities)
    c. diversities (differences)
    d. care (caring)
    e. health (wellness)
15. a. families headed by single women
    b. the elderly
    c. future generations of those now in poverty
16. a. The cultural background of each participant.
    b. The expectations and beliefs of each about health care.
    c. The cultural context of the encounter.
    d. The degree of agreement between the two persons' sets of beliefs and values.

# C h a p t e r   9

## Matching

1. i   2. f   3. d   4. a   5. c   6. b   7. e   8. g
9. h   10. j   11. e   12. a   13. f   14. c   15. g   16. b
17. i   18. d   19. h

## Multiple Choice

1. c   2. b   3. b   4. d   5. c   6. a   7. d   8. d
9. a   10. c

## Completion

1. a. Optimal functioning in all dimensions.
   b. Normal growth and development.
   c. Normal reactions to physical and emotional stress.
   d. Ability to tolerate changing situations.
2. Phase 1: bleeding is controlled by vasoconstriction of blood vessels at the site. Histamines are released and capillary permeability increases, allowing increased blood flow and white blood cells into the area. Phase 2: exudate is released from the wound. Phase 3: damaged cells are repaired by either regeneration or formation of scar tissue.
3. resistance
4. alarm reaction
5. exhaustion
6. An individual substitutes what is perceived as good or a strength for a perceived weakness.
7. An individual refuses to acknowledge the presence of a condition that is disturbing.
8. An individual's own undesirable impulses are attributed to another person or object.
9. An individual returns to an earlier method of behaving.
10. An individual consciously expresses an unacceptable or impossible impulse or feeling in a more acceptable way.

## Sequencing

1. Step 2: Lists alternatives.
2. Step 3: Chooses from among alternatives.
3. Step 1: Identifies the problem.
4. Step 4: Implements a plan.
5. Step 5: Evaluates.

# C h a p t e r   1 0

## Matching

1. b   2. a   3. e   4. c   5. d   6. e   7. d
8. b   9. a   10. c

## Multiple Choice

1. c   2. a   3. d   4. b   5. d   6. a   7. c

## Correct the False Statements

1. false—genetic heredity
2. true
3. true
4. false—isolation
5. false—the ethic of care

## Completion

1. Growth and development are orderly and sequential and are also continuous and complex.
2. Growth and development follows regular and predictable trends.
3. Growth and development are both differentiated and integrated.
4. Different aspects of growth and development occur at different stages, at different rates, and can be modified.
5. The pace of growth and development is specific for each individual person.
6. The four major concepts are:
   a. stages of development
   b. developmental goals or tasks
   c. psychosocial crises
   d. the process of coping
7. Selfishness
8. Goodness
9. Nonviolence
10. The six functions are:
    a. affective (meeting psychosocial needs)
    b. socialization
    c. reproduction
    d. family coping
    e. economics
    f. providing physical necessities
11. undifferentiated faith
12. intuitive-projective faith
13. mythical-literal faith
14. synthetic-conventional faith
15. individuative reflective faith
16. conjunctive faith
17. universalizing faith
18. superego
19. identity vs role confusion
20. formal operations stage
21. synthetic-conventional faith

# Chapter 11

## Matching

| 1. h | 2. g | 3. a | 4. b | 5. d | 6. c | 7. i | 8. e |
|---|---|---|---|---|---|---|---|
| 9. f | 10. j | 11. a | 12. b | 13. d | 14. f | 15. c | 16. e |

## Multiple Choice

| 1. b | 2. c | 3. a | 4. d | 5. b | 6. a | 7. c | 8. d |
|---|---|---|---|---|---|---|---|
| 9. b | 10. b | | | | | | |

## Correct the False Statements

1. false—toddler
2. true
3. false—adolescents
4. false—gonorrhea
5. true

## Completion

1. Heart rate: over 200 (2); Respiratory effort: good, crying (2); Muscle tone: active motion (2); Reflex irritability: vigorous cry (2); Color: completely pink (2) = normal newborn.
2. a. Nicotine doubles the risk of low birth weight.
   b. Fetal alcohol syndrome causes birth defects, including retarded growth, developmental delay, and impaired intellectual abilities.
   c. Increase the probability of congenital anomalies, low birth weight, and withdrawal syndrome. Crack causes lethargy, hypersensitivity to stimuli, diarrhea, inability to visually focus.
3. The areas assessed are:
   a. gross motor behavior/skills
   b. fine motor behavior/skills
   c. language acquisition
   d. personal/social interaction
4. The six psychosocial needs are:
   a. Learning the physical and psychologic changes of pregnancy.
   b. Accepting his supportive role in meeting maternal dependency needs.
   c. Understanding alterations in sexual need and activity during pregnancy.
   d. Exploring feelings about the developing infant.
   e. Learning about the birthing process.
   f. Accepting his own feelings about the actual birth.
5. Child abuse is the intentional, nonaccidental physical or sexual abuse of a child by a parent or other caregiver entrusted with his or her care (Freiberg, 1987).
6. a. Associate common accidents to developmental level.
   b. Encourage relaxed feeding and regular burping to prevent aspiration.
   c. Emphasize that bottles should not be propped and left with an unattended infant.
   d. Emphasize the use of bumper pads and keeping crib side rails up at all times.
   e. Teach the correct use of infant car seats.
   f. Emphasize never leaving an infant unattended on a table, chair, or regular bed.
   g. Teach proper positioning for sleeping; discourage the use of pillows.
7. a. Sex education needs to begin at age 7 or 8.
   b. Families need encouragement to talk about sex at home.
   c. Caregivers need encouragement to answer questions honestly and correctly.
   d. Menstruation needs to be discussed by at least age 8 (some girls menstruate as young as age 9).
8. a. Fatty tissue redistributed; men tend to develop abdominal fat; women thicken in the middle; weight gain.
   b. Dry skin; wrinkle lines appear; gray hair appears; men may begin to lose hair on the head.
   d. Gradual decrease in muscle mass, strength, and agility; loss of calcium from bone—especially in postmenopausal women.
   e. Changes in near vision (presbyopia); diminished hearing acuity.
   f. Decreasing hormone production, resulting in menopause/andropause.

# C h a p t e r   1 2

## Matching

1. a   2. e   3. c   4. b   5. d

## Multiple Choice

1. c   2. b   3. a   4. d   5. b   6. c   7. a   8. d
9. c   10. d

## Completion

1. individuals over 75 years old
2. a. Adjusting to declining physical strength and health.
   b. Adjusting to retirement and reduced income.
   c. Adjusting to changes in health of one's spouse.
   d. Establishing an explicit affiliation with one's age group.
   e. Adopting and adapting social roles in a flexible way.
   f. Establishing satisfactory physical living arrangements.
3. a. heart disease
   b. cancer
   c. hypertension
   d. arthritis
   e. diabetes mellitus
4. hip fracture surgery
5. Five normal physiologic changes are:
   a. Slower response to multiple stimuli.
   b. Decreased rate of reflex response.
   c. Less efficient temperature regulation and pain perception.
   d. Declining sense of balance; more difficult fine movements.
   e. Shorter sleep at night; awakens more easily.
6. Questions include:
   a. What time do you go to bed?
   b. What time do you get up?
   c. What do you do before you go to bed?
   d. How many hours do you sleep each night?
   e. What time of day do you take naps?

# Chapter 13

## Matching

1. j  2. a  3. i  4. b  5. h  6. c  7. g  8. d
9. f  10. e  11. b  12. a  13. d  14. c  15. e

## Multiple Choice

1. b  2. c  3. a  4. d  5. c

## Completion

1. Schultz' clinical symptoms of grief are:
   a. repeated somatic distress
   b. tightness in the chest
   c. choking or shortness of breath
   d. sighing
   e. empty feeling in the abdomen
   f. loss of muscular power
   g. intense subjective distress
2. The five personal questions are:
   a. If I could control the events that result in my own death, where would I want to be? What cause of death would I choose? Whom would I want to have present during my terminal illness?
   b. What fears do I have about death?
   c. How would I answer these same questions for a terminally ill client for whom I am caring?
   d. How could I improve the quality of care for a terminally ill client for whom I am caring?
   e. If I were a member of the client's family, what things would I want the nurse to do for me?
3. hearing
4. The dying client's physical needs are:
   a. personal hygiene
   b. pain control
   c. nutritional and fluid needs
   d. movement
   e. elimination
   f. respiratory care
5. The circumstances are:
   a. accident
   b. suicide
   c. homicide
   d. illegal therapeutic procedure
6. a. individual
   b. circulatory
   c. respiratory
   d. brain
   e. brainstem
7. Some needs of grieving families are participating:
   a. in some way in what is happening.
   b. by giving some form of care.
   c. by feeling free to either stay at or leave the bedside.
   d. by sharing in mutual decision-making with the health-care staff and the loved one.

# C h a p t e r   1 4

## Matching

1. c    2. e    3. a    4. d    5. b

## Multiple Choice

1. a    2. d    3. d    4. b    5. a

## Correct the False Statements

1. false—nursing process
2. true
3. false—Yura and Walsh
4. true
5. false—nursing process
6. true
7. false—scientific method

## Completion

1. a. Systematic: Each nursing process is part of an ordered sequence of activities.
   b. Dynamic: There is a great interaction and overlapping among the five steps.
   c. Interpersonal: Nurses are client-centered rather than task-centered.
   d. Goal-oriented: Nurses and clients work together to identify specific goals related to wellness promotion, disease/illness prevention, health restoration and coping with altered functioning.
   e. Universally applicable: Once nurses have a working knowledge of the nursing process, they can practice nursing in any type of setting.
2. a. Scientifically based, holistic, individualized care.
   b. The opportunity to work collaboratively with nurses.
   c. Individualized care.
   d. Continuity of care.
3. a. 1972: New York State Nurse Practice Act identified diagnosing as belonging to the legal domain of professional nursing.
   b. 1973: American Nurses Association Standards of Practice included diagnosing as a function of professional nursing.
   c. 1973: First National Conference on Classification of Nursing Diagnosis.

## Sequencing

1. (3) planning
2. (5) evaluating
3. (1) assessing
4. (4) implementing
5. (2) diagnosing

# C h a p t e r   1 5

## Matching

1. c    2. a    3. b    4. f    5. e    6. d    7. a    8. b
9. a    10. a    11. b    12. b    13. b    14. a    15. c

## Multiple Choice

1. d    2. c    3. a    4. a    5. d    6. b    7. d

## Correct the False Statements

1. false—data base assessment
2. false—only data directly related to the planned health care of the client
3. true
4. true
5. true
6. false—person
7. true
8. false—objective data
9. false—functional abilities of the client

## Completion

1. a. introduction
   b. termination
   c. preparatory phase
   d. working phase
2. a. inspection
   b. palpation
   c. percussion
   d. auscultation
3. a. client
   b. support persons
   c. client record
   d. health care professionals
   e. nursing and other health care literature
4. a. health orientation of the client
   b. developmental stage of client
   c. client's need for nursing
5. a. Identify potentially relevant factors in advance of collection. Practice interview strategies.
   b. Determine specific purpose of data collection for each client. Consider existing data before initiating collection. Consider modifying data collection tool or selecting alternative.
   c. Review and practice communication techniques discussed in Chapter 20. Role play several explanations of purposes of data collection. Identify general data desired before collection.
   d. Recollect that it is impossible to give quality care without knowledge of changes in client's status. Ongoing data collection is critical to the deletion or modification of old problems and the identification of new ones.
   e. Sharpen observation skills by independently observing the same situation with a peer and compare notes afterward. Role play several validation techniques.

# C h a p t e r   1 6

## Matching

1. h   2. g   3. a   4. c   5. d   6. b   7. f   8. e
9. (c) Identifying a problem with a client.
10. (a) Recognizing significant data; comparing data to standards.
11. (b Recognizing data clusters rather than single cues.
12. (d) Reaching conclusions; i.e., no problem.
13. (a) Recognizing significant data; comparing data to standards.
14. (c) Identifying a strength in a client.
15. (d) Reaching conclusions; i.e., clinical problem other than nursing diagnosis.

## Multiple Choice

1. c   2. b   3. b   4. a   5. c

## Completion

1. Using legally inadvisable language.
2. √
3. dentifying responses not necessarily unhealthy.
4. √
5. Both clauses say the same thing.
6. √
7. Including value judgment.
8. Identifying responses not necessarily unhealthy.
9. √
10. Including medical diagnosis.
11. Identifying problems as signs and symptoms.
12. Reversing clauses.
13. √
14. Both clauses say the same thing.
15. Identifying problems/etiologies that cannot be altered.
16. Both clauses say the same thing.
17. √

18. Mr. Klinetob, aged 86, has been seriously depressed since the death of his wife of 52 years, 6 months ago. While he suffers from <u>degenerative joint disease</u> and has talked for years about having "just a touch of arthritis," this never kept him from being up and about. Recently, however, <u>he spends all day sitting in a chair</u> and seems to have no desire to engage in self-care activities. He tells the visiting nurse that <u>he doesn't get washed up anymore because he's "too stiff" in the morning to bathe</u> and <u>"just doesn't seem to have the energy."</u> The visiting nurse notices that <u>his hair is matted and uncombed, his face has traces of previous meals, and he has a strong body odor.</u> His adult children have complained that their normally fastidious father seems not to care about personal hygiene any longer.

> *Nursing Diagnosis:* Bathing/Hygiene Self-Care Deficit, related to decreased strength and endurance, discomfort, and depression, as evidenced by matted and uncombed hair, new beard, food particles on face, and strong body odor.

19. Miss Ebenezer sustained a right-sided cerebral infarct that resulted in <u>left hemiparesis</u> (paralysis on left side of body) and <u>left "neglect."</u> <u>She ignores the left side of her body</u> and actually denies its existence. <u>When asked about her left leg, she stated that it belonged to the woman in the next bed</u>—this while she was in a private room. This patient was previously quite active; <u>she walked for 45–60 minutes four or five times a week and was an avid swimmer.</u> At present she <u>cannot move either her left arm or leg.</u>

> *Nursing Diagnosis:* Body Image Disturbance, related to left hemiparesis (paralysis), as evidence by her ignoring the left side of her body following her inability to move it.

20. . . . Rosemary informs the nurse in her pediatrician's office that she is concerned about how all this is affecting her family. <u>"Ted and I both love Sarah and would do nothing to hurt her,</u> but I am so angry about this whole situation that I am afraid I may be taking it out on her." Questioning reveals that Rosemary has found herself <u>yelling at Sarah for minor disobediences and spanking her—something she rarely did before.</u> Both Ted and Rosemary had commented before about Sarah's striking physical resemblance to the fertility specialist but attributed this to coincidence. <u>"Whenever I see her now I can't help but see Dr. Clowser and everything inside me clenches up and I want to scream."</u> Both Ted and Rosemary express great remorse that Sarah, who is innocent, is bearing the brunt of something that is in no way her fault.

> *Nursing Diagnosis:* Parental Role Conflict, related to unexpected discovery about their daughter's biological father, as evidenced by parental concern about increased incidence of parental yelling and spanking and the anger the child evokes in her parents because of her physical resemblance to the fertility specialist who deceived them.

# Chapter 17

## Matching

1. b    2. a    3. d    4. c    5. f    6. e

## Multiple Choice

1. c    2. a    3. b    4. c

## Completion

1. a. Deriving nursing measures from nursing diagnoses.
   b. Identifying options.
   c. Selecting from options.
   d. Writing nursing orders.
2. a. Clear and concise description of nursing action.
   b. Dated when written and reviewed.
   c. Signed by nurse prescribing the order.
   d. Uses abbreviations accepted by institute.
   e. Refers nurse to agency's procedure manual or other literature for steps of routine, lengthy procedures.
3. a. Nursing care related to basic human needs.
   b. Nursing care related to nursing diagnoses.
   c. Nursing care related to medical care of plan.
4. a. Goals stated too generally.
   b. Goals not developed from specific nursing diagnosis.
   c. Nursing orders not written clearly.
   d. Not involving client in planning process.
   e. Failure to update plan of care.
5. Mrs. Myers learns one lesson on nutrition per day, beginning 2/16.
6. After viewing a film on smoking, Mrs. Gray identifies three dangers of smoking.
7. √
8. √
9. By next visit client will list three benefits of psychotherapy
10. √
    Sample answers for 11–15 follow; other goals may also be correct:
11. By 11/2, client will reestablish fluid balance as evidenced by (1) an approximate balance between fluid intake and fluid output—to average approximately 2500 ml; and (2) a urine specific gravity within the normal range—1.010–1.025.
12. By next visit, client will report a resumption of usual level of sexual activity following her acceptance of her new body image.
13. By 6/4, client will report a decrease in the number of stress incontinent episodes (less than one per day), following her use of Kegel's exercises.
14. By 8/10, client reports that he has sufficient energy to carry out the priority activities identified 8/2.
15. By end of shift, client reports better pain management (pain decreased to less than 3 on a scale of 10), related to new administration schedule.

## Sequencing

1. Step 2
2. Step 4
3. Step 1
4. Step 3

# C h a p t e r  1 8

## Matching

1. a   2. b   3. a   4. c   5. b   6. c   7. c   8. a
9. b   10. a   11. c   12. b   13. f   14. d   15. g   16. a
17. c   18. e   19. b

## Multiple Choice

1. c   2. a   3. d   4. b   5. b

## Correct the False Statements

1. true
2. false—problem oriented
3. false—protocals
4. true
5. true
6. false—documentation
7. true

## Completion

1. a. Determining the need for assistance.
   b. Promoting self-care; teaching, counseling, and advocacy.
   c. Assisting clients to meet health goals.
2. a. client variables
   b. nurse variables
   c. resources
   d. current standards of care
   e. research findings
3. a. concise, comprehensive nursing assessment
   b. up-to-date care plan individualized to client
   c. narrative notes
   d. flow sheets
   e. graphic sheets
   f. medical records
   g. discharge summary
4. a. reporting
   b. conferring
   c. referring

# Chapter 19

## Matching

1. a　2. b　3. b　4. a　5. a　6. b　7. a　8. a
9. c　10. c　11. b

## Multiple Choice

1. b　2. c　3. a　4. c　5. d　6. b　7. c　8. d
9. d　10. a

## Completion

1. a. Terminate the plan of care.
   b. Modify the plan of care.
   c. Continue the plan of care.
2. a. Decision on how well the goal was achieved.
   b. All client data or behavior that supports the data.
3. a. *Structure:* focuses on environment in which care is provided.
   b. *Process:* focuses on the nature and sequence of activities carried out by the nurse implementing the nursing process.
   c. *Outcome:* focuses on measurable changes in health status of the client or results of nursing care.
4. a. Develop evaluative criteria.
   b. Collect data and compare it to standards.
   c. Summarize findings and make interpretations.
   d. Identify courses of action.
   e. Take corrective action based on findings.

# C h a p t e r   2 0

## Matching

| | | | | | | | |
|---|---|---|---|---|---|---|---|
| 1. b | 2. c | 3. a | 4. a | 5. c | 6. b | 7. f | 8. c |
| 9. e | 10 h | 11. b | 12. d | 13. a | 14. g | 15. b | 16. c |
| 17. a | 18. e | 19. d | | | | | |

## Multiple Choice

1l.c    2. b    3. b    4. d    5. a    6. c

## True or False

1. T
2. F—Nonverbal communication is more likely to be involuntary.
3. T
4. F—More than one person must be involved in the communication process.
5. F—Communication is influenced by the way people feel about themselves and others.
6. T
7. T
8. F—Past experiences influence what is sent and received.
9. T
10. T

## Completion

1. a. touch
   b. eye contact
   c. facial expression
   d. gait
   e. posture
   f. gestures
   g. general physical appearance
   h. mode of dressing
   i. sounds
   j. silences
2. a. dynamic
   b. purposeful and time-limited
   c. The person providing the assistance assumes the dominant role.
3. a. warmth and friendliness
   b. openness
   c. empathy
   d. competence
   e. consideration of client variables
4. The following are sample answers; other answers may also be acceptable.
   a. Read written word on chart, verbal history, written communication in Kardex and chart, and verbal and nonverbal interaction.
   b. Communication to other nurses and to client;, written communication of diagnosis in Kardex and chart.
   c. Verbal communication with client and other nurses; written communication of plan in Kardex and chart.
   d. Verbal and nonverbal communication in care, e.g., teaching, counseling, supporting, coordinating, written communication in chart.
   e. Verbal and nonverbal feedback to client re: goal achievement; written documentation of client goal achievement in the client record.

# C h a p t e r   2 1

## Matching

| | | | | | | | |
|---|---|---|---|---|---|---|---|
| 1. c | 2. b | 3. a | 4. d | 5. b | 6. a | 7. d | 8. c |
| 9. b | 10. d | 11. f | 12. e | 13. d | 14. a | 15. c | 16. g |
| 17. b | 18. h | 19. a | 20. b | 21. g | 22. e | 23. d | 24. c |
| 25. f | | | | | | | |

## Multiple Choice

| | | | | | | |
|---|---|---|---|---|---|---|
| 1. c | 2. a | 3. a | 4. d | 5. b | 6. d | 7. c |

## Correct the False Statements

1. false—psychomotor
2. false—counseling
3. true
4. false—developmental
5. true
6. true
7. true

## Completion

1. a. the knowledge, attitudes or skills the client/family needs to independently manage health care
   b. readiness to learn
   c. ability to learn
   d. learning strengths
2. a. promoting wellness
   b. preventing illness
   c. restoring health
   d. facilitating coping
3. a. Cognitive Domain: categorizes, defines, explains, lists, states
   b. Affective Domain: chooses, defends, helps, justifies, shares
   c. Psychomotor Domain: arranges, assembles, constructs, shows
4. a. short-term counseling
   b. long-term counseling
   c. motivational counseling

# Chapter 22

## Matching

1. c   2. f   3. b   4. e   5. a   6. d   7. b   8. a
9. b   10. c   11. a

## Multiple Choice

1. a   2. d   3. c   4. b   5. d   6. a

## Correct the False Statements

1. false—mentorship
2. true
3. false—traditional
4. true
5. false—dependent
6. true
7. true

## Completion

1. a. Threat to self: List the advantages of proposed change both for individuals and members of the group.
   b. Lack of understanding: Explain proposed change to all affected persons in simple, concise language.
   c. Limited tolerance for change: Introduce change gradually. Involve everyone affected by change in design and implementation of process.
   d. Disagreement about benefits of change: Relate proposed changes to existing beliefs and values of person or group.
   e. Fear of increased responsibility: Provide incentives for committee to change; for example, money, status, time off, etc.
2. a. Unfreezing—need for change recognized.
   b. Moving—change initiated after careful process of planning.
   c. Refreezing—change becomes operational.
3. a. communication skills
   b. problem solving skills
   c. management skills
   d. self-evaluation skills
4. a. Durable power of attorney for health care: An advance directive which appoints an agent an individual trusts to make decisions about health care in the event of the appointing person's incapacity.
   b. Living will: Nonbinding document expressing a client's desire not to have life sustained by artificial life support systems or heroic efforts.
5. Sample Answers:
   a. Using therapeutic touch findings to guide use of touch in practice. Using research findings on the special needs of rape victims to develop a protocal for rape victims.
   b. Identifying which factors place clients at risk for falls. Identifying factors that enhance nursing satisfaction and decrease staff turnover.
   c. Participating in the evaluation of research proposal. Ensuring that client consent to participate in treatment is truly informed.
6. Sample Answers:
   a. Patient Situation: A 37-year-old female; recently arrived in U.S. from Guatemala and diagnosed with ovarian cancer; does not speak English.
   Nursing Advocacy Response: Obtain a translator and make sure the client understands her diagnosis, prognosis, and treatment options.
   b. Patient Situation: An 88-year-old client, post-stroke, refuses surgical repair of hernia.
   Nursing Advocacy Response: Make sure the patient understands the consequences of refusing treatment, and communicate her wishes to the doctor. If the patient wants to formulate an advance directive, offer to secure legal assistance.

# C h a p t e r   2 3

## Matching

1. e   2. a   3. c   4. b   5. d   6. g   7. h   8. f
9. a   10. b   11. i   12. c   13. e   14. d   15. i   16. f
17. d   18. a   19. b   20. g   21. j   22. h   23. e   24. c
25. e   26. g   27. a   28. b   29. c   30. f   31. h   32. i
33. j   34. d

## Multiple Choice

1. c   2. d   3. a   4. d   5. d   6. c   7. a   8. b
9. c   10. b   11. d   12. a   13. c   14. b   15. d

## Correct the False Statements

1. False—1 1/2 inches
2. False—systolic
3. True
4. False—60–100
5. True
6. False—independent

## Completion

1. a. radiation
   b. convection
   c. evaporation
   d. conduction
2. a. loss of appetite
   b. headache
   c. dry, hot skin
   d. flushed face
   e. thirst
   f. general malaise
3. a. long, thin
   b. blunt
4. a unconscious
   b. irrational
   c. seizure-prone
   d. infants/young children
   e. diseases of the oral cavity
   f. surgery of the mouth or nose
5. The space between the fifth and the sixth ribs, about 8 cm (3 inches) to the left of the median line and slightly below the nipple.
6. Can feel own pulse instead of client's pulse.
7. 1:4
8. In a sitting or standing position, gravity lowers organs in the abdominal cavity, which fall away from the diaphragm. This gives more room for the lungs to expand in the chest, thus allowing them to take in more air with each breath.
9. a. peripheral resistance
   b. pumping action of the heart
   c. blood volume
   d. viscosity of blood
   e. elasticity of vessel walls
10. a. manometer
    b. cuff
11. a. low
    b. low
    c. high
    d. low
    e. high

# C h a p t e r   2 4

## Matching

| | | | | | | | |
|---|---|---|---|---|---|---|---|
| 1. f | 2. a | 3. c | 4. d | 5. g | 6. b | 7. e | 8. c |
| 9. a | 10. b | 11. e | 12. g | 13. d | 14. h | 15. f | 16. c |
| 17. a | 18. b | 19. e | 20. d | 21. d | 22. a | 23. e | 24. i |
| 25. f | 26. c | 27. b | 28. h | 29. g | | | |

## Multiple Choice

| | | | | | | | |
|---|---|---|---|---|---|---|---|
| 1. a | 2. b | 3. d | 4. c | 5. b | 6. d | 7. a | 8. c |
| 9. d | 10. d | | | | | | |

## Correct the False Statements

1. false—inspection
2. false—hirsutism
3. true
4. true
5. false—before
6. false—palpation
7. true
8. true
9. true
10. false—expressive

## Completion

1.  a. Establish a nurse-client relationship.
    b. Gather data about the client's general health status, integrating physiologic, psychologic, cognitive, socio-cultural, developmental, and spiritual dimensions.
    c. Identify client strengths.
    d. Identify actual or potential health problems.
    e. Establish a base for the nursing process.
2.  a. supine
    b. prone
    c. erect
    d. sitting
    e. dorsal recumbent
    f. Sims
    g. lithotomy
    h. knee-chest
3.  a. shape
    b. size
    c. consistency
    d. surface
    e. mobility
    f. tenderness
    g. pulsatile
4.  a. soft
    b. medium
    c. loud
    d. very loud
    e. loud
5.  a. carotid
    b. brachial
    c. radial
    d. femoral
    e. posterior tibial
    f. dorsalis pedis
    g. popliteal
6.  a. pitch
    b. loudness
    c. quality
    d. duration
7.  a. Olfactory–sensory: sense of smell
    b. Optic–sensory: sense of vision
    c. Oculomotor–motor: constrict pupils, raise eyelids
    d. Trochlear–motor: downward and inward eye movements
    e. Trigeminal–motor and sensory: chewing, mastication, sensation of the face and neck
    f. Abducens–motor: lateral eye movements
    g. Facial–motor and sensory: move facial muscles, sense of taste on anterior two thirds of the tongue
    h. Acoustic–sensory: sense of hearing
    i. Glossopharyngeal–motor and sensory: movement of pharynx, swallowing, sense of taste
    j. Vagus–motor: swallowing, speaking
    k. Spinal accessory–motor: moving shoulder muscles
    l. Hypoglossal–motor: tongue movement and strength
8.  a. lub
    b. mitral
    c. tricuspid
    d. ventricular
    e. $S_1$
    f. apical
    g. $S_2$
    h. systole
    i. aortic
    j. pulmonic
    k. dub
    l. one
9.  a. age
    b. changes in breast tissue
    c. pain
    d. discharge from the nipple
    e. knowledge and practice of breast self-examination
10. a. eye opening
    b. motor response
    c. verbal response
11. a. petechiae, freckle
    b. mole
    c. hive, mosquito bite
    d. herpes simplex
    e. acne, impetigo
    f. athlete's foot
    g. common blackhead
    h. common mole
12. a. cecum
    b. appendix
    c. right ovary and fallopian tube (females)
    d. right ureter and lower kidney pole
    e. right spermatic cord (males)

# Chapter 25

## Matching

| | | | |
|---|---|---|---|
| 1. d | 2. g | 3. e | 4. a |
| 5. f | 6. c | 7. b | 8. a |
| 9. b, c | 10. b, c | 11. a, b, c | 12. e |
| 13. a | 14. b | 15. d | 16. c |

## Multiple Choice

1. c    2. d    3. b    4. a    5. b    6. c    7. c    8. a
9. d    10. b    11. a    12. c    13. a

## Correct the False Statements

1. false—incident report
2. true
3. true
4. false—children
5. false—20 pounds
6. true
7. false—stop, drop and roll

## Completion

1. Sample Answers
   a. Developmental considerations: Each age group has its own particular risks. Education to promote awareness of potentially dangerous situations must begin as early as possible and continue throughout the life span.
   b. Life style: Certain occupations, environments, and recreational activities place individuals in more hazardous situations than others. Stress may precipitate unhealthful life styles involving drug or alcohol abuse. Certain areas where crime is prevalent may threaten physical as well as emotional well-being.
   c. Mobility: Any limitation in mobility is potentially unsafe. An elderly client with an unsteady gait is prone to falling. Injuries that limit mobility necessitate the use of supportive devices, and careful instruction and preparation are required for safe use of these devices.
   d. Sensory perception: Any impairment in sight, hearing, smell, taste, or sense of touch can reduce sensitivity to the environment, predisposing the client to falls. An insensitivity to fire alarms, reduction in ability to detect gas or smoke, and the ingestion of tainted food can be directly related to alterations in sensory perception.
   e. Knowledge: An awareness of safety precautions is crucial in promoting and maintaining wellness.
   f. Ability to communicate: Fatigue, stress, medication, aphasia, and language barriers are examples of situations that can affect personal interchange and interfere with an accurate perception of events.
   g. Health state: When an individual is chronically ill or in a weakened health state, the focus of health care includes preventing accidents as well as promoting wellness and restoring the client to a healthy state.
   h. Psychosocial state: Stressful situations tend to narrow an individual's attention span and make him more prone to depression. Depression may result in confusion and disorientation, accompanied by reduced awareness or concern about environmental hazards.

2. a. Age greater than 65.
   b. Previous falls are documented.
   c. Vision or sense of balance is impaired.
   d. Medication regimen includes diuretics, tranquilizers, sedatives/hypnotics, analgesics.
   e. Postural hypotension is recorded.
   f. Reaction time is slowed.
   g. Confusion or disorientation is apparent.
   h. Mobililty is impaired.

3. a. High risk for injury related to refusal to use child safety seat.
   b. High risk for poisoning related to reduced vision.
   c. High risk for suffocation related to child left unattended in bathtub.
   d. High risk for trauma related to history of previous falls.
   e. Impaired home maintenance management related to insufficient finances.

4. a. Thorough orientation to surroundings.
   b. Careful survey of physical surroundings for hazards.
   c. Bed wheels locked and bed in low position.
   d. Call bell and personal articles within client's reach.
   e. Examination of client's footwear.
   f. Use of restraints when alternative measures have failed.

5. a. To restrict the movement of an extremity when an infusion is running.
   b. To help prevent unconscious or delerious clients from pulling at wound dressings and tubings leading from the body.
   c. To help prevent clients who are unsteady and at risk of falling when trying to get out of bed or up in a chair.

6. a. danger of suffocation from improperly applied vests
   b. impaired circulation
   c. altered skin integrity
   d. pressure sores and contractures
   e. dehydration
   f. incontinence
   g. sensory deprivation
   h. emotional distress

7. a. **R**escue the client
   b. sound the **A**larm
   c. **C**onfine the fire
   d. **E**xtinguish it or **E**vacuate

8. a. Allow greatest degree of mobility possible.
   b. For restraint applied to extremity, ensure that two fingers can be inserted between the restraint and client's wrist or ankle.
   c. Pad bony prominences.
   d. Maintain restrained extremity in normal anatomic position.
   e. Use appropriate knot.
   f. Fasten restraint to bed frame and not to the side rail; site should not be readily accessible to the client.

9. a. Kitchen: Checking the condition of the pilot light and securing the stove knobs out of the reach of children; chairs should be at proper height and in good condition; storage areas should be easily reached; floor should be in good condition; knives and sharp instruments should be kept out of reach of children; cleaning chemicals should be kept out of reach of children; make sure electrical outlets are grounded.

   b. Living Room: Stairways should be secured from children falling; rooms should be uncluttered to permit easy mobility; electrical outlets should be covered by childproof devices.

   c. Bedroom: Checking the accessibility of light switches; adequacy of lighting; bed and chairs should be of adequate height; young children should have appropriate size bed and railings.

   d. Bathroom: Placing mat or skidproof strips in tub/shower; illuminate medicine cabinet and secure from access by children; make sure electrical outlets by sink have grounds and automatic shut-off.

   e. Porch and Yard: Checking to see that sidewalks and steps are in good repair, with handrails securely fastened; there should be adequate lighting; holes and wells should be filled in; pools should have locked fence to keep small children out.

10. Sample Answers

   a. Kitchen: cleaners, medicines, insecticides.

   b. Bedroom: cosmetics, diet pills, vitamins.

   c. Laundry Room: bleaches, detergents, disinfectants.

   d. Bathroom: medicines, deodorizers, drain openers.

   e. Garage/basement: antifreeze, gasoline, paint stripper.

   f. Living Room: cigarette butts, plants, lamp oil.

11. a. Use equipment only for the use for which it was intended.

   b. Do not operate equipment with which you are unfamiliar.

   c. Handle equipment with care to prevent damaging it.

   d. Use three-prong electric plugs whenever possible.

   e. Do not twist or bend electric cords. The wires in the cords might break.

   f. Be alert to signs that indicate that equipment is faulty, such as breaks in electric cords, sparks, smoke, electric shocks, loose or missing parts, and unusual noises or odors. Report signs of trouble immediately.

   g. Make certain that electric cords are not in a position to be trapped as beds are raised or lowered. This can strip insulation covering the electric wires.

   h. Be alert for wet surfaces on areas where electric cords or connections are present.

## Sequencing

1. a. 3
   b. 1
   c. 9
   d. 7
   e. 6
   f. 8 or 4
   g. 5
   h. 2
   i. 4 or 8

# Chapter 26

## Matching

| | | | |
|---|---|---|---|
| 1. i | 2. g | 3. c | 4. a |
| 5. l | 6. h | 7. j | 8. d |
| 9. f | 10. e | 11. b | 12. k |
| 13. c | 14. a | 15. d | 16. b |
| 17. d | 18. a | 19. c | 20. b |
| 21. e | 22. c | 23. a | 24. c |
| 25. b, c | 26. d | 27. e | 28. a |
| 29. c | 30. d | 31. b | |

## Multiple Choice

| | | | | | | |
|---|---|---|---|---|---|---|
| 1. c | 2. d | 3. a | 4. b | 5. a | 6. c | 7. a |
| 8. d | 9. a | 10. b | | | | |

## Correct the False Statements

1. false—sterilization
2. false—medical asepsis
3. true
4. true
5. true
6. false—disease specific isolation
7. true

## Completion

1. a. Infectious agent: Some of the most prevalent agents capable of causing infection include bacteria, viruses and fungi.
   b. Reservoir: The reservoir for growth and multiplication of microorganisms is the natural habitat of the organism. Possible reservoirs include other humans and animals, as well as food, water, milk, and inanimate objects.
   c. Portal of exit: The portal of exit from the reservoir is the point of escape for the organism. Common escape routes include respiratory, gastrointestinal and genitourinary tracts, as well as breaks in the skin.
   d. Means of transmission: An organism may be transmitted from its reservoir via direct contact, indirect contact, vehicles, airborne routes, or vectors.
   e. Portal of entry: The portal of entry is the point at which organisms enter a host. The urinary, respiratory, gastrointestinal tracts, and the skin are common entry points.
   f. Susceptible host: For microorganisms to continue to exist, they must find a source that is acceptable and overcome any resistance mounted by the host's defenses.

2. a. Direct contact: Direct contact involves close proximity between the susceptible host and an infected person or carrier, such as occurs in touching, kissing, or sexual intercourse.
   b. Indirect contact: Indirect contact requires personal contact with an inanimate object, such as a contaminated instrument.
   c. Vectors: Vectors such as mosquitoes, ticks, and lice are nonhuman carriers that transmit organisms from one host to another.
   d. Airborne route: Microorganisms can be spread via the airborne route by droplet nuclei when coughing, sneezing, and talking, or by becoming attached to dust particles.
   e. Vehicles: Contaminated blood, food, or inanimate objects are vehicles for routes of transmission.

3. Sample Answers—other answers may also be correct.
   a. Intact skin and mucous membranes protect the body against microbial invasion.
   b. The normal pH levels of gastric secretions, and of the genitourinary tract, help ward off microbial invasion.
   c. The body's white blood cells influence resistance to certain pathogens.
   d. Immunization, natural or acquired, acts to resist infection.
   e. Fatigue, climate, nutritional and general health status, the presence of preexisting illnesses, and some kinds of medicines play a part in the susceptibility of a potential host.
   f. Stress may adversely affect the body's normal defense mechanisms.

4. Sample Answers—other answers may also be correct.
   a. Client will use appropriate cleansing and disinfecting techniques.
   b. Client will demonstrate an awareness of the necessity of proper immunizations.
   c. Client will demonstrate proper hand washing.
   d. Client will demonstrate proper disposal of soiled articles.

5. Sample Answers—other answers may also be correct.
   a. Home: Wash hands before preparing food or eating. Keep foods refrigerated, especially those containing mayonnaise
   b. Using public facilities: Wash hands after using any public bathroom. Use tongs to lift food from common service trays in cafeterias, food stores, or salad bars.
   c. Community: Food handlers should be examined for evidence of disease. Sterilized combs and brushes should be used in barber and beauty shops.

6. a. Escherichia coli
   b. Staphylococcus aureus
   c. Streptococcus faecalis
   d. Pseudomonas aeruginosa
   e. Klebsiella

7. a. Constant surveillance by infection control committees and nurse epidemiologists.
   b. Having written infection prevention practices for all agency personnel.
   c. Using practices to help promote and keep clients in the best possible physical condition.
8. a. Transient bacteria: Transient bacteria, normally picked up by the hands in the usual activities of daily living, are relatively few on clean and exposed areas of the skin. They are attached loosely to the skin, usually in grease, fats and dirt, and are found in greater numbers under the fingernails. They can be removed with relative ease by thorough and frequent hand washing.
   b. Resident bacteria: Resident bacteria, normally found in creases in the skin, are relatively stable in number and type. They cling tenaciously to the skin by adhesion and adsorption, and considerable friction with a brush is required to remove them.
9. a. Nature of organisms present: Some organisms are destroyed easily while others are able to withstand certain commonly used sterilization and disinfection methods.
   b. Number of organisms present: The more organisms present on an item, the longer it takes to destroy them.
   c. Type of equipment: Equipment with small lumens, crevices or joints require special care. Certain articles may be damaged by various sterilization and disinfection methods and require special handling.
   d. Intended use of equipment: The need for medical or surgical asepsis influences the preparation and cleansing of equipment.
   e. Available means for sterilization and disinfection: The choice of chemical or physical means of sterilization or disinfection is made on the basis of the nature and number of organisms, the type and intended use of the equipment, and the availability and practicality of the means.
   f. Time: Time is a key factor. Failure to observe recommended time periods is grossly negligent.

10. a. Wear gloves when contact with body substances, mucous membranes, or nonintact skin is likely.
    b. Wear a gown or plastic apron to prevent soiling of clothing from bodily substances.
    c. Wear masks and/or eyegear to protect mucous membranes of eyes, nose and mouth from splattering of body substances.
    d. Use good hand-washing technique before, after, and between each client contact.
    e. Place uncapped needles and sharp instruments in puncture-proof containers.
    f. Bag soiled linen securely before transporting to laundry area. Dispose of trash in plastic bags according to agency policy.

## Sequencing

1. a. 3
   b. 6
   c. 11
   d. 7
   e. 9
   f. 1
   g. 4
   h. 2
   i. 10
   j. 8
   k. 5

# Chapter 27

## Matching

1. d  2. a  3. e  4. b  5. c  6. f  7. g  8. i
9. d  10. k  11. a  12. c  13. j  14. h  15. f  16. l
17. b  18. e

## Multiple Choice

1. a  2. c  3. d  4. a  5. b  6. d  7. c  8. d

## Completion

1. a. Obtaining consent: The physician is responsible for obtaining a signed consent form prior to any diagnostic test. The client has the right to know what the test involves, any risks or complications, and any other available options.
   b. Scheduling tests: The nurse may be responsible for scheduling diagnostic tests with another hospital departments. The nurse must have a thorough understanding of the procedure and know the proper sequence when multiple tests have been ordered.
   c. Preparing the client: The nursing care plan should incorporate physical and psychologic preparation of the client. Generally, the nurse follows written protocols for physical preparation. The nurse needs to recall personal experiences and rely on interpersonal communication to help client deal with the test psychologically.
   d. assembling the equipment: Responsibility for assembling equipment for the test will vary, depending on the setting. The nurse is usually responsible for gathering supplies when the examination is performed at the client's bedside or in a nearby treatment room. If the procedure is sterile, the nurse maintains surgical asepsis. Protective equipment must be available.
2. a. Collecting baseline data: The nurse is responsible for informing the physician of any manifestation that may threaten life that has caused difficulty in the past. Undue anxiety should be noted.
   b. Evaluating the client: The nurse focuses on physical reaction and emotional state during the procedure. The nurse needs to be alert for significant deviations from baseline vital signs, nausea or vomiting, pallor, unusual pain, or excessive anxiety.
   c. Supporting the client: The nurse respects the client's sense of privacy and provides a drape or cover to ensure warmth. The nurse may have to touch therapeutically to assist the client to hold steady in an uncomfortable position. Holding a client's hand may provide comfort during stressful or painful moments.
   d. Assisting the examiner: The nurse may be responsible for handing equipment to the physician and providing additional supplies as needed in addition to maintaining a sterile field and using whatever protective equipment is required.

3. a. Assessing the client: Baseline data should be available for comparison and may indicate the onset of any adverse reactions. Some tests require frequent assessments recorded on a flowsheet at the client's bedside.
   b. Assisting the client: In addition to being aware of clinical implications after the study, the nurse is concerned about the client's comfort. Supportive measures that provide warmth, relieve pain, or provide direction and explanations are effective nursing interventions.
   c. Preparing for specimens and caring for equipment: Any specimen obtained during a test must be properly identified and delivered to the appropriate laboratory. The label should include client name, identification number, date, and nature of specimen. Reusable equipment must be rinsed of blood and body fluids and prepared for sterilization. Disposable equipment needs to be discarded in proper receptacles.
   d. Documenting the procedure: After a procedure is completed, the nurse needs to record the date and time, the type of diagnostic study, whether a specimen was obtained, and the client's response.
4. a. Procedure: A liver biopsy is the needle aspiration of a sample of liver tissue. The procedure is brief and may be administered at bedside. The client assumes a supine position with right hand placed under the head. Client is asked to hold breath 10 seconds after exhalation. Using sterile technique physician inserts needle between two of the right lower ribs or below the right rib cage, obtains biopsy specimen and removes needle. Client should resume breathing and a pressure dressing should be applied.
   Nursing responsibilities: Collecting baseline data and reviewing pertinent laboratory reports, reporting abnormalities to physician, explaining to the client details and instructions for the procedure, assessing client after the procedure, being alert for complications.
   b. Procedure: A lumbar puncture is the insertion of a needle into the subarachnoid space in the spinal canal to obtain fluid for analysis, relieve pressure, inject drugs, or inject dyes. The client is positioned on the side with knees flexed and head bent forward with chin touching chest.
   Nursing responsibilities: Observe the client's reaction during the procedure; note color, pulse rate, and respiratory rate and report abnormalities to physician. Place client in recumbent position following procedure and offer fluids. Observe client's general physical reaction to the procedure and report unusual reactions such as twitching, vomiting, or slow pulse.
   c. Procedure: Surgical asepsis is observed to withdraw fluid from the peritoneal cavity. A sterile trocar and cannula are used to enter the peritoneal cavity near the midline of the abdomen, approximately halfway between the umbilicus and the pubis.
   Nursing responsibilities: Weigh client and measure abdominal girth prior to and after the procedure. Record baseline vital signs and encourage client to void before procedure. Place client in sitting position. During and after procedure observe client for untoward reactions associated with electrolyte imbalance. Note client's color, blood pressure, pulse and respiratory rate. Note type and amount of drainage present. Place sterile, heavy dressing over incision.

d. Procedure: Thoracentesis is the entering and aspirating of fluid from the pleural cavity in order to obtain a specimen or remove accumulated fluids. The procedure is done at bedside, sitting on a chair or edge of bed. After a local anesthetic is administered, the needle is inserted between the ribs through the intercostal muscles and fascia and into the pleura. The needle is removed and a small sterile dressing is placed over entry site.

Nursing responsibilities: Collect baseline data prior to the examination, instruct client to lie very still. Observe client for color, pulse rate, and respiration, and report any deviation from the norm to physician. Watch for signs of punctured lung such as blood in sputum and respiratory distress.

e. Procedure: The electrical activity of the heart is received through electrodes placed on the skin on various places on the body. Normal and abnormal findings are recognized for each placement of leads. The ruled paper for an EKG is calibrated to assist in reading it. The horizontal lines represent the measurement of voltage and the vertical lines measure time. When the heart is diseased, the waves may be abnormal in size, form, or position.

Nursing responsibilities: Explain the purpose and technique to the client and instruct him to lie quietly while the tracing is being recorded. Explain electricity will not be transferred to the body.

f. Procedure: Radiography is the use of X-rays to secure data about health status. An X-ray is a high energy electromagnetic wave capable of penetrating solid matter and acting on photographic film. X-rays determine the size, shape, and functioning of some organs, the characteristics of bones, and detect of masses.

Nursing responsibilities: Teach and prepare persons as necessary. Food and fluid restrictions will vary. Nurse is responsible for monitoring the client's condition and recording observations when the diagnostic procedure is completed.

g. Procedure: Magnetic and radio-frequency waves produce cross-sectional images of body tissues on a computer screen to provide unique information about the chemical make-up of tissues. MRI is a noninvasive procedure that requires client to be placed head first in the supine position into a narrow tunnel-like machine. All metal objects must be removed from client.

Nursing responsibilities: Prepare client for the claustrophobic experience of an MRI scan. Suggest client close eyes. Client needs to remain still. Client should empty bladder prior to test for comfort. No observations are necessary after test.

h. Procedure: Ultrasonography is a noninvasive procedure that involves the use of ultrasound to produce an image or photograph of an organ or tissue. A transducer converts energy from one form to another, produces the ultrasound waves and converts the reflected waves into electrical energy. The electrical energy produces an image on a viewing screen which can be recorded. The person will be asked to remain quiet during the procedure.

Nursing responsibilities: No special preparations are necessary except for abdominal ultrasonography which requires food and fluid restrictions. There is no discomfort with this procedure.

# C h a p t e r   2 8

## Matching

1. e   2. c   3. b   4. a   5. d

## Multiple Choice

1. d   2. c   3. a   4. b   5. d

## Correct the False Statements

1. true
2. false—highest
3. false—remains at the hospital
4. true
5. false—physician's order

## Completion

1. a. Include discharge planning in the care of any person admitted to any type of health-care setting.
   b. Collaborate with other health team members in meeting needs of the client and family in all settings and in all levels of health.
   c. Involve the client and his/her family in the planning process.
2. a. Recognize and take necessary steps to reduce anxiety.
   b. Remember that the medical or surgical condition for which the client is being treated is only one part of his/her life.
   c. Communicate with the client as an individual so that he or she can maintain a personal identity.
   d. Take time to learn who the client being admitted is.
   e. Provide for client/family participation and decision-making in all aspects of care.
3. A systematic process of preparing the client to leave the health-care facility and for maintaining continuity of care.
4. Have the client sign a form releasing the hospital and physician from responsibility for any ill effects that may result from such action. Client's signature must be witnessed; financial arrangements must be completed.
5. a. Are there barriers that inhibit function?
   b. Are there assistive devices in the bathroom?
   c. Is hot water, heat, and space needed for supplies available?
   d. Is the community rural or urban?
   e. Is health care accessible and readily available?
   f. Is transportation available?
   g. Are there any known hazards in the environment?

# C h a p t e r   2 9

## Matching

| | | | | | | | |
|---|---|---|---|---|---|---|---|
| 1. b | 2. e | 3. d | 4. m | 5. l | 6. i | 7. h | 8. g |
| 9. a | 10. c | 11. k | 12. f | 13. j | 14. d | 15. e | 16. a |
| 17. c | 18. b | 19. f | 20. b | 21. a | 22. e | 23. d | 24. c |

## Multiple Choice

| | | | | | | | |
|---|---|---|---|---|---|---|---|
| 1. b | 2. d | 3. a | 4. c | 5. d | 6. c | 7. b | 8. a |
| 9. c | 10. a | | | | | | |

## Correct the False Statements

1. true
2. false—ischemia
3. true
4. true
5. false—outer canthus
6. false—mouth
7. true
8. false—close
9. true

## Completion

1. a. The skin protects the body: Invasion of the body by bacteria is prevented by the skin. Injury to underlying tissues and organs is decreased by intact skin.
   b. The skin helps regulate body temperature: The production of perspiration and its loss by evaporation help cool the body. Much heat is lost from the body by radiation and by conduction when the blood supply to the skin is increased by vasodilation.
   c. The skin is a sense organ: There are receptors for pain, touch, pressure, and temperature in the skin that help the body receive stimuli from the environment.
   d. The skin is an excretory organ: Water, salts, and nitrogenous wastes are lost from the skin, although in much smaller quantities than are lost from the kidneys.
   e. The skin helps maintain water and electrolyte balance: The escape of excess water and electrolytes from the body is prevented by the skin.
   f. The skin produces and absorbs vitamin D: A precursor for vitamin D is present in skin, which in conjunction with ultraviolet rays from the sun produces vitamin D.
2. a. Shortly after awakening, the client is assisted with toileting, if necessary, and then provided comfort measures designed to refresh the client, and in preparation for breakfast (or diagnostic tests).
   b. After breakfast, the nurse completes morning care. Depending on the client's self-care abilities, the nurse offers assistance with toileting, oral care, bathing, back massage, special skin care measures, hair care, cosmetics, dressing, and positioning for comfort. Agency policies are followed in refreshing or changing bed linens, and the client's bedside area is tidied.
   c. Since clients frequently receive visitors in the afternoon or evening, or use this time to rest when not scheduled for tests, the nurse should ensure the client's comfort after lunch and offer assistance to nonambulatory clients with toileting, hand washing and oral care. Straightening bed linens and helping clients with mobility problems to reposition themselves comfortably are other welcome measures.
   d. Shortly before client retires, the nurse offers assistance with toileting, washing of face and hands, and oral care. Many clients find that a back massage helps them to relax. Soiled bed linens or clothing should be changed and the client positioned comfortably. Protective devices should be checked and the call light and other objects the client needs should be placed within easy reach.
   e. As needed care: The nurse offers individual hygiene measures as needed. Clients who are diaphoretic may need their clothing and bed linens changed several times a shift.
3. Elements of a safe bedside unit include the following: client call light functioning and always within reach; bed positioned properly and at the appropriate height; side rails and restraints safely used when indicated; principles of medical asepsis followed; electrical equipment safely grounded; and uncluttered walk space. Factors providing a comfortable bedside unit include attention to ventilation, odors, room temperature, lighting, and noise.

4. Sample Answers
   a. Bathe less frequently, especially when the outdoor temperature and humidity are low.
   b. Avoid defatting agents, such as alcohol, on dry and easily injured skin.
   c. Add moisture to the air through a humidifier.
   d. Use an emollient to soften and soothe, and protect dry skin after it is cleansed.
   e. Increase fluid intake.

5. Sample Answers
   a. Client's lips, oral mucosa, gums, and tongue are intact, moist, and free of inflammation and lesions.
   b. The client demonstrates the ability to masticate and swallow food.
   c. Client verbalizes the importance of fluoride use and regular dental examinations.

6. a. Clean the eye from the inner canthus to the outer canthus, using a wet, warm washcloth, cotton ball, or compress to soften crusted areas. Use artificial tear solution or normal saline at least every four hours when the blink reflex is decreased or absent. Offer correct eyeglasses, contact lens, or artificial eye care instruction.
   b. Clean the external ear with a washcloth-covered finger, instructing client never to insert objects into the ear for cleaning purposes. Assist with the softening and removal of excessive wax deposits. Offer hearing aid teaching and care.
   c. Clean the nose by instructing the client to blow the nose while both nares are patent, unless contraindicated. Remove crusted secretions around the nose and keep this tissue intact by applying a non-water soluble ointment.

7. a. Stage one: The primary sign is redness. The skin doesn't return to a normal color when the pressure is relieved, but there is no induration; the skin and underlying tissues remain soft.
   b. Stage two: Redness persists, usually accompanied by edema and induration. The epidermis may blister or erode.
   c. Stage three: There is an open lesion and a crater, exposing subcutaneous tissue. You may be able to see fascia at the base of the ulcer.
   d. Stage four: Necrosis will extend through the fascia and may even involve the bone. Eschar is a common finding. Bone destruction can lead to periostitis, osteitis, and osteomyelitis.

## Chapter 29: Case Study

1. Objective data are underlined; subjective data are bold-faced.

Mrs. Chijioke, <u>an 88-year-old woman</u> who lived alone for years, was brought to the hospital after neighbors found her lying at the bottom of her cellar steps. She <u>broke her hip</u> and is now <u>three days after hip repair surgery</u>. The nurse assigned to care for Mrs. Chijioke noticed during the patient's bath that the <u>skin of her coccyx, heels and elbows was reddened</u>. The <u>skin did return to a normal color when pressure was relieved in these areas</u>. There was <u>no edema, nor was there induration or blistering</u>. While Mrs. Chijioke was able to be lifted out of bed into a chair, <u>she spent most of the day in bed, lying on her back with an abductor pillow between her legs</u>. At <u>5', 89 pounds,</u> Mrs. Chijioke looked lost in the big hospital bed. Her <u>eyes were bright</u> and she usually <u>attempted a warm smile, but she had little physical strength and would lie seemingly motionless for hours</u>. Her <u>skin was wrinkled and paper thin and her arms were already bruised from unsuccessful attempts at initiating intravenous therapy</u>. Dehydrated on admission since **she had spent almost 48 hours crumpled at the bottom of her steps before being found by her neighbors,** Mrs. Chijioke was clearly in need of nutritional, fluid, and electrolyte support. A long-time diabetic, Mrs. Chijioke is now spiking a <u>temperature (39.0°C–102.2°F)</u>, which concerns her nurse.

## 2. Nursing Process Worksheet

**Health Problem:**
High risk for impaired skin integrity.

**Etiology:**
Immobility, effects of aging, dehydration, and effects of illness.

**Signs & Symptoms (Defining Characteristics):**
Skin of her coccyx, heels and elbows is reddened — returns to normal color when pressure is relieved; lies on back motionless when unattended; skin is wrinkled and thin; elevated temperature: 39.0°C

**Client Goal:**
Whenever observed, the client's skin appears clean and intact (no redness, blistering, indurations).

**Nursing Interventions:**
1. Reposition client in correct alignment at least every 1 to 2 hours and ensure protection of pressure points where possible; examine skin for signs of breakdown with each position change.
2. Massage pressure points and keep skin clean and dry.
3. Keep bed linens dry and free of wrinkles.
4. Monitor high risk factors: dehydration, effects of illness.

**Evaluative Statement:**
10/6/93: Goal met. Client's skin is clean and intact and shows no signs of breakdown. Continue prevention program.

*M. Wong, RN*

3. *Client strengths:* Concerned neighbors; until now has been able to care for herself and keep herself in good health.
*Personal strengths:* Ability to recognize clients at high risk for problems such as impaired skin integrity. Strong commitment to meeting the needs of geriatric clients. Experienced clinician.

4. 10/6/93: Client remains on a 2-hour positioning regimen. The protective heel and elbow pads have resulted in intact skin in these areas—no redness. The skin on her coccyx appears reddened after she lies on her back but the redness disappears when the pressure is relieved. No constant redness, edema or induration. Skin remains dry—lotion applied with each position change.

*M. Wong, RN*

# C h a p t e r   3 0

## Matching

1. 1   2. a   3. g   4. o   5. d   6. k   7. b   8. n
9. c   10. m   11. j   12. h   13. e   14. i   15. f   16. d
17. b   18. c   19. a   20. a   21. b   22. d   23. c
24. e (joints between the atlas and axis)
25. a (shoulder and hip joints)
26. f (joint between carpezium and metacarpal of thumb)
27. b (wrist joint)
28. c (carpal bones of wrist)
29. d (elbow, heel, and ankle joints)
30. o   31. n   32. i   33. f   34. h   35. a   36. c   37. d
38. m   39. j   40. k   41. l   42. b   43. e   44. g   45. g
46. d   47. h   48. a   49. f   50. b   51. e   52. c

## Multiple Choice

1. a   2. d   3. b   4. c   5. d   6. d   7. a   8. c
9. b   10. a   11. d   12. d   13. a

## Correct the False Statements

1. false—shape
2. true
3. false—tendons
4. false—point of insertion
5. true
6. true
7. true
8. false—isometric
9. true
10. false—elevation
11. false—quadriplegia
12. true

## Completion

1. See Table on next page.

| Body System | Effects of Exercise | Effects of Immobility |
|---|---|---|
| **Cardiovascular** | ↑ efficiency of heart<br>↓ resting heart rate, blood pressure<br>↑ blood flow and oxygenation—body parts | ↑ cardiac workload<br>↑ risk of, orthostatic hypotension<br>↑ risk of venous thrombosis |
| **Respiratory** | ↑ depth of respiration<br>↑ respiratory rate<br>↑ gas exchange at alveolar level<br>↑ rate carbon dioxide excretion | ↓ depth of respiration<br>↓ rate of respiration<br>pooling of secretions<br>impaired gas exchange |
| **Gastrointestinal** | ↑ appetite<br>↑ intestinal tone | disturbance in appetite<br>altered protein metabolism, digestion |
| **Urinary** | ↑ blood flow to kidneys<br>↑ efficiency maintaining fluid and acid base balance<br>↑ efficiency in excreting body wastes | ↑ urinary stasis<br>↑ risk of renal calculi<br>↓ bladder muscle tone |
| **Musculoskeletal** | ↑ muscle efficiency<br>↑ coordination<br>↑ efficiency of nerve impulse transmission | ↓ muscle size, tone, and strength<br>↓ joint mobility<br>↓ flexibility<br>bone demineralization<br>↓ endurance, stability<br>↑ risk of contractures |
| **Metabolic** | ↑ efficiency of metabolic system<br>↑ efficiency of body temperature regulation | ↑ risk of electrolyte imbalance<br>altered exchange of nutrients and gases |
| **Integument** | improved tone, color<br>turgor from improved circulation | ↑ risk of skin breakdown and formation of pressure ulcers |
| **Psychological Well-Being** | energy, vitality<br>general well-being<br>improved sleep<br>improved appearance<br>improved self-concept<br>positive health behaviors | ↑ sense of powerlessness<br>↓ self-concept<br>↓ social interaction<br>↓ sensory stimulation<br>altered sleep-wake pattern<br>↑ risk of depression |

2. a. It supports the soft tissues of the body.
   b. It protects the delicate structures of the body.
   c. It furnishes surfaces for the attachments of muscles, tendons and ligaments which in turn pull on the individual bones and produce movement.
   d. It serves as storage areas for mineral salts and fat.
   e. It produces blood cells.
3. a. Body alignment or posture: Permits optimal musculoskeletal balance and operation and promotes healthy physiologic functioning. No undue strain on joints, muscles, tendons, or ligaments while balance is maintained.
   b. Balance: A body in correct alignment is balanced. An object is balanced when its center of gravity is close to its base of support, the line of gravity goes through the base of support, and the object has a wide base of support.
   c. Coordinated body movement: Using major muscle groups rather than weaker ones takes advantage of the body's natural levers and fulcrums.
4. a. Improved cardiopulmonary function
   b. Decreased blood pressure
   c. Increased bone mineral content
   d. Increased muscle strength, coordination, and joint range of motion
   e. Improved fat and carbohydrate metabolism
5. a. The nurse would assess Mrs. Mulherin's general ease of movement: are body parts fluid, voluntarily controlled, coordinated; gait—is head erect, vertebrae straight, knees and feet forward, arms swinging freely in alternation with leg swings; alignment—in standing position, can a straight line be drawn from the ear through the shoulder and hip, and in bed, are the head, shoulders, and hips aligned; joint structure and function—are there joint deformities, is there a full range of motion; muscle mass, tone and strength—are they adequate to accomplish movement/work; endurance—is she able to turn in bed, maintain correct alignment when sitting and standing, ambulate and perform self-care activities?
   b. Activity intolerance related to decreased muscle mass, tone, and strength. Impaired physical mobility related to muscle atrophy (contractures) and limited joint mobililty (ankylosis).
   c. Do range of motion exercises twice a day regularly to build up muscle and joint capabilities. Use quadriceps drills two or three times each hour, four to six times a day. Do gluteal settings twice a day and push-ups three or four times a day.

6. a. Rocking bed: The bed is adjusted to rock at the frequency of client's respiration. The rocking aids respiration by shifting the abdominal viscera, which in turn helps move the diaphragm up and down, helping air to be forced into and out of the lungs.
   b. Chair bed: permits the client to be in a semi-sitting position, which may aid the client's cardiac output.
   c. Circular bed: The direction of support can be changed so the client can be placed in a variety of positions; especially helpful for client who will be completely helpless for an extended period.
   d. Stryker frame: The client can be alternated between the supine and prone positions without changing alignment; useful for totally immobilized client.
   e. Footboards: Helps avoid footdrop by providing a firm surface against which the feet of the bed-fast client can be placed for proprioceptor stimulation.
   f. Sandbags: Sandbags immobilize an extremity and support body alignment.
   g. Trochanter rolls: Used to support the hips and legs so that the femurs do not rotate outward.
   h. Trapeze bar: The client can grasp the bar with one or both hands and then raise the trunk from the bed. It can also be used to perform exercises.
7. a. Fowler's position: Calls for the head of the bed to be elevated from 45–60 degrees. This position promotes cardiac and respiratory functioning because abdominal organs drop in this position and provide maximal space in the thoracic cavity.
   b. Supine or dorsal recumbent position: The client lies flat on the back with the head and shoulders slightly elevated with a pillow. The feet and neck are in need of attention in this position.
   c. Side-lying or lateral position: The client lies on the side and the main weight of the body is borne by the lateral aspect of the lower scapula and the lateral aspect of the lower ilium. It relieves pressure on the scapulae, sacrum, and heels, and allows the legs and feet to be comfortably flexed.
   d. Prone position: The client lies on the abdomen with the head turned to the side; client is straightened out in this position. This position helps to prevent flexion contractures of the hips and knees.
8. a. Walker: A lightweight metal frame with four legs. It provides a sense of security and support.
   b. Canes: Three variations—single-ended canes with a half-circle handle, single-ended canes with straight handles, canes with three or four prongs to provide a wide base of support.
   c. Braces: Braces that support weakened leg muscles are available in many variations and must be fitted properly.
   d. Crutches: Underarm or axillary crutches are most commonly used. They must be measured and client must be taught to use them.
9. Sample Answers:
   a. Client will demonstrate correct execution of isometric/isotonic exercise program.
   b. Client will perform activities of daily living with greatest degree of independence possible.
   c. Client will independently (or with the use of adaptive devices) demonstrate correct alignment, transfers, and ambulation.

## Chapter 30: Case Study

1. Objective data are underlined; subjective data are bold-faced.

Robert Witherspoon, a <u>42-year-old university professor</u>, presented for his first "physical" shortly after his father's death. His father died of complications of coronary artery disease. Mr. Witherspoon is <u>5 feet 9 inches tall, weighs 235 pounds</u>, has a decided "<u>paunch</u>," and reports that **until now, he has made no time for exercise because he preferred to utilize any free time he had reading or listening to classical music. He enjoys French cuisine, including rich desserts**, and has a cholesterol level of 310 mg/dl [normal is 150mg-250mg/dl]. He expresses being **frightened by his father's death** and is appropriately concerned about his elevated cholesterol level. **"I guess I've never given much thought to my health before. . . but my dad's death changed all that. I know coronary artery disease runs in families and I can tell you that I'm not ready to pack it all in yet.** Tell me what I have to do to fight this thing." He admits that he used to tease a colleague—who lowered his cholesterol from 290 to 200 by diet and exercise alone—by accusing him of being a fitness freak. **"Now I'm recognizing the wisdom of his health behaviors and wondering if diet and exercise won't do the trick for me**. Can you help me design an exercise program that will work?"

2. **Nursing Process Worksheet**

**Health Problem:**
Altered health maintenance; lack of exercise program.

**Etiology:**
Low value placed on fitness and self-care behaviors in the past.

**Signs & Symptoms (Defining Characteristics):**
5'9" tall; 235 lbs; until now "no time" for exercise; "I've never given much thought to my health before"; "Tell me what I have to do to fight this thing—Can you help me design an exercise program that will work?"

**Client Goal:**
At next visit, 10/27/93, client reports adherence to the exercise program developed.
9/30/93 [additional goals will describe desired changes in weight and cholesterol level].

**Nursing Interventions:**
1. Explore the client's fitness goals, interests, skills, exercise opportunities, and exercise capacity.
2. Assist the client in obtaining medical clearance for exercise.
3. Explore feasible exercise activities with the client, considering health benefits sought, time involved, need for special equipment, precautions, and risk.
4. Develop an exercise program that specifies warm-up and cool-down activities and three or four major exercise activities from which the client can choose. Specify frequency, duration, and intensity.
5. Encourage the client to complement the exercise program with everyday activities that require exercise.
6. Try to identify with the client potential threats to the exercise program's successful implementation. Plan support strategies.

**Evaluative Statement:**
10/27/93: Goal partially met; client reports that the second week into his program his "jogging buddy" got sick and that without the support of his friend he stopped exercising regularly; wants to resume. Revision: explore new strategies to strengthen resolve/adherence.
*J. McKeough, RN*

3. *Client strengths:* Client is highly motivated to develop new self-care behaviors as a result of his father's death—asking for help.
*Personal strengths:* Good understanding of the relationship between self-care behaviors (exercise, nutrition) and health; experienced in designing exercise programs; knowledge of benefits/risks associated with exercise; strong interpersonal/counseling skills .

4. 10/27/93: Whereas the client left the last session "enthusiastic" about beginning an exercise program, he reported today that he "feels like a failure" since he wasn't faithful to the goals he set for himself. After losing his exercise buddy, he found it easy to "skip runs," and he hasn't found another racquetball partner. We identified and reinforced the progress he has made and developed new goals that are less dependent on external support.
*J. McKeough, RN*

# Chapter 31

## Matching

1. h    2. g    3. c    4. a    5. d    6. e    7. b    8. f
9. b    10. h    11. i    12. e    13. g    14. f    15. d    16. k
17. j    18. c    19. a

## Multiple Choice

1. b    2. c    3. d    4. a    5. c    6. d    7. b    8. c
9. a    10. b

## Completion

1. Sample Answers
   a. How many hours of sleep do you usually get in a day? Do you usually go to bed and wake up about the same time each day?
   b. How have you been sleeping? Do you wake up frequently during the night?
   c. In what way does the sleep you get each day affect your everyday living? Has this sleep disturbance caused any change in your sex life?
   d. Do you feel rested and ready to start the day when you wake up? Are you having difficulty concentrating?
   e. Describe what you usually do to help yourself fall asleep. Do you take any medications to help you sleep?
   f. Tell me about your sleep problems. Do you recall changing your position frequently during the night?
2. Sample Answers
   a. Difficulty remaining asleep related to noise of hospital environment and need for periodic treatment.
   b. Excessive daytime sleeping related to effects of biologic aging.
   c. Altered sleep-wake patterns related to frequent rotations of shift.
   d. Premature wakening related to alcohol dependency.
   e. Difficulty falling asleep related to worries about family.
3. a. Regular sleep: Muscle tonus low, eyelids closed and still, respirations 36 breaths/min., even, and regular rhythm.
   b. Irregular sleep: Muscle tonus greater, movements follow no sequence, frequent grimaces, intermittent gross mouthing, respirations irregular, mean rate is greater than during regular sleep.
   c. Periodic sleep: Respiratory rates periodic—bursts of rapid shallow breathing alternate with bursts of deep, slow respirations.

   d. Drowsiness: Less activity than irregular or periodic but more activity than in regular sleep, eyes dull or glazed, open and close intermittently, just before closing may roll upward, generally regular respirations may become tachypneic, may be high-pitched squeal.
   e. Alert inactivity: Eyes are open and bright and make conjugate movements in vertical and horizontal plane, face relaxed, respirations more variable and faster than regular sleep, not seen before 3 1/2 weeks.
   f. Crying: Vocalization accompanied by gross motor activity, open or closed eyes, tears can be seen as early as 24 hours after birth.
4. a. Toddlers: averages from 10–15 hours sleep, two naps per day common, awakens two or three times during night, should manifest individual pattern of night sleep, naps, and awake time in 24-hour period.
   b. School-aged children: Normally require average of 8–10 hours sleep, varies with each individual.
   c. Adolescents: unusual sleep-wakefulness pattern, sleep needs vary.
   d. Young adults: Many factors influence the need for rest and sleep, generally 7–8 hours sleep but some can do with less, percentage of time in each stage of sleep decreases with age except for stage I REM which maintains stable psychologic balance in each individual.
   e. Middle adults: Total sleep time decreases with particular decrease in amount of stage IV sleep. Number of sleep arousals increases and time in bed spent awake increases.
   f. Older adults: Sleep-wakefulness patterns altered in the aged, difficulty falling asleep and more easily awakened once asleep. Stage I time increases with less time being spent in stages III and IV. Amount of REM sleep decreases because the length of each episode shortens.
5. a. Stage I: Transitional stage between wakefulness and sleep; person in relaxed state but aware of surroundings; involuntary muscle jerking; stage normally only lasts for minutes; person aroused easily; comprises about 5 percent of total sleep.
   b. Stage II: Person falls into state of sleep; can be aroused with relative ease; comprises 50–55 percent of sleep.
   c. Stage III: Depth of sleep increases and arousal becomes increasingly difficult; comprises about 10 percent of our sleep.
   d. Stage IV: Greatest depth of sleep—delta sleep, arousal difficult, physiologic changes in body; comprises about 10 percent of our sleep.
6. a. Eyes: dart back and forth quickly.
   b. Muscles: small-muscle twitching, such as on the face, large-muscle immobility, resembling paralysis.
   c. Respirations: irregular; sometimes interspersed with apnea.
   d. Pulse: rapid and/or irregular.
   e. Blood pressure: increases or fluctuates.
   f. Gastric secretions: increase.
   g. Metabolism: increases, body temperature increases.
   h. Brain waves: encephalogram tracings active.
   i. Sleep cycle: REM sleep enters from stage II of NREM sleep and reenters NREM sleep at stage II: arousal from sleep difficult.

7.

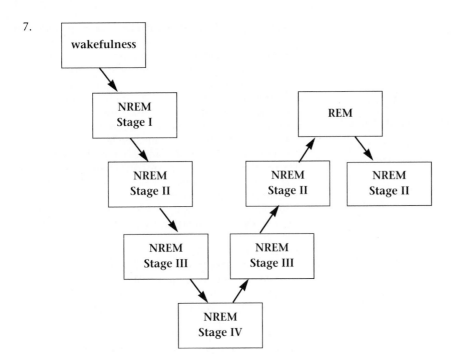

8. Sample Answers
   a. Prepare a restful environment.
   b. Promote bedtime rituals.
   c. Offer appropriate bedtime snacks and beverages.
   d. Promote relaxation.
   e. Promote comfort.

## Chapter 31: Case Study

1. Objective data are underlined; subjective data are bold-faced.

Gina Cioffi, a <u>23-year-old graduate nurse,</u> is <u>three months in her new position as a critical care staff nurse in a large tertiary care medical center.</u> **"I was so excited about working three twelve-hour shifts a week when I started this job, thinking I'd have lots of time for other things I want to do, but I'm not so sure anymore. I've been doing extra shifts when we're short-staffed because the money is so good, and right now it seems I'm always tired and all I think about all day long is how soon I can get back to bed. Worst of all, when I do finally get into bed, I often can't fall asleep—especially if things have been busy at work and someone "went bad." Does everyone else feel like me?"** Looking at Gina, you notice <u>dark circles under her eyes</u> and are suddenly struck by the change in her appearance from when she first started working. At that time, she <u>"bounced into work" looking fresh each morning and her features were always animated.</u> Now her <u>skin color is pale, her hair and clothes look rumpled, and the "brightness" that was so characteristic of her earlier is strikingly absent.</u> With some gentle questioning, you discover that **she frequently goes out with new friends she has made at the hospital when her shift is over, and sometimes goes for 48 hours without sleep. "I know I've gotten myself into a rut . . . How do I get out of it? I used to think my sleep habits were bad at school, but this is a hundred times worse, because there never seems to be time to crash . . . I have to just keep on going."**

### 2. Nursing Process Worksheet

**Health Problem:**
Sleep-pattern disturbance: altered sleep-wake patterns.

**Etiology:**
Twelve hour shift work and stress of new job.

**Signs & Symptoms (Defining Characteristics):**
Works three twelve hour shifts plus two to three ''extra'' shifts/week; ''right now it seems like I am always tired and all I think about all day long is how soon I can get back to bed . . . when I do finally get into bed I often can't fall asleep.'' Dark circles under eyes; pale skin; sometimes goes 48 hours without sleep; reports being less animated.

**Client Goal:**
By this time next month (7/22/93) client reports she is sleeping soundly for a minimum of 6-7 hours/night, at least 6 days a week, as evidenced by her feeling "less fatigued" and more "in control" of sleep situation.

**Nursing Interventions:**
1. Instruct client to keep a sleep diary for 7 days and analyze its contents at the end of that week
2. Counsel client about the need to reevaluate priorities (e.g., working extra shifts).
3. Develop stress management strategies, including relaxation exercises.
4. Identify and reduce (where possible) factors interfering with sleep.

**Evaluative Statement:**
10/6/93 Goal Met: Sleeping 7–8 hours per night, and generally feels refreshed upon awakening.
*N. McLoughlin, RN*

3. *Client strengths:* Strongly motivated at present to address this problem.
*Personal strengths:* Comprehensive knowledge of the physiology of sleep and sleep requirements and patenrs; familiarity with the stresses of clinical nursing—especially for the graduate nurse; strong interpersonal skills; creative problem-solver.

4. 10/6/93: Client "bounced into the office" with the vigor and enthusiasm she displayed when she first started working. Her skin had regained its usual coloring and glow and her face was animated. She expressed gratitude for my "helping her recover her old self" and reported that she is sleeping 7–8 hours/night, and usually wakes up refreshed and ready to tackle the new day. On questioning, she expressed new appreciation for the need to balance rest and activity and appears to have developed a workable plan for ensuring adequate rest.
*N. McLoughlin, RN*

# Chapter 32

## Matching

1. j   2. g   3. d   4. a   5. b   6. e   7. h   8. f
9. c   10. i   11. c   12. d   13. b   14. a   15. c   16. a
17. b   18. c   19. j   20. h   21. f   22. c   23. b   24. m
25. k   26. g   27. d   28. a   29. e   30. i   31. l   32. n

## Multiple Choice

1. a   2. c   3. d   4. b   5. c   6. a   7. d   8. b
9. a   10. c

## Correct the False Statements

1. true
2. false—prostaglandins
3. false—delta fibers
4. true
5. false—rhizotomy
6. true
7. false—central pain syndrome
8. false—shifting
9. false—intermittent
10. true
11. false—affective

## Completion

1. a. See table below for sample answers.
   b. Sample Answers
      *Situation A:* Pain—Acute migraine, related to unrelieved stress asmanifested by furrowed brows, nausea and anxiety.
      *Situation B:* Pain—related to animal scratch and fear, as manifested by pulling back from cat, swelling and redness around scratch, and exaggerated weeping.
      *Situation C:* Pain—acute postoperative, related to cesarean section as manifested by refusal to move, muscle tension, and rigidity and helplessness.
      *Situation D:* Chronic pain—related to degenerative joint disease as manifested by grimacing, refusal to walk, increased blood pressure, and exaggerated restlessness.
2. Sample Answers
   a. Family will demonstrate ability to discuss pain experience and offer emotional support to client.
   b. Client will demonstrate ability to perform ADLs while using pain control methods as taught.
   c. Client will describe a gradual reduction in pain, using a scale of 0–10.
   d. Client will demonstrate willingness to take prescribed analgesic by asking for medication without prompting from staff.
   e. Client will demonstrate means of controlling pain while continuing to cough and deep breathe.

| Situation | Behavioral | Physiological | Affective |
|-----------|------------|---------------|-----------|
| A | furrowed brows | nausea | anxiety |
| B | crying | swelling and redness on scratched area | fear |
| C | refusal to move | muscle tension<br><br>rigidity | helplessness |
| D | grimacing, refusal to walk | increased blood pressure | exaggerated restlessness |

3. See table below.
4. Sample Answers
   a. the client's verbalizataion and description of the pain
   b. duration of the pain
   c. location of the pain
   d. quality of the pain
   e. chronology of the pain
   f. aggravating factors
   g. behavioral responses
   h. impact of pain experience on activities and life style

| Medication | Action | Major Side Effect | Narcotic (Y/N) |
|------------|--------|-------------------|----------------|
| a. Morphine | CNS mechanism, blocks pain stimulus to brain | n/v, sedation, respiratory depression | yes |
| b. Demerol | CNS mechanism, blocks pain stimulus to brain | n/v, sedation, respiratory depression | yes |
| c. Aspirin | blocks prostaglandin synthesis | n/v, gastric distress, inhibits coagulation | no |

## Chapter 32: Case Study

1. Objective data are underlined; subjective data are bold-faced.

Tabitha Wilson is a <u>24-month old infant with AIDS who is hospitalized, this admission, with infectious diarrhea.</u> She is well known to the pediatric staff and there is real concern that she might not pull through this admission. She has suffered many of the complications of AIDS and is no stranger to pain. At the present time, the <u>skin on her buttocks is raw and excoriated and tears stream down her face whenever she is moved. Her blood pressure also shoots up when she is touched.</u> The severity of her illness has left her <u>extremely weak and listless</u>, and her **foster mother reports that she no longer recognizes her child.** When alone in her crib, <u>she seldom moves and moans softly.</u> Several nurses have expressed great frustration caring for Tabitha, because they find it hard to perform even simple nursing measures—like turning, diapering, and weighing her—when they see how much pain these procedures cause.

**2. Nursing Process Worksheet**

**Health Problem:**
Pain.

**Etiology:**
Excoriated skin on buttocks and debilitating effects of illness.

**Signs & Symptoms (Defining Characteristics):**
Tears stream down face when moved and blood pressure shoots up; moans; skin on buttocks is raw and excoriated.

**Client Goal:**
By 2/15/93 client's behaviors indicate that pain is sufficiently relieved for client to rest comfortably—even during procedures.

**Nursing Interventions:**
1. Report pain assessment to M.D. and collaborate on designing effective pain management program.
2. Ensure that the analgesia administration schedule produces consistent comfort.
3. Collaborate with wound care specialist in implementing program for healing of lesions on buttocks.

**Evaluative Statement:**
2/15/93: Goal partially met, client's behavior (absent tears, decreased moaning, decreased BP) indicate some pain relief but procedures that involve moving the client still result in great discomfit. *Revision:* reconsult with physician.

*E. Daniel, RN*

3. *Client strengths:* Client and her parents are greatly liked by the staff; parents show great willingness to be involved in care.
*Personal strengths:* Knowledge of pain experience; experience in designing and monitoring pain management regimens; experience with pain management in infants and children; good rapport with wound and skin care specialist; strong interpersonal skills.

4. Tabitha's response to procedures is markedly improved since the new analgesic regime has been implemented. However, while she no longer "tears up" when touched and her blood pressure is more stable during procedures, she continues to cry during her bath and during procedures that involve more movement. Will speak with MD about modifying analgesic regimen.

*E. Daniel, RN*

# Chapter 33

## Matching

1. i   2. m   3. e   4. c   5. a   6. d   7. g   8. b
9. f   10. h   11. k   12. l   13. j
14. c—oysters
15. g—whole grains
16. a—liver
17. j—organ meats
18. d—shellfish
19. b—iodized salt
20. e—nuts
21. f—fluoridated water
22. i—liver
23. h—wheat
24. f—whole grain
25. a—milk
26. g—salt
27. b—poultry
28. e—salt
29. c—green leafy vegetables
30. d—meat
31. k—dark green, leafy vegetables
32. i—milk
33. f—meat
34. h—liver
35. a—citrus fruits
36. d—yeast
37. b—pork
38. g—salmon
39. j—vegetable oils
40. c—eggs
41. e—asparagus

## Multiple Choice

1. c   2. a   3. b   4. c   5. b   6. c   7. a   8. d
9. c   10. b   11. c   12. a   13. d

## Correct the False Statements

1. true
2. false—hemoglobin
3. false—soft diets
4. true
5. true
6. true
7. false—20 percent
8. true
9. false—4
10. true
11. true

## Completion

1. a. $170 \times 10 = 1,700$; $170 \times 5 = 850$; $1,700 + 850 = 2,500$ cal.
   b. $170 \times 15 = 2,550$ cal.
   c. $170 \times 21 = 3,570$ cal.
2. a. Eat a variety of foods.
   b. Maintain healthy weight.
   c. Choose low fat dairy products, lean meats, and foods prepared with little or no fat.
   d. Limit salt, alcohol, and caffeine.
   e. Choose a diet with plenty of vegetables, fruits, and grain products.
3. a. Fruits and vegetables—4–5 servings
      Grains—3–5 servings
      Milk and milk products—2–4 servings
      Meat, poultry, and fish—2 servings.
   b. Bread, cereal, grains, and pasta—6–11 servings
      Vegetables—3–5 servings
      Fruits—2–4 servings
      Milk, yogurt, and cheese—2–3 servings
      Meat, poultry, fish, dry beans, eggs, and nuts—2–3 servings
      Fats, oils, sweets—use sparingly.
4. a. Dietary data—screen 24-hour food recall, food frequency record.
   b. Medical-socioeconomic data—screen brief personal and family history.
   c. Anthropometric data—screen height, weight, IBW, UBW.
   d. clinical data—screen and in-depth observation for signs and symptoms of malnutrition.
   e. biochemical data—screen serum hemoglobin, hematocrit, and albumin; total lymphocyte count.
5. a. Aspirate 10–20 ml of gastrointestinal fluid.
   b. Measure the pH of aspirated gastrointestinal fluid.
   c. Inject 10–20 ml of air into the tube while simultaneously auscultating over the epigastric area with a stethoscope.
   d. Ask the client to talk or hum. A large-bore tube in the trachea would prohibit the client from speaking but the smaller tubes do not usually interfere with speech.
6. a. Members of certain age groups (infants, adolescents, pregnant and lactating women, and the elderly).
   b. Those who smoke, abuse alcohol, or use medications on a long-term basis.
   c. Those who are chronically ill, either physically or psychologically.
   d. Those who are poor or finicky eaters, like chronic dieters, strict vegetarians, and food faddists.
7. a. Drugs that change the pH of the GI tract.
   b. Drugs that increase GI mobility.
   c. Drugs that damage intestinal mucosa.
   d. Drugs that bind with nutrients, rendering them unavailable to the body.
8. Sample Answers
   a. Inadequate food intake, fad dieting, numerous food intolerances or allergies.
   b. NPO with simple IV therapy for longer than three days.
   c. Inadequate tube feedings.
   d. Changes in taste, smell, or appetite.

9. Sample Answers
  a. Serve small, frequent meals to avoid overwhelming the client with large amounts of food.
  b. Solicit food preferences and encourage food from home, if possible.
  c. Offer alternatives for items the client cannot or will not eat.
  d. Encourage or provide good oral hygiene.
  e. Be sure the client's tray looks attractive.
10. a. By way of a tube inserted through the nose and into the stomach—nasogastric feeding.
  b. By way of a tube surgically inserted directly into the stomach—gastrostomy tube.
  c. By way of a tube inserted directly into the intestine by way of a tube through the nose (nasoduodenal or nasojejunal) or a tube surgically inserted into the small intestine (jejunostomy).

11. Percutaneous endoscopic gastrostomy tubes have become the standard method for accessing the GI tract when long-term nutritional support is necessary. A PEG tube is threaded via an endoscope through the esophagus into the stomach and then pulled through a stab wound made in the abdominal wall.
12. a. Dehydration, diarrhea, and intestinal cramping: these symptoms can be controlled by reducing strength of the formula and by introducing it more slowly.
  b. Spilling of glucose in the urine and frequent urination: these symptoms can usually be relieved by reducing the strength of the formula and by introducing it more slowly.
  c. Nausea: the feedings should be stopped and the patient examined for gastric residual. Slowing the rate of the administration of the nourishment is ordinarily indicated.
  d. Aspiration of nourishment: it can usually be prevented by keeping the client in a semisitting position so that the nourishment is less likely to enter the esophagus and be aspirated.
  e. Vomiting: vomiting tends to occur when the nourishment does not leave the stomach. The gastric residual should be checked and the amount of feedings reassessed.

## Chapter 33: Case Study

1. Objective data are underlined; subjective data are bold-faced.

Mr. Church, a <u>74 year-old white male</u>, is being admitted to the geriatric unit of the hospital for a diagnostic work-up. He was <u>diagnosed as having Alzheimer's disease four years ago</u> and just <u>one year ago was admitted to a long-term care facility</u>. His wife of 49 years is extremely devoted and informed the nurse taking the admission history that she instigated his admission to the hospital because **she was alarmed with the amount of weight he was losing.** Assessment revealed a <u>six foot-tall, emaciated male, who weighed 149 pounds</u>. **His wife reported he lost 20 pounds in the last two months**. The staff at the long-term care facility report that <u>he was eating his meals and his wife validated that this was the case</u>. No one seemed sure, however, of the caloric content of his diet. His wife nodded her head vigorously when asked if her husband seemed more agitated and hyperactive recently. Mr. Church has <u>dull, sparse hair, pale, dry skin, and dry mucous membranes.</u>

## 2. Nursing Process Worksheet

**Health Problem:**
Altered nutrition: Less than body requirements.

**Etiology:**
Imbalance between energy expenditure and caloric intake.

**Signs & Symptoms (Defining Characteristics):**
6 feet, 149 pounds; appears "emaciated"; 20-pound weight loss over 2 months; is "eating meals"; more "hyperactive and agitated" than usual; dull, sparse hair; pale, dry skin; dry mucous membranes.

**Client Goal:**
By one month (1/20/93) client will demonstrate signs of ingesting adequate calories to meet energy needs as evidenced by 5–10 pound weight gain.

**Nursing Interventions:**
1. Do a 72-hour diet history to determine the average number of calories the client ingests daily.
2. Provide whatever assistance the client needs with feeding. Add high-caloric snacks to the client's diet, increasing calories progressively until the pattern of weight loss is replaced by weight gain.
3. Until the desired weight is regained and maintained, weigh the client daily and keep an accurate fluid I & O and calorie intake record.
4. Explore nursing strategies to reduce agitation and hyperactivity, e.g., music, balanced solitude and social interaction, rest periods, etc.

**Evaluative Statement:**
1/20/93: Goal met, client gained 8 pounds over last month and seems to enjoy high-caloric snacks.
*M. Bendyna, RN*

3. *Client strengths:* Client has a very supportive wife. *Personal strengths:* Sound knowledge of nutrition and of Alzheimer's disease. Experienced in working with persons with Alzheimer's disease and their families. Experienced gerontological nurse.

4. Over the past month, the client's diet has been increased by 2000 cal/daily. He enjoys high-calorie snacks of peanut butter and jelly sandwiches, milk shakes, dried fruit and nuts, pasta salads, and an occasional Snicker's bar. He has regained 8 of 20 pounds he lost and his wife is delighted. He remains hyperactive but scheduled walks have decreased some of his agitation. Will continue to monitor his nutritional needs.
*M. Bendyna, RN*

# C h a p t e r   3 4

## Matching

| 1. d | 2. h | 3. a | 4. e | 5. b | 6. c | 7. g | 8. f |
|------|------|------|------|------|------|------|------|
| 9. c | 10. a | 11. c | 12. d | 13. b | 14. c | 15. b | 16. c |
| 17. d | 18. c | 19. a | 20. b | 21. f | 22. e | 23. a | 24. b |
| 25. g | 26. c | 27. d |

## Multiple Choice

| 1. c | 2. d | 3. b | 4. a | 5. a | 6. c | 7. d | 8. c |
|------|------|------|------|------|------|------|------|
| 9. a | 10. b | 11. c | 12. c | 13. a |

## Correct the False Statements

1. true
2. false—stress incontinence
3. true
4. false—acidic
5. false—woman
6. true
7. false—dorsal recumbent (or side-lying for women)
8. true

## Completion

1. a. Developmental considerations: Infants are born with no urinary control. Most children develop urinary control between the ages of 2 and 5 years. Physiologic changes that accompany normal aging may affect urination in the elderly.
   b. Food and fluid: The kidneys should preserve a careful balance of fluid intake and output. Caffeine-containing beverages have a diuretic effect and increase urine production. Alcohol produces the same effect by inhibiting the release of the antidiuretic hormone. Foods high in water content may increase urine production. High sodium foods and beverages cause sodium and water reabsorption and retention.
   c. Life style: Individual, family, and sociocultural variables influence a person's normal voiding habits.
   d. Psychologic variables: Individuals experiencing stress often find themselves needing to void smaller amounts of urine at more frequent intervals. Stress can also interfere with the ability to relax perineal muscles and the external urethral sphincter.
   e. Activity and muscle tone: Exercise increases metabolism and optimal urine production and elimination. With prolonged periods of immobility, decreased bladder and sphincter tone can result in poor urinary control and urinary stasis.
   f. Pathologic conditions: Certain renal or urologic problems can affect both the quantity and quality of urine produced.
   g. Medication: Medications have numerous effects on urine production and elimination. Nephrotoxic drugs are a grave concern. Abuse of analgesics can result in nephrotoxicity. Certain drugs cause urine to change color.
2. a. Measuring urine output.
   b. Collecting urine specimens.
   c. Determining the existence of abnormal constituents in the urine.
   d. Assisting with diagnostic procedure.
3. a. Retention or Foley catheter: indwelling catheter used for the gradual decompression of an overextended bladder, intermittent bladder drainage and irrigation, and continuous bladder drainage.
   b. Intermittent catheter: used to drain bladder for shorter periods of time; can be inserted by patient.
   c. Suprapubic catheter: used for continuous drainage; inserted through small incision above pubic area.
   d. Condom catheter: soft, pliable plastic or rubberized material device applied externally to penis when voluntary control of urine is not possible.
4. a. Relieve urinary retention.
   b. Obtain sterile specimen from a woman.
   c. Measure amount of residual urine in bladder.
   d. Obtain urine specimen when one cannot be secured satisfactorily by other means.
   e. Empty the bladder for surgery and diagnostic examinations.
5. An ileal conduit is a surgical diversion of the ureter to the ileum, rather than to the bladder. This separated section of the small intestine is then brought to the abdominal wall, where urine is excreted through a stoma.
6. a. prepuce
   b. glans clitoris
   c. labia majora
   d. urethral orifice (meatus)
   e. vagina
   f. vestibule
   g. labia minora
   h. perineum
   i. anus
7. a. bladder
   b. ureter
   c. kidney
   d. urethra

## Chapter 34: Case Study

1. Objective data are underlined; subjective data are bold-faced.

Mr. Eisenberg, <u>age 84</u>, was hurriedly admitted to a nursing home when his wife of 62 years died. He has <u>two adult children</u>, neither of whom feel prepared to care for him the way his wife did. **"We don't know how mom did it year after year. After he retired from his law practice, he was terribly demanding and it just seemed nothing she did for him pleased him. His Parkinson's disease does make it a bit difficult for him to get around, but he's able to do a whole lot more than he is letting on. He's always been this way."** You are talking with his son and daughter because the aides have reported to you that he is <u>frequently incontinent of both urine and stool during the day as well as during the night</u>. He is <u>alert</u> and appears <u>capable of recognizing the need to void or defecate and signaling for any assistance he needs</u>. His son and daughter report that this was never a problem at home—that <u>he was able to go into the bathroom with assistance</u>. He has been depressed about his admission to the home and seldom speaks, even when directly approached. He has refused to participate in any of the floor social events since his arrival.

## 2. Nursing Process Worksheet

### Health Problem:
Toileting self-care deficit.

### Etiology:
Depression on entering nursing home and decreased will to live.

### Signs & Symptoms (Defining Characteristics):
Incontinent of both urine and stool during both the day and night (need to determine the frequency); alert and capable of recognizing and signaling the need to void/defecate; able to walk to bathroom with assistance.

### Client Goal:
Within two weeks (6/17/93) client will communicate the need to void/defecate appropriately, as evidenced by reduction of incontinent episodes to "one accident" daily.

### Nursing Interventions:
1. Initiate a regular toileting schedule with the client where he is assisted to the bathroom; utilize these interactions to reinforce the importance of his maintaining his independence.
2. Refrain from using adult incontinent pads or in any way communicating that incontinence is "ok."
3. Call an interdisciplinary conference to develop a strategy to ease his transition to the home.

### Evaluative Statement:
6/17/93: Goal partially met; when assisted to the bathroom the client voids/defecates—but if the staff neglect to offer their assistance the client will not use his call light to request assistance, and incontinent episodes continue (greater than one per day on some days). Revision: Continue to counsel regarding transition to the home and importance of independence.

*P. Wu, RN*

3. *Client strengths:* Client is alert and capable of communicating his needs for assistance. Is mobile with assistance. *Personal strengths:* Good knowledge of gerontological nursing and experience in caring for the elderly. Experienced counselor and teacher of appropriate selfcare measures.

4. 6/15/93: A review of the client's record reveals three incontinent episodes in the last 24 hours (2 urine, 1 stool). When questioned about why he did not ask for assistance to the bathroom, the client refused to answer. Generally he cooperates with the toileting regimen, and when taken to the bathroom voids/defecates as needed. Will continue to counsel regarding the importance of his independently managing his toileting needs. Will reevaluate his ability to recognize the need to void/defecate and ability to ask for assistance.

*P. Wu, RN*

# Chapter 35

## Matching

| | | | | | | | |
|---|---|---|---|---|---|---|---|
| 1. d | 2. h | 3. a | 4. f | 5. g | 6. e | 7. i | 8. j |
| 9. k | 10. b | 11. m | 12. l | 13. c | 14. c | 15. a | 16. d |
| 17. b | 18. d | 19. a | 20. e | 21. b | 22. c | 23. g | 24. f |
| 25. a | 26. m | 27. h | 28. b | 29. n | 30. c | 31. i | 32. q |
| 33. o | 34. r | 35. d | 36. l | 37. p | 38. e | 39. k | 40. j |

## Multiple Choice

| | | | | | | | |
|---|---|---|---|---|---|---|---|
| 1. b | 2. d | 3. a | 4. c | 5. a | 6. d | 7. a | 8. b |
| 9. d | | | | | | | |

## Correct the False Statements

1. false—esophagogastroduodenoscopy
2. false—barium enema or lower gastrointestinal examination
3. true
4. true
5. false—diarrhea
6. true
7. true
8. true
9. false—fecal impaction
10. true

## Completion

1. A. sigmoid colostomy
   B. descending colostomy
   C. transverse (Single B) colostomy
   D. ascending colostomy
   E. ileostomy
2. Sample Answers
   a. Developmental considerations: Age affects in part what a person eats and the body's ability to digest nutrients and eliminate wastes.
   b. Daily patterns: Most people have regular patterns of bowel elimination, which include frequency, timing considerations, position, and place. Changes in any of these may upset a person's routine and cause constipation.
   c. Food and fluid: Both the type and amount of foods eaten and the amount of foods ingested affect elimination. Healthy elimination is facilitated by a high fiber diet and a daily fluid intake of 2,000 ml to 3,000 ml.

d. Activity and muscle tone: Regular exercise improves gastrointestinal motility and muscle tone, while inactivity decreases both.
   e. Life style: Individual, family, and sociocultural variables influence a person's usual elimination habits. Feelings about bowel elimination, daily schedules, and leisure activities contribute to a habit of regular defecation.
   f. Psychologic variables: Emotional stress may have a direct effect on gastrointestinal motility, and diarrhea can be expected during any periods of high anxiety.
   g. Pathologic conditions: Changes in stool characteristics or frequency may be one of the first clinical manifestations of a disease, and their evaluation may lead to the diagnosis of the disease.
   h. Medications: medications are available either to promote or inhibit peristalsis. Other types of medication may affect bowel elimination or stool characteristics.
3. a. inspection
   b. auscultation
   c. percussion
   d. palpation
4. Sample Answers
   a. Void first because the laboratory study may be inaccurate if the stool contains urine.
   b. Use a clean or sterile bedpan or the bedside commode, depending on the specific specimen required.
   c. Defecate into the required container rather than the toilet bowel because the laboratory study may be hindered by the water in the bowel.
   d. Do not place toilet tissue in the bedpan or specimen container because contents in the paper may influence laboratory results.
5. Sample Answers
   a. The client will have a soft, formed bowel movement every one to three days without discomfort.
   b. The client will explain the relationship between bowel elimination and dietary fiber, fluid intake, and exercise.
6. a. timing
   b. positioning
   c. privacy
   d. nutrition
   e. exercise
7. a. change in bowel elimination pattern
   b. blood in the stools
   c. rectal or abdominal pain
   d. change in the character of the stool
   e. sensation of incomplete emptying after bowel movement

## Sequencing

1. 5
2. 7
3. 1
4. 3
5. 6
6. 4
7. 2

## Chapter 35: Case Study

1. Objective data are underlined; subjective data are bold-faced.

Ms. Elgaresta, age 54, a single, Hispanic woman, is being followed by a cardiologist who monitors her heart arrhythmia. Last month, she was started on a new heart medication. This visit, she complains to the nurse practitioner who works with the cardiologist; **"Right after I started taking that medication, I got terribly constipated and nothing seems to help. I'm desperate and about ready to try dynamite unless you can think of something else!" She reports a change in her bowel movements from one soft formed stool daily to one to two hard stools weekly—stools that cause much straining.** The nurse practitioner realizes that regulating Ms. Elgaresta's heart is difficult and that her best cardiac response to date has been with the medication now causing the constipation. Reluctant to suggest substituting another medication too quickly, she asks more questions and discovers the following. **"I've never been much of a drinker. Two cups of coffee in the morning and maybe a glass of wine at night. Water? Almost never. And I don't drink juices or soft drinks."** Analysis of her diet reveals a diet low in fiber; **"I never was one much for vegetables, and they can just keep all this bran stuff that's out on the market! Coffee and a cigarette. That's for me!"** Ms. Elgaresta is a workaholic computer programmer who has little leisure time and who spends what she has watching TV. She reports **tiring after walking one flight of stairs, and states that she avoids all forms of vigorous exercise.**

## 2. Nursing Process Worksheet

**Health Problem:**
Constipation

**Etiology:**
New medication, deficient fiber and fluid intake, and insufficient exercise.

**Signs & Symptoms (Defining Characteristics):**
Change in bowel habits: from one soft, formed stool daily to 1–2 hard stools per week and straining.

**Client Goal:**
One month after new regime begins (5/4/93) client reports one soft, formed stool every one-two days.

**Nursing Interventions:**
1. Counsel client about the relationship between diet (fiber intake and fluids) and bowel elimination, and exercise and bowel elimination.
2. Assess client's willingness and motivation to make life style changes and develop workable plan.
3. Reinforce importance of continuing medication.

**Evaluative Statement:**
5/4/93: Goal met. Client now passing soft, formed stool almost every day.

*B. Shevorkis, RN*

3. *Client strengths:* Client is highly motivated to learn new self-care behaviors.
*Personal strengths:* Knowledge of the physiology of elimination; experienced client educator and counselor; excellent role model of healthy self-care behaviors.

4. 5/4/93: Client in for one-month follow-up and expressed delight with effects of new self-care behaviors! (1) decreased fat consumption and increased fiber in diet, (2) increased fluid intake—especially water, (3) increased exercise, and (4) 30-minute periods of aerobic exercise per week. Constipation problem is resolved: passes soft stool almost every day—and she reports having much more energy for work. Progress reinforced.

*B. Shevorkis, RN*

# C h a p t e r   3 6

## Matching

1. b  2. e  3. i  4. d  5. j  6. f  7. h  8. g
9. c  10. a  11. g  12. j  13. h  14. i  15. e  16. f
17. c  18. a  19. d  20. b
21. g—2400–3000 ml
22. a—500 ml
23. h—5500 ml
24. b—3500–4300 ml
25. d—1200–1500 ml
26. c—1200–1500 ml
27. e—4000–4800 ml
28. f  29. c  30. a  31. b  32. d  33. e

## Multiple Choice

1. b  2. d  3. a  4. c  5. a  6. b  7. d  8. c
9. a  10. d  11. c  12. a  13. b  14. c  15. c  16. d
17. d

## Correct the False Statements

1. false—auscultation
2. true
3. true
4. false—suppressants
5. true
6. false—vibration
7. false—cigarette smoking
8. true
9. false—nasal catheter
10. true
11. false—endotracheal tube

## Completion

1. **A** is for Airway: Tip the head and check for breathing.
The respiratory tract must be opened so air can enter.
**B** is for Breathing: If the victim does not start to breathe
spontaneously after the airway is opened, give two slow,
full breaths.
**C** is for Circulation: Check the pulse. If the victim is
pulseless, artificial circulation must be started with
breathing.
2. Sample Answers
   a. Client will demonstrate effective respiratory rate and
   rhythm.
   b. Client will identify possible contributing factors.
   c. Client will evaluate adaptive coping mechanisms
   when dealing with stress and/or anxiety.
3. Sample Answers
   a. "I never feel as though I am getting enough air." A
   70-year-old man with 20-year history of COPD, recent
   development of pneumonia. He is pale with circum-
   oral cyanosis. Respiratory rate is 40 per minute and
   shallow. Rhonchi are auscultated bilaterally. Coughing
   episodes produce little sputum.

   b. "Lately I've been experiencing shortness of breath,
   nausea, and swollen ankles." A cyanotic 50-year-old
   male using pursed-lip breathing while sitting in emergency room stretcher. Sitting hunched forward with
   overbed table supporting him. Altered blood gases
   show respiratory acidosis.
   c. "I have a tingling feeling in my fingers." Hyperventilating, tachypnea (40 min).
4. Sample Answers:
   a. Usual patterns of respiration: "How would you
   describe your breathing patterns?" "Do you smoke?"
   b. Cough: "What is your cough like?" (dry, bubbly,
   hoarse.) "Are you exposed to dust, fumes?"
   c. Chest pain: "Is the pain worse with inspiration? expiration? coughing?" "Does the pain radiate?"
   d. Dyspnea: "Is it constant, or remittent, or related to
   any activity?" "Have you ever been told that you have
   asthma? Emphysema? Tuberculosis? Heart disease?"
   e. Fatigue: "Are you getting your normal amount of
   sleep at night?" "Has your sleep at night been affected
   by any difficulty breathing?"
5. a. The integrity of the airway system to transport air to
   and from the lungs.
   b. Properly functioning alveolar system in the lungs to
   oxygenate venous blood and to remove carbon dioxide from the blood.
   c. A properly functioning cardiovascular system to carry
   nutrients and wastes to and from body cells.
6. a. Inhalation, the active phase, involves movement of
   muscles and thorax to bring air into the lungs.
   b. Exhalation, the passive phase, is the movement of air
   out of the lungs.
7. a. Levels of health: Persons with renal or cardiac disorders often demonstrate a compromise in respiratory
   functioning due to fluid overload. Persons with
   chronic illnesses often have muscle wasting and poor
   muscle tone, including those of the respiratory system.
   b. Development: Physical changes, e.g., scoliosis, will influence breathing patterns so air trapping occurs. Obese
   people are often short of breath with activity and alveoli
   at base of lungs are rarely stimulated to expand fully.
   c. Life style: Sedentary activity patterns do not encourage the expansion of alveoli and the development of
   pulmonary exercise patterns. Persons who exercise
   regularly are better able to respond to stressors to respiratory health. Cigarette smoking is a major contrib-
   utor to lung disease.
   d. Environment: There is a direct correlation between air
   pollution and cancer and lung diseases. Persons who
   have experienced an alteration in respiratory functioning in the past are often unable to continue self-
   care activities in polluted environments.
   e. Psychologic health: individuals responding to stress
   might demonstrate excessive sighing or hyperventilation breathing patterns.
8. a. Avoid open flame in client's room.
   b. Place "No Smoking" signs in conspicuous places in
   the client's room.
   c. Check to see that electric equipment used in the
   room—such as electric bell cords, razors, radios, and
   suctioning equipment—is in good working order and
   emits no sparks.
   d. Avoid wearing and using synthetic fabrics that build
   up static electricity.
   e. Avoid using oils in the area.

## Chapter 36: Case Study

1. Objective data are underlined; subjective data are bold-faced.

Toni is a <u>14-year-old</u> who is on the adolescent mental health unit following a suicide attempt. Her chart reveals that on several occasions when her mother was visiting, she began <u>hyperventilating (increased respiratory rate [42] and increased depth)</u>. Gasping for breath on these occasions, she nevertheless pushed away all who approached her to assist. Her mother confided that she and her husband are in the midst of a divorce and that it hasn't been easy for Toni at home. **"I know she's been having a rough time at school and I guess I've been too caught up in my own troubles to be there for her."** When you attempt to discuss this with Toni and mention her mother's concern, she begins <u>hyperventilating again.</u>

## 2. Nursing Process Worksheet

**Health Problem:**
Ineffective breathing patterns.

**Client Goal:**
By her second week in the unit (3/22/93), Toni will demonstrate an effective respiratory rate and rhythm (not to exceed 24) during her mother's visits.

**Etiology:**
Anxiety.

**Nursing Interventions:**
1. Use interview questions directed to Toni and her mother to determine the nature of the problem, its probable cause, and its effect on lifestyle.
2. Demonstrate conscious controlled breathing and encourage client to use it during periods of anxiety or activity.
3. Maintain a "safe" environment. Same nurses always work with this client. Maintain eye contact during conversation.
4. If fear is the cause, encourage client to ventilate concerns. Reduce cause of fear, if feasible.
5. If there is a strong emotional component, discuss with client the development of effective coping skills with professional counseling.

**Signs & Symptoms (Defining Characteristics):**
Periods of hyperventilation (increased RR—42—and increased depth)—associated with situations which are stressful (mother).

**Evaluative Statement:**
3/22/93: Goal partially met; on two occasions, Toni has remained in control of her breathing during her mother's visits. On at least one occasion, she hyperventilated.

*K. O'Leary, RN*

3. *Client strengths:* The client's strengths still need to be identified; Mother seems to be gaining an appreciation of her needs.
*Personal strengths:* Good understanding of the effects of stress and experienced in helping clients replace maladaptive coping strategies with adaptive strategies.

4. 3/22/93: This morning, Toni began talking about the difficult situation at home. When asked about her relationship with her mother she began gulping for air, but "caught herself" and quickly reestablished control of her breathing, consciously decreasing her rate and depth. Whereas she has shown no signs of hyperventilation on two of her mother's last visits, she had one episode where she hyperventilated and totally "lost control," and needed sedation. She stated she feels like she is making progress—but still has a long way to go before she will feel comfortable at home and in control of simple, everyday things, like breathing.

*K. O'Leary, RN*

# C h a p t e r   3 7

## Matching

| | | | | | | | |
|---|---|---|---|---|---|---|---|
| 1. i | 2. f | 3. a | 4. c | 5. g | 6. d | 7. j | 8. e |
| 9. b | 10. h | 11. f | 12. a | 13. d | 14 b | 15. g | 16. e |
| 17. c | 18. g | 19. b | 20. a | 21. i | 22. h | 23. c | 24. e |
| 25. d | 26. f | 27. b | 28. a | 29. d | 30. c | | |

## Multiple Choice

| | | | | | | | |
|---|---|---|---|---|---|---|---|
| 1. b | 2. c | 3. a | 4. a | 5. a | 6. b | 7. d | 8. c |
| 9. b | 10. a | 11. d | 12. b | 13. c | 14. b | | |

## Correct the False Statements

1. false—hypovolemia
2. true
3. false—third space fluid shift
4. false—hypercalcemia
5. true
6. true
7. false—hypermagnesemia
8. true
9. true
10. true
11. false—NA$^+$
12. true

## Completion

1. a. Osmosis—the process by which the solvent water passes from an area of lesser solute concentration to an area of greater solute concentration until equilibrium is established.
   b. Diffusion—the tendency of solutes to move freely throughout a solvent. The solute moves from an area of higher concentration to an area of lower concentration until equilibrium is established.
   c. Active transport—the process that requires energy for the movement of substances through a cell wall, from an area of lesser concentration to an area of higher concentration.
   d. Filtration—the passage of fluid through a permeable membrane from an area of high pressure to one of lower pressure.
2. a. ingested liquids
   b. water in food
   c. water from metabolic oxidation
3. a. buffers
   b. respiratory mechanisms
   c. renal mechanisms
4. a. Clients with acute and chronic illness (e.g., diabetes mellitus, congestive heart failure, renal failure).
   b. Clients with abnormal losses of body fluids (e.g., prolonged or severe vomiting and diarrhea, draining wounds, fistulas).
   c. Clients with burns and traumas.
   d. Clients undergoing therapies with the potential to disrupt fluid and electrolyte balance (e.g., medications such as diuretics and steroids, treatments such as intravenous therapy, and total parenteral nutrition).
5. a. Increased hematocrit values: found in severe dehydration and shock.
   b. Decreased hematocrit: found with acute, massive blood loss, and with hemolytic reaction following transfusion of incompatible blood.
   c. Increased levels of hemoglobin: found in hemo-concentration of the blood.
   d. Decreased levels of hemoglobin: found with severe hemorrhage and following a hemolytic reaction.
6. a. Accurate administration consistent with manufacturer's guidelines.
   b. Knowledge of the intended therapeutic effect and evaluation.
   c. Observation for adverse effects.
   d. Observation for drug reactions.
   e. Teaching the client appropriate health care behaviors.
7. a. Accessibility of a vein.
   b. Condition of the vein.
   c. Type of fluid to be infused.
   d. Anticipated duration of infusion.

8. a. Blood transfusion—the infusion of whole blood or a blood component, such as plasma, red blood cells, or platelets, into the venous circulation.
   b. Typing—the laboratory examination to determine a person's blood type.
   c. Crossmatching—the process of determining compatibility between blood specimens.
   d. Antigen—a substance that causes the formation of antibodies.
   e. Antibody—a protein substance developed in the body in response to the presence of an antigen that has in some way gained access to the body.
   f. Agglutinin—an antibody that causes a clumping of specific antigens.
   g. Rh factor—an inherited antigen in human blood.
   h. RhoGam—an anti-Rh gamma globulin.
9. Sample Answers
   a. The client will enter surgery in fluid balance as evidenced by stable body weight, urine output of 30–50 ml per hour, and urine specific gravity of 1.010 to 1.025. The client will enter surgery in electrolyte balance, as evidenced by normal laboratory values for sodium, chloride, potassium, and bicarbonate.
   b. The client will maintain approximately equal fluid intake and output, maintain urine output of 30–50 ml/hour, maintain stable body weight, maintain stable vital signs, and be free of signs indicating fluid, electrolyte, or acid-base disturbances.
10. a. Careful pretransfusion assessment of the client.
    b. Accurate identification and matching of the blood to be transfused with its intended recipient.
    c. Ongoing monitoring of the client throughout the transfusion for transfusion reactions.
11. a dextrose
    b. amino acids
    c. select electrolytes and minerals capable of reestablishing positive nitrogen balance and weight gain

12. a. Phlebitis: Discontinue the infusion immediately, apply warm moist compresses to the affected site, avoid further use of the vein, restart the infusion in another vein.
    b. Speed shock: Discontinue the infusion immediately, report symptoms to physician, monitor vital signs, use the proper IV tubing, carefully monitor the rate of fluid flow, check the rate frequently for accuracy.
    c. Fluid overload: Slow the rate of infusion, notify the physician immediately, monitor vital signs, check the rate frequently for accuracy.
    d. Allergic reaction: Stop transfusion immediately and KVO with normal saline, notify physician stat, administer antihistamine parenterally as necessary.
    e. Bacterial reaction: Stop infusion immediately, obtain culture of client's blood and return blood bag to lab, monitor vital signs, notify physician, administer antibiotics stat.
13. metabolic alkalosis
14. respiratory acidosis with renal compensation
15. metabolic acidosis with partial respiratory compensation
16. respiratory alkalosis
17. respiratory acidosis
18. See Table on next page.

## Sequencing

1. Step 3
2. Step 6
3. Step 8
4. Step 1
5. Step 4
6. Step 2
7. Step 5
8. Step 7

18.

| pH | PCO2 | HCO3 | Nature of Disturbance | Comp. Present? Yes | No | If Yes Renal | Respiratory | If Yes Partial | Complete |
|------|------|------|------------------------|-----|-----|-------|-------------|---------|----------|
| 7.28 | 63 | 25 | respiratory acidosis | | x | | | | |
| 7.20 | 40 | 14 | metabolic acidosis | | x | | | | |
| 7.52 | 40 | 35 | metabolic alkalosis | | x | | | | |
| 7.48 | 30 | 31 | resp. & met. alkalosis | | | | | | |
| 7.16 | 82 | 30 | respiratory acidosis | x | | x | | x | |
| 7.36 | 68 | 35 | respiratory acidosis | x | | x | | | x |
| 7.56 | 23 | 26 | respiratory alkalosis | | x | | | | |
| 7.40 | 40 | 26 | none | | | | | | |
| 7.56 | 23 | 26 | respiratory alkalosis | | x | | | | |
| 7.26 | 70 | 25 | respiratory acidosis | | x | | | | |
| 7.52 | 44 | 38 | metabolic alkalosis | | x | | | | |
| 7.32 | 30 | 18 | metabolic acidosis | x | | | x | x | |
| 7.49 | 34 | 26 | respiratory alkalosis | | x | | | | |
| 6.98 | 84 | 18 | resp. & met. acidosis | | x | | | | |

## Chapter 37: Case Study

1. Objective data are underlined; subjective data are bold-faced.

Rebecca is a <u>college freshman</u> who, on the night she had her wisdom teeth removed, had an <u>oral temperature of 39.5°C (103.1°F).</u> She had a sore throat several days prior to the extraction, but neglected to mention this to the oral surgeon. Because of the **soreness in her throat she reported that she had greatly decreased both her food and fluid intake.** Friends that night gave her some Tylenol, which brought her temperature down, and encouraged her to drink more fluids. When they checked on her in the morning her <u>temperature was elevated again </u>and **she said she had felt too weak during the night to drink.** She was brought to the student health service where the admitting nurse noticed her <u>dry mucous membranes, decreased skin turgor, and rapid pulse.</u> At <u>5'2" and 98 pounds,</u> Rebecca was always petite but she had lost **four pounds in the last week.**

### 2. Nursing Process Worksheet

**Health Problem:**
Fluid volume deficit.

**Etiology:**
Decreased fluid intake (sore throat and weakness) and loss of water and electrolytes in fever.

**Signs & Symptoms (Defining Characteristics):**
Elevated temperature (39.5°C), 4 pounds weight loss in one week, dry mucous membranes, decreased skin turgor, and rapid pulse.

**Client Goal:**
By 3/19/93 client demonstrates corrected fluid volume deficit as evidenced by (1) balanced fluid intake/output averaging 2500 ml fluid; (2) urine specific gravity within a normal range of 1.010–1.025; (3) moist mucous membranes and adequate skin turgor; (4) pulse returns to baseline.

**Nursing Interventions:**
1. Assess for worsening of fluid volume deficit.
2. Give oral fluids that are non-irritating if tolerated.
3. If not tolerated, confer with M.D. regarding IV replacement therapy.
4. Monitor response to fluid therapy: V.S., urinary volume and specific gravity, increased skin turgor, moist mucous membranes, increased body weight.

**Evaluative Statement:**
3/19/93: Goal met. Client has corrected fluid volume deficit; fluid intake and output averaging 2700 ml fluid; vital signs returned to baseline; increased skin turgor and moist mucous membranes.

*J. Barclay, RN*

3. *Client strengths:* Previously healthy; concerned friends, highly motivated to correct deficit.
   *Personal strengths:* Strong knowledge of fluid, electrolyte, and acid-base balance; good interpersonal skills.

4. 3/19/93: Client tolerating oral replacement fluids and understands importance of increasing fluids until the deficit is corrected. Friends are reminding her to drink at frequent intervals. Vital signs returned to baseline. Yesterday's fluid intake was 2900 ml fluid with 2500 ml output. Improved skin turgor and moist mucous membranes. Gained back 2 lbs.

*J. Barclay, RN*

# C h a p t e r   3 8

## Matching

| | | | | | | | |
|---|---|---|---|---|---|---|---|
| 1. a | 2. e | 3. d | 4. b | 5. g | 6. f | 7. c | 8. b |
| 9. a | 10. b | 11. a | 12. c | 13. c | 14. d | 15. b | 16. c |
| 17. a | 18. d | 19. b | 20. c | 21. b, d | | | |

## Multiple Choice

| | | | | | |
|---|---|---|---|---|---|
| 1. d | 2. c | 3. b | 4. b | 5. c | 6. c |

## Completion

1. a. significance
   b. competence
   c. virtue
   d. power
2. a. Encourage clients to identify their strengths.
   b. Replace self-negation with positive thinking.
   c. Notice and reinforce client strengths.
   d. Encourage clients to will for themselves the strengths they desire and try them on.
3. a. Body will change, but client keeps the old body boundary.
   b. Client changes a body boundary even though his body remains intact.
4. a. developmental considerations
   b. culture
   c. internal and external resources
   d. history of success and failure
   e. stressors
   f. aging, illness, or trauma
5. Sample Answers
   a. Assist her to find meaning in the experience, to regain mastery to the extent that this is possible, and to realistically evaluate the adequacy of her coping strategy.
   Teach her to develop a game plan for confronting anxiety-producing situations.
   Help to identify and secure interventions for treatable depressions.
   Remedy treatable causes of self-identity disturbances, such as pain or substance abuse.
   b. Notice and affirm positive physiologic characteristics of the client.
   Teach preventive self-care measures that reduce discomforting signs of aging.
   Explore new activities (including hobbies) which are within the changing physical capabilities of the client.
   c. Assist client to identify and utilize personal strengths.
   Communicate that you value the client, simply for who he is; know and use the name he prefers; ask him questions about his life, interests, values.
   Engage client in activities in which he can be successful.
   Empower client to meet his needs; provide necessary knowledge, teach new behaviors, instill the belief that he can change.
   d. Explore with client the many roles she has fulfilled throughout her lifetime; invite reminisences.
   Facilitate grieving over valued roles that are no longer able to be performed.

## Sequencing

1. Step 3
2. Step 6
3. Step 5
4. Step 2
5. Step 4
6. Step 1

## Chapter 38: Case Study

1. Objective data are underlined; subjective data are bold-faced.

An English teacher asks you, the school nurse, to see one of her students whose <u>grades have recently dropped</u> and who <u>no longer seems to be interested in school</u>—or anything else. "She was one of my best students and I can't figure out what's going on. She seems reluctant to talk about this change." When Julie, a <u>16-year-old junior</u>, walks into your office you are immediately struck by her <u>stooped posture, unstyled hair, and sloppy appearance</u>. Julie is <u>attractive, but at 5 feet 3 inches and 150 pounds, she is overweight.</u> Although Julie is initially reluctant to talk, she breaks down at one point and confides that for the first time in her life she feels **"absolutely awful"** about herself. **"I've always concentrated on getting good grades and achieved this easily. But right now this doesn't seem so important. I don't have any friends.** All I hear the girls talking about is boys and <u>I was never even asked out by a boy</u>—which I guess isn't surprising. Look at me. . . ." After a few questions, it becomes clear that Julie has new expectations for herself based on what she observes in her peers, and she finds herself falling far short of her new, ideal self. Julie admits that in the past, **once she set a goal for herself she was always able to achieve it, because she is strongly self-motivated.** Although she has withdrawn from her parents and teachers, she admits that she does have trusted adults who have been a big support to her in the past. "If only I could become the kind of teenager other kids like and have lots of friends!"

## 2. Nursing Process Worksheet

**Health Problem:**
Situational low self-esteem.

**Etiology:**
Perceived inability to meet newly accepted peer standards regarding socialization/dating.

**Signs & Symptoms (Defining Characteristics):**
Feels "absolutely awful" about herself; 5'3", 150 lbs; "I don't have any friends"; never dated; grades have dropped recently; new lack of interest/vitality; stooped posture; unstyled hair; sloppy appearance.

**Client Goal:**
In one month, 10/10/93, client will report she feels "better" about herself, based on new socialization experiences with peers and improved body image.

**Nursing Interventions:**
1. Assist client to develop workable self-care strategies to decrease weight and enhance physical appearance.
2. Explore client's interest in activities that will serve two goals: enable client to develop friendships while improving body image, e.g., sports, dancing, hiking clubs.
3. Counsel client about peer relationships/sexuality/dating.

**Evaluative Statement:**
10/10/93: Goal partially met; client states she feels great about losing weight (150, down to 145) and likes her "new look" but still feels shy with peers and no dates. Revision: celebrate new self-care behaviors and re-evaluate efforts to enhance peer relationships.
*M. Stenulis, RN*

3. *Client strengths:* Physically attractive; past history of achieving personal goals; strongly self-motivated; trusting relationships with adults (parents and teachers). *Personal strengths:* Ability to establish trusting nurse-client relationship with high school students; knowledge of teen social "norms"; successful history of motivating teens to develop and take pride in healthy self-care behaviors.

4. 10/10/93: Met with client one month after initial meeting. In that time, she lost 5 pounds, which she attributes to decreased snacking and increased activity (joined field hockey team). She walked into the office with erect posture and exhibited more interest/vitality than in last meeting. She reports still feeling very shy with her peers and is uncomfortable with boys. She is very interested, however, in participating in group activities where she can overcome her shyness, and will hopefully make new friends.
*M. Stenulis, RN*

# C h a p t e r   3 9

## Matching

1. a   2. c   3. d   4. b   5. c   6. d   7. b   8. a

## Correct the False Statements

1. true
2. false—sensory perception
3. true
4. true
5. false—emotional response
6. true
7. true
8. false—sensorineural
9. false—presbyopia

## Completion

1. Sample Answers
   a. Developmental considerations: Different types of sensory stimulation are needed for growth as sensory receptors, organs, and the nervous system mature. Although newborns are capable of rudimentary perceptual discriminations at birth, many neural pathways are immature and must be stimulated to develop, become refined, and function adequately. Sensory functioning may progressively decline during adulthood as the result of aging or chronic illness. Adults may need to compensate for the loss of one type of stimulation by increasing other sources of sensory stimulation.
   b. Culture: Culture may dictate the amount of sensory stimulation considered normal. Ethnic norms, religious norms, income group norms and the norms of subgroups within a culture all influence the amount of sensory stimulation sought by an individual.
   c. Personality/lifestyle: Different personality types demand different levels of stimulation. Lifestyle choices can dramatically influence the quantity and quality of stimuli received by an individual.
   d. Stress: Increased sensory stimulation may be sought during periods of low stress simply to maintain cortical arousal. During high-stress periods, multiple stressors may already be overloading the sensory system and decreased sensory stimulation is desired.
   e. Illness/medications: Illness can affect the reception of sensory stimuli and their transmissions and perception. Medications can alert or depress the central nervous system and interfere with the perception of sensory stimuli.
2. a. Stimulate as many senses as possible.
   b. Explain procedures to client.
   c. Be aware of client's need for sensory aids and prostheses.
   d. Teach client sensory self-stimulation.
3. a. Be careful what is said in person's presence—hearing is believed to be the last sense lost in an unconscious person.
   b. Assume person can hear you and talk with him/her in a normal tone of voice.
   c. Speak to the person before touching him/her.
   d. Keep environmental noise low.
4. a. Sensory perceptional alteration: Sensory deprivation related to parents' inability to provide a developmentally stimulating environment for infant.
   b. Sensory perceptional alteration: Chronic sensory deprivation related to effects of aging and institutionalization.
5. a. sensory status
   b. level of mobility
   c. preferred stimulation level
   d. sensory, perceptual, and social environments
   e. mental status
   f. behavioral changes
   g. personal resources

## Chapter 39: Case Study

1. Objective data are underlined; subjective data are bold-faced.

Mr. Gibson, an <u>81-year-old married African-American,</u> with much prodding from his wife, reluctantly reports that **he seems not to be hearing as well as he used to be. "I don't know what the trouble is. I'm in perfect health—always have been. More and more people just seem to be mumbling instead of talking."** You notice that <u>he is seated on the edge of his chair and strains toward you when you speak to him.</u> His wife reports that <u>he has stopped going out and pretty much stays in his room whenever people come to the house to visit</u>—because **he is embarrassed** by his inability to hear. "This is really a shame because <u>George was always the life of the party."</u> You ask Mr. Gibson if he has ever had his hearing evaluated and he tells you, <u>"no,"</u> that until now **he's been trying to convince himself that nothing's wrong with his hearing.**

## 2. Nursing Process Worksheet

**Health Problem:**
Sensory/perceptual alteration: auditory.

**Etiology:**
Reluctance to accept that he has an auditory problem and to seek help.

**Signs & Symptoms (Defining Characteristics):**
Leans forward to hear speaker; attempts to deny hearing loss and attributes problem to others who are "mumbling"; has greatly reduced opportunities for conversation; has not sought help until now.

**Client Goal:**
After medical evaluation of hearing loss, and treatment, client demonstrates better coping with auditory problem by increasing time he spends socializing with others.

**Nursing Interventions:**
1. Explain that hearing loss often accompanies aging and that a medical evaluation is important to secure the proper treatment.
2. Assist the client to make an appointment for evaluation.
3. Explore strategies to improve his communication abilities and prevent social isolation.

**Evaluative Statement:**
12/5/93: Goal partially met; hearing aid has enabled client to comprehend most one-on-one communication, but ability to hear well in groups is still impaired. Is willing to investigate possibility of learning to lip read. No longer avoids company—especially if one or two.

*D. Mason, RN*

3. *Client strengths:* Healthy until now; wife is supportive; previous history of strong interactional skills.
*Personal strengths:* Recognize significance of sensory/perceptual alterations; ability to distinguish changes in perceptual abilities normally related to aging from those indicating treatable medical problem; ability to establish trusting nurse-patient relationship with older clients.

4. 12/5/93: Client presents after auditory examination revealed a partial sensorineural loss, which was distorting his perception of certain frequencies, and which was partially correctable with amplification. Client still leans close to speaker, but in a one-on-one conversation, his responses demonstrate his ability to correctly interpret most of what the speaker communicates. He reports he still has great difficulties listening in groups. His wife noted with delight that he seems more like "his old self" when one or two friends come to visit. He expresses interest in learning how to lip read.

*D. Mason, RN*

# C h a p t e r   4 0

## Matching

| | | | | | | | |
|---|---|---|---|---|---|---|---|
| 1. f | 2. a | 3. i | 4. b | 5. e | 6. h | 7. c | 8. g |
| 9. d | 10. d | 11. j | 12. g | 13. a | 14. i | 15. b | 16. h |
| 17. e | 18. c | 19. f | 20. g | 21. k | 22. i | 23. l | 24. a |
| 25. c | 26. e | 27. j | 28. h | 29. b | 30. d | 31. f | 32. j |
| 33. a | 34. f | 35. b | 36. h | 37. c | 38. i | 39. d | 40. g |
| 41. e | | | | | | | |

## Multiple Choice

| | | | | | | | |
|---|---|---|---|---|---|---|---|
| 1. d | 2. a | 3. c | 4. b | 5. a | 6. c | 7. d | 8. a |
| 9. b | 10. c | | | | | | |

## Completion

1. a. confrontation
   b. documentation
   c. written complaint
   d. government complaint
2. a. permission giving
   b. limited information
   c. specific suggestions
   d. intensive therapy

3. a. developmental considerations
   b. culture
   c. religion
   d. ethics
   e. life style
4. a. Provide information to the client regarding examination.
   b. Teach the client.
   c. Provide support for client during exam.
   d. Assist examiner, if appropriate, with any procedure or laboratory study.
5. Sample Answers
   a. Natural family planning
   Advantages: methods can be effective in avoiding pregnancy if mutual understanding, support, and motivation exist between the woman and her partner. There are no side effects, like the ones that can be experienced in hormonal methods, and no messy devices to insert.
   Disadvantages: requires abstinence during ovulation, requires complete understanding of the woman's signs and symptoms of ovulation.
   b. Barrier methods
   Advantages: condoms help to prevent STDs, appropriate for women with sensitivity to the pill, effective when used correctly, relatively inexpensive methods.
   Disadvantages: Devices must be applied prior to intercourse; not all women can wear a cervical cap due to anatomical differences and there is evidence a cervical cap can cause cervical inflammation and increase risk of pelvic infection; spermicides are not effective alone; vaginal sponge carries some risk of toxic shock syndrome.
   c. Intrauterine devices
   Advantages: high effectiveness rate; little care or motivation on part of client is necessary; excellent method for women who have completed their families and are not ready for sterilization.
   Disadvantages: many serious side effects and resulting complications.
   d. Hormonal methods
   Advantages: many beneficial noncontraceptive effects, such as protecting women against development of breast, ovarian, and endometrial cancer; almost 100 percent effective if taken as directed.
   Disadvantages: cost may be prohibitive to some women; compliance is necessary; some women should not take the pill in the presence of certain physiologic disorders or diseases.
   e. Sterilization
   Advantages: after initial surgery and recheck, no further compliance is necessary; almost 100 percent effective.
   Disadvantages: should be considered permanent and irreversible.

## Sequencing

1. Step 3
2. Step 2
3. Step 4
4. Step 1

## Chapter 40: Case Study

1. Objective data are underlined; subjective data are bold-faced.

Anthony Piscatelli, a <u>6-foot tall, well-muscled, healthy, 19-year-old college freshman in the school of nursing</u>, confides to his nursing advisor that **"everything is great"** about college life—with one exception. **"All of a sudden I find myself questioning the values I learned at home about sex and marriage.** My mom was really insistent that each of her sons should respect women and that intercourse was something you saved until you were ready to get married. If she told us once she told us a hundred times that we'd save ourselves, the girls in our lives, and her and dad a lot of heartache if could just learn to control ourselves sexually. Problem is that no one here seems to subscribe to this philosophy. **I feel like I'm abnormal in some way to even think like this.** There's a lot of sexual activity in the dorms and no one even thinks you're serious if you talk about virginity positively. What do you think? Did my mom sell me a bill of goods? Is it true that if you take the proper precautions no one gets hurt and everyone has a good time?" Tony reports that **he is a virgin** and that he **does really miss his close family back home. "I do get lonely at times, and would love to just cuddle with someone or even give and get a big hug—but no one seems to understand this."**

## 2. Nursing Process Worksheet

**Health Problem:**
High risk for altered sexuality patterns.

**Etiology:**
Discrepancy between his family's values about sex and marriage and those he is discovering in peer group.

**Signs & Symptoms (Defining Characteristics):**
"All of a sudden I find myself questioning the values I learned at home about sex and marriage"; feels like he is "abnormal" in some way to value virginity; lonely—wants intimacy; "Is it true that if you take the proper precautions, no one gets hurt and everyone has a good time?"

**Client Goal:**
By next meeting, 11/17/93, client reports personal satisfaction with the results of his reevaluation of his beliefs/values concerning sex and marriage.

**Nursing Interventions:**
1. Assess client's knowledge of sexual development and needs for intimacy and belonging and correct any misinformation.
2. Explore with the client the source of the beliefs/values he learned at home and assist the client to determine the role he wants these beliefs/values to play in his life.
3. Compare and contrast the options of abstinence and becoming sexually active and perform related sexual teaching.
4. Refer to appropriate on-campus sexuality classes, counseling center, seminars, as indicated.

**Evaluative Statement:**
11/17/93: Goal not met. Client reports that his confusion has only deepened and he now feels like his "head is warring with his body." Reports sleeping with his girlfriend but feeling very guilty afterwards—now ignores this girl. Revision: see if he's willing to talk with peer or professional counselor regarding sexual concerns.
*R. LeBon, RN*

3. *Client strengths:* Healthy; caring family; ability to voice his concern; very "likeable" person.
*Personal strengths:* Sound knowledge of sexuality; respect for and appreciation of sexuality; understanding of developmental challenges of young adults and self-identity and intimacy needs; ability to create trusting relationships with young adults.

4. 11/17/93: Client states he is "more confused now" than when we last met. He yielded to peer pressure and slept with girlfriend; used condom. While he "enjoyed this experience" he has been "wracked with guilt" ever since. He cannot reconcile this behavior with what he learned at home and continues to feel "unsure" of who he wants to be. He definitely wants some resolution of this conflict and is interested in speaking with professional sexuality counselor. Referral made.
*R. LeBon, RN*

# C h a p t e r   4 1

## Matching

| | | | | | | | |
|---|---|---|---|---|---|---|---|
| 1. f | 2. a | 3. b | 4. c | 5. d | 6. e | 7. c | 8. a |
| 9. d | 10. b | 11. e | 12. h | 13. f | 14. g | 15. b | 16. j |
| 17. a | 18. i | 19. c | 20. f | 21. h | 22. d | 23. e | 24. g |

## Multiple Choice

| | | | | | | |
|---|---|---|---|---|---|---|
| 1. a | 2. d | 3. d | 4. c | 5. c | 6. a | 7. d |

## Completion

1. Sample Answers
   a. A 30-year-old male client in advanced stages of AIDS states: "I can't believe how little time I have when I have left so many things in my life undone."
   b. A 20-year-old female client grieves for an aborted fetus and the loving relationship that could have prevented her suffering. She states: "Why did he have to walk out on me when I told him I was having his baby? I can't live without him and would give up motherhood to have him back."
   c. A 68-year-old male client who believes he will always carry the guilt of a failed relationship with his wife states: "If only I had been there when she needed me. Now work means nothing to me without Carol at my side."
2. Sample Answers
   a. A 50-year-old agnostic man wants nothing to do with a God who would let his wife die in a car accident. He states that if there is a God, he must be cruel and merciless.
   b. A 72-year-old Roman Catholic woman who is used to walking to church for Mass every morning is admitted to a nursing home. There is only a nondenominational service available to clients on Sunday.
   c. A 68-year-old Jewish man, who practiced his religion on occasion, is recovering from a massive myocardial infarction. He questions whether God has abandoned him because he wasn't good enough during his lifetime.
   d. A 22-year-old Protestant woman marries an atheist and abandons her family and religion. After a serious illness she questions who she is and what God means to her.
   e. A 32-year-old woman with terminal cancer is unable to accept her prognosis and blames God for letting this happen to her.
   f. A 40-year-old father of two girls who was diagnosed with Parkinson's Disease questions why God let this happen to him when he led a good life, lived by the rules of his religion and had a loving relationship with his wife and children.
   g. A retired maintenance man with no family support feels that no one cares about him and God has forgotten him.
3. a. Offer compassionate presence.
   b. Assist in struggle to find meaning and purpose in the face of suffering, illness, and death.
   c. Foster relationships with God/humans that nurture the spirit.
   d. Facilitate client's expression of religious/spiritual beliefs and practices.
4. a. Make counselor feel welcome.
   b. Answer any questions about the client.
   c. Direct the counselor to the client and make sure the client is ready to receive the counselor.
   d. Prepare the client's room for the visit.

## Chapter 41: Case Study

1. Objective data are underlined; subjective data are bold-faced.

Jeffrey Stein is a <u>31-year-old attorney</u> who is presently in a step-down unit following his transfer from cardiac care unit, where he was <u>treated for a massive heart attack.</u> "<u>Bad hearts run in my family</u> but **I never thought it would happen to me.** <u>I jog several times a week and work out at the gym, eat a low fat diet, and I don't smoke.</u>" Jeffrey is <u>5 feet 7 inches, weighs about 150 pounds, and is well-built.</u> His second night in the step-down unit, <u>he is unable to sleep</u> and tells the nurse, "**I've really got a lot on my mind tonight. I can't stop thinking about how close I was to death.** If I wasn't with someone who knew how to do CPR when I keeled over, I probably wouldn't be here today." Gentle questioning reveals that Mr. Stein is worried about what would have played out had he died. "**I don't think I've ever thought seriously about my mortality and I sure don't think much about God.** <u>My parents were semi-observant Jews but I don't go to synagogue myself. I celebrate the holidays</u> but that's about all. **If there is a God, I wonder what he thinks about me.**" He asks if there is a rabbi or anyone he can talk with in the morning who could answer some questions for him and perhaps help him get himself back on track. "For the last couple of years, **all I've been concerned about is paying off my school debts and making money.** I guess there's a whole lot more to life, and maybe this was my invitation to sort out my priorities."

## 2. Nursing Process Worksheet

**Health Problem:**
Spiritual distress: spiritual anxiety.

**Etiology:**
Challenged belief and value system.

**Signs & Symptoms (Defining Characteristics):**
Recent massive heart attack; unable to sleep x 1; raised in semi-observant Jewish family but "for the last couple years only concerned about making money and paying off school debts"; questions about afterlife.

**Client Goal:**
After meeting with Rabbi White 2/12/93, client reports feeling "less anxious" about his religious belief system and reevaluated sense of priorities.

**Nursing Interventions:**
1. Encourage client to continue to share concerns about his religious beliefs and value system.
2. Arrange for client to talk with the hospital's Jewish chaplain in the morning.
3. Normalize this experience by sharing with the client that serious illness often prompts life review.
4. Recommend that the client begin to list the things in life that are most important to him.

**Evaluative Statement:**
Client slept last two nights after meeting with Rabbi White and reports being "less anxious" about "religion." He says there are some things he wants to change about his life and this is a good time to start.

*T. Michael Gray, RN*

3. *Client strengths:* Healthy; practices healthy self-care behaviors; strongly motivated to attain life goals. Knows himself well enough to "name his problems" and cares enough about himself to seek the assistance he needs. *Personal strengths:* Belief that meeting spiritual needs is an important component of good nursing; excellent rapport with the hospital's pastoral care department; history of establishing therapeutic relationships with clients.

4. 2 AM, 2/14/93: Before client fell asleep, he thanked me for arranging for him to meet with Rabbi White. "I guess I did what a lot of people do . . . forget all about God while they try to make a living." He appears less anxious about his religious beliefs and feels that his "recent bout with death" was a timely reminder to evaluate his priorities in life and make some needed changes. Sleeping peacefully at present.

*T. Michael Gray, RN*

# C h a p t e r   4 2

## Matching

| | | | | | | | |
|---|---|---|---|---|---|---|---|
| 1. c | 2. g | 3. i | 4. k | 5. a | 6. e | 7. j | 8. l |
| 9. b | 10. d | 11. f | 12. h | 13. h | 14. a | 15. d | 16. f |
| 17. b | 18. g | 19. c | 20. i | 21. e | 22. m | 23. a | 24. o |
| 25. c | 26. n | 27. b | 28. k | 29. e | 30. i | 31. l | 32. d |
| 33. h | 34. f | 35. g | 36. j | 37. k | 38. a | 39. j | 40. b |
| 41. h | 42. g | 43. c | 44. d | 45. f | 46. e | 47. i | 48. f |
| 49. g | 50. a | 51. d | 52. e | 53. b | 54. c | | |

## Multiple Choice

| | | | | | | | |
|---|---|---|---|---|---|---|---|
| 1. c | 2. b | 3. d | 4. a | 5. d | 6. b | 7. c | 8. a |
| 9. c | 10. d | 11. b | 12. b | 13. a | 14. d | 15. c | |

## Correct the False Statements

1. 1. false—body surface area formula
   2. true
   3. false—parenteral
   4. false—reconstitution
   5. true
   6. true
   7. false—intramuscular
   8. true
   9. true
   10. false—rectus femoris
   11. true
   12. false—3ml
   13. false—intravenous
   14. false—piggyback
   15. true
   16. true
   17. true
   18. false—sclera
   19. true

## Completion

1. a. 1.5 cc
   b. tab i
   c. 0.5 tab
   d. 3 tabs
   e. 0.5 tab
   f. 3 tabs
   g. 0.5 tab (1/2 tab)
   h. 0.5 tab (1/2 tab)
   i. 2 tabs
   j. 4 cc

2. See Table below.

|  | Xanax | Zantac | Cipro |
|---|---|---|---|
| Dosage | 0.25–.5 mg | 150–300 mg | 250–750 mg |
| Route of administration | P.O. | P.O. | P.O. |
| Frequency/schedule | tid | bid | bid |
| Desired effects | relief of anxiety | cure/relief peptic ulcer | cure/treat infection |
| Possible adverse effects | drowsiness lightheadedness dry mouth constipation | malaise rash G.I. upset | G.I. upset nausea diarrhea |
| S&S of toxic drug effects | diminished reflexes somnolence confusion | tachycardia G.I. upset | CNS stimulation |
| Special instructions | no alcohol | none | no antacids |
| Recommended course of action with problems | gastric lavage | none | none |

See Figure below.

## Medical Administration Record

| RD DATE | PRN | MEDS. | |
|---|---|---|---|
| /24/93 | Dalmane 30 mg | **DATE** | |
| | PO hs prn | **TIME** | |
| | | **INIT** / **SITE** | |
| /24/93 | Tylenol with codeine #2 | **DATE** | 2/24/93 |
| | PO q4h prn | **TIME** | 10 AM |
| | | **INIT** / **SITE** | CL/PO |

### SINGLE ORDERS—PREOPERATIVES

| RD DATE | MEDICATION—DOSAGE—ROUTE OF ADMIN | DATE/TIME  SITE/INITITALS |
|---|---|---|
| /24/93 | Regular Insulin U-100 | 2/24/93  11 AM  Ⓡ thigh/CL |
| | 10U SQ STAT | |

**INJECTION SITES MUST BE CHARTED**

### ROUTINE MEDICATIONS

| RD DATE | MEDICATION—DOSAGE—ROUTE OF ADMIN | HR | 2/25 | 2/26 | 2/27 | 2/28 | 3/1 | 3/2 | 3/3 |
|---|---|---|---|---|---|---|---|---|---|
| /24/93 | Tenormin 50 mg PO od | 10AM | CL | | | | | | |
| | | | | | | | | | |
| /24/93 | Hydrodiuril 50 mg PO od | 10AM | CL | | | | | | |
| | | | 130/90 | | | | | | |
| /24/93 | NPH Insulin U-100 45U | 7:30 AM | CL | | | | | | |
| | SQ daily in AM | | Ⓛ arm | | | | | | |
| | | | | | | | | | |
| /24/93 | Cipro 500 mg PO q12h | 10AM | CL | | | | | | |
| | | 10PM | | | | | | | |
| | | | | | | | | | |
| /24/93 | Timoptic 0.25%  † gtt | 10AM | CL | | | | | | |
| | OD bid | 6PM | | | | | | | |
| | | | | | | | | | |
| /24/93 | Nitropaste 1/2' q8h | 8AM | CL  130/90 | | | | | | |
| | to chest wall | 4PM | | | | | | | |
| | | 12M | | | | | | | |
| | | | | | | | | | |
| /24/93 | Colace 100 mg PO od | 10AM | CL | | | | | | |

C  Claire Long, RN

4. a. Three "checks":
   when the nurse reaches for the container
   immediately prior to pouring the medication
   when replacing the container to the drawer or shelf
   b. Five rights:
   right medication
   right client
   right dosage
   right route
   right time

5. a. route of administration
   b. viscosity of the solution
   c. quantity to be administered
   d. body size
   e. type of medication
6. a. Ampules—An amplule is a glass flask containing a single dose of medication for parenteral administration.
   b. Vials—A vial is a glass bottle with a self-sealing stopper through which medication is removed. The single-dose, rubber-capped vial is usually covered with a soft, metal cap that can be easily removed.
   c. Prefilled cartridges—Provides a single-dose of medication. The nurse inserts the cartridge into a reusable holder.
7. See Table below.

| Route | Term Used to Describe Route |
|---|---|
| Given by mouth. | oral administration |
| Given via respiratory tract | inhalation |
| Given by injection (types of injections) | subcutaneous injection<br>intramuscular injection<br>intradermal injection<br>intravenous injection<br>intra-arterial injection<br>intracardial injection<br>intraperitoneal injection<br>intraspinal injection<br>intraosseous injection |
| Given on skin or mucous membrane (types of administration) | vaginal administration<br>rectal administration<br>sublingual administration<br>buccal administration<br>inunction<br>instillation<br>irrigation |

8. a. aa
   b. ac
   c. bid
   d. c̄
   e. cap
   f. hs
   g. IM
   h. IV
   i. qod
   j. PO
   k. prn
   l. qd
   m. qh
   n. qid
   o. stat

9. a. Subcutaneous tissue lies between the epidermis and the muscle. Sites for these injections are: outer aspect of the upper arm; anterior aspect of the thigh; lower abdominal wall; and upper back.
   b. Located in the buttocks; the posterior superior iliac spine and greater trochanter are palpated. An imaginary line is drawn between the posterior superior iliac spine and the greater trochanter. The site is lateral and slightly superior to the midpoint of the line.
   c. Involves the gluteus medius and gluteus minimus muscles in the hip area. Place the palm of the hand over the greater trochanter with fingers facing client's head. Place index finger on anterior superior iliac spine and the middle finger extends dorsally. Palpate the crest of the ileum. A triangle is formed, injection is in center of triangle.
   d. A thick muscle that covers the anterolateral aspect of the thigh, bounded by the midanterior thigh on the front of the leg and the midlateral thigh on the side. Divide the thigh into thirds horizontally and vertically; give injection in outer middle third.
   e. On the anterior part of the thigh; used only when other areas are countraindicated.
   f. Located in the lateral aspect of the upper arm. Locate by palpating the lower edge of the acromion process. A triangle is formed at the midpoint in line with the axilla on the lateral aspect of the upper arm.

10. a. Z-track technique: Used to administer medications that are highly irritating to subcutaneous tissues. The dorsogluteal or vastus lateralis sites can be used. The skin is pulled to one side, about 1 inch laterally, and held in this position with the non-dominant hand. The needle is inserted and aspirated for blood. The solution is injected. Light, steady pressure is applied over the site. Displaced tissue is allowed to return to normal position after needle is removed.
    b. Heparin lock: Used for a client who requires intermittent intravenous medication but not a continuous intravenous infusion. It consists of a needle or catheter connected to a short length of tubing capped with a sealed injection port. Needle and tubing are anchored to client's arm.

## Sequence

1. Step 6
2. Step 9
3. Step 7
4. Step 1
5. Step 10
6. Step 2
7. Step 8
8. Step 4
9. Step 11
10. Step 5
11. Step 3

# C h a p t e r   4 3

## Matching

| 1. i | 2. b | 3. e | 4. a | 5. j | 6. c | 7. g | 8. d |
|------|------|------|------|------|------|------|------|
| 9. f | 10. h | 11. e | 12. a | 13. b | 14. d | 15. c | |

## Multiple Choice

| 1. b | 2. a | 3. c | 4. a | 5. d | 6. d | 7. c |
|------|------|------|------|------|------|------|
| 8. a | 9. c | 10. b | | | | |

## Correct the False Statements

1. true
2. false—granulation tissue
3. false—primary
4. true
5. false—retention sutures
6. true
7. false—binder
8. true
9. true
10. false—vasodilation

## Completion

1. a. The body's ability to handle tissue trauma is influenced by the extent of the damage and by the person's general health.
   b. The body's response to injury is more effective if proper nutrition has been maintained.
   c. The body responds systematically to trauma in any of its parts.
   d. The blood transports substances to and from injured tissue.
   e. Intact skin and mucous membranes serve as first lines of defense against microorganisms.
   f. Normal healing is promoted when the wound is free of foreign bodies, including bacteria.
2. a. 21
   b. 2 years
   c. collagen
   d. stronger
   e. blood vessels
   f. scar
3. a. Large amounts of subcutaneous tissue and tissue fat may slow wound healing; fatty tissue is more difficult to suture, more prone to infection, and takes longer to heal.
   b. Impairs circulation, which decreases healing.
   c. Smoking decreases oxygenation of tissues, which decreases healing.
4. a. purulent drainage
   b. increased drainage
   c. pain
   d. redness
   e. swelling
   f. increased body temperature
   g. increased white blood cell count

5. a. slipped suture
   b. dislodged clot from stress at the suture line/operative site
   c. infection
   d. erosion of a blood vessel by a foreign body
6. Cover wound area with sterile towels soaked in saline; notify the physician immediately.
7. A = Airway
   B = Breathing
   C = Circulation
8. a. physical status of the client
   b. cause of the wound
   c. location, size, and severity of the wound
   d. support systems available
   e. social and work history of the client
9. a. How long will the heat or cold be applied?
   b. What body part is involved?
   c. Is the skin intact?
   d. How large is the area?
   e. What is the client's age?
   f. What is the client's physical condition?
10. a. Promote wound healing.
    b. Relieve pain.
    c. Relieve muscle tension and joint stiffness.
    d. Warm a part of the body.
    e. Reduce edema.
11. a. Relieve pain.
    b. Limit inflammation and suppuration.
    c. Control bleeding.
12. a. There is a danger of electric shock if a pin touches a wire in the heating pad.
    b. Moisture may cause short-circuiting of the heating element and electric shock may occur.
    c. The area should be clean and dry to prevent burning (moisture increases transfer of heat).
    d. Moist heat evaporates and cools rapidly, so an additional source of heat is required.
    e. Covers on ice bags provide comfort from the cold and also absorb moisture that may accumulate on the outside of the bag.
    f. Draping during a sponge bath prevents shivering, which would increase temperature.
    g. Evaporation of moisture on the skin further helps to reduce body temperature.
13. a. Absorb drainage and help promote wound healing.
    b. Protect the wound from mechanical injury.
    c. Promote homeostasis, help prevent hemorrhage, aid in wound edge approximation (when used as a pressure dressing).
    d. Splint or immobilize the wound, facilitating healing and preventing further trauma.
    e. Prevent contamination from environment.
    f. Provide physical, psychologic, and aesthetic comfort.

# C h a p t e r   4 4

## Matching

| | | | | | | | |
|---|---|---|---|---|---|---|---|
| 1. c | 2. a | 3. c | 4. b | 5. a | 6. b | 7. a | 8. a |
| 9. b | 10. a | 11. b | 12. e | 13. c | 14. f | 15. a | 16. d |
| 17. b | 18. c | 19. d | 20. a | 21. f | 22. f | 23. d | 24. b |
| 25. a | 26. g | 27. c | 28. e | | | | |

## Multiple Choice

1. c    2. a    3. d    4. b    5. c

## Correct the False Statements

1. false—sensory
2. true
3. false—infants and older adults
4. false—larger
5. true
6. true
7. false—side-lying
8. true
9. true
10. true

## Completion

1. a. confused
   b. unconscious
   c. sedated
   d. mentally incompetent
   e. a minor
2. a. adrenal steroids
   b. anticoagulants
   c. tranquilizers
   d. antibiotics
   e. diuretics
3. a. Induction: Begins with administration of the anes-
      thetic agent and continues until the client is ready for
      the incision.
   b. Maintenance: From the incision until near the end of
      the procedure.
   c. Emergence: Starts as client begins to emerge from the
      anesthesia and ends when the client is ready to leave
      the operating room.
4. Cardiovascular
   a. decreased cardiac output, heart rate, cardiac reserve
   b. decreased peripheral circulation
   c. increased vascular rigidity
5. Respiratory
   a. reduced vital capacity
   b. diminished cough reflex
   c. decreased oxygenation of blood
6. Neurologic
   a. sensory deficit
   b. decreased reaction time
7. Renal
   a. decreased renal blood flow
   b. reduced bladder capacity

8. Integument
   a. decreased vascularity
   b. dry, inelastic skin
9. a. fear of the unknown
   b. fear of pain or death
   c. fear of changes in body image and self-concept
10. a. Client will be physically and emotionally prepared for
       surgery.
    b. Client will demonstrate turning, coughing, and deep-
       breathing exercises.
    c. Client will verbalize understanding of postoperative
       pain control.
    d. Client will maintain fluid intake and nutritional bal-
       ance to meet needs.
11. a. Hyperventilate the alveoli and prevent their recol-
       lapse.
    b. Improve lung expansion and volume.
    c. Help expel anesthetic gases and mucus.
    d. Facilitate oxygenation of tissues.
12. a. Improves venous return.
    b. Improves respiratory function.
    c. Improves gastrointestinal peristalsis.
13. a. To serve as baseline data for the intraoperative period
       and to report any abnormal findings.
    b. To allow postoperative assessment of skin and
       nailbeds for circulation and oxygenation of tissues.
    c. Dentures may cause respiratory obstruction during
       anesthesia.
    d. To prevent loss or injury from swelling during or after
       surgery.
14. a. To alleviate anxiety and facilitate anesthesia induc-
       tion.
    b. To decrease pulmonary and oral secretions, and to
       prevent laryngospasms.
    c. To facilitate sedation and relaxation, and to reduce
       the amount of anesthesia needed.
    d. To decrease gastric acidity and volume in order to
       decrease danger of aspiration if vomiting occurs.
15. a. Assess and monitor physical and emotional status of
       clients.
    b. Promote physical and psychological comfort and
       safety.
    c. Prevent complications.
    d. Facilitate coping with alterations in structure and
       function.
    e. Promote a return to health and maximize wellness.